T0231102

Recent Progress in Alzheimer's and Parkinson's Diseases

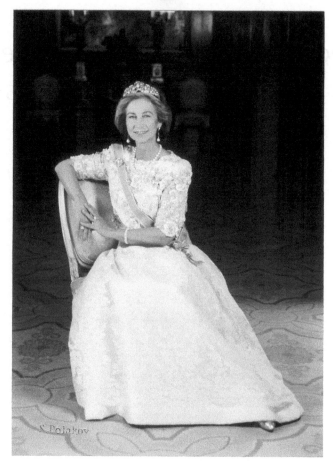

Her Majesty Queen Sophia of Spain

Recent Progress in Alzheimer's and Parkinson's Diseases

Edited by

Israel Hanin PhD
Professor and Chairman Emeritus, Department of Pharmacology and Experimental Therapeutics
Loyola University Medical Center
Maywood, Illinois, USA

Ramón Cacabelos MD PhD DMSci
President and Chief Executive Officer
EuroEspes, Santa Marta de Babío
La Coruña
Spain

Abraham Fisher PhD
Senior Scientist
Israel Institute for Biological Research
Ness-Ziona
Israel

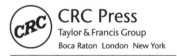

CRC Press
Taylor & Francis Group
Boca Raton London New York

CRC Press is an imprint of the
Taylor & Francis Group, an **informa** business

CRC Press
Taylor & Francis Group
6000 Broken Sound Parkway NW, Suite 300
Boca Raton, FL 33487-2742

© 2005 by Taylor & Francis Group, LLC
CRC Press is an imprint of Taylor & Francis Group, an Informa business

No claim to original U.S. Government works

This book contains information obtained from authentic and highly regarded sources. Reasonable efforts have been made to publish reliable data and information, but the author and publisher cannot assume responsibility for the validity of all materials or the consequences of their use. The authors and publishers have attempted to trace the copyright holders of all material reproduced in this publication and apologize to copyright holders if permission to publish in this form has not been obtained. If any copyright material has not been acknowledged please write and let us know so we may rectify in any future reprint.

Except as permitted under U.S. Copyright Law, no part of this book may be reprinted, reproduced, transmitted, or utilized in any form by any electronic, mechanical, or other means, now known or hereafter invented, including photocopying, microfilming, and recording, or in any information storage or retrieval system, without written permission from the publishers.

For permission to photocopy or use material electronically from this work, please access www.copyright.com (http://www.copyright.com/) or contact the Copyright Clearance Center, Inc. (CCC), 222 Rosewood Drive, Danvers, MA 01923, 978-750-8400. CCC is a not-for-profit organization that provides licenses and registration for a variety of users. For organizations that have been granted a photocopy license by the CCC, a separate system of payment has been arranged.

Trademark Notice: Product or corporate names may be trademarks or registered trademarks, and are used only for identification and explanation without intent to infringe.

Visit the Taylor & Francis Web site at
http://www.taylorandfrancis.com

and the CRC Press Web site at
http://www.crcpress.com

Contents

List of contributors

H Akiyama MD PhD
Tokyo Institute of Psychiatry
Department of Psychogeriatrics
2-1-8 Kamikitazawa
Setagaya-ku
Tokyo 156-8585
Japan

GM Alley BS
Department of Psychiatry and Neurology
Institute of Psychiatric Research
Indiana University School of Medicine
791 Union Drive, Rm PR-313
Indianapolis, IN 46202-4887
USA

C Alves da Costa PhD
Institut de Pharmacologie Moléculaire et Cellulaire
UMR6097 CNRS/UNSA
660 Route des Lucioles
06560 Valbonne
France

H Arai MD PhD
Department of Geriatrics
Tohoku University School of Medicine
Sendai 980-8578
Japan

N Ariel
Department of Biochemistry and Molecular Genetics
Israel Institute for Biological Research
Ness-Ziona 74100
Israel

J Avila PhD
Centro de Biología Molecular "Severo Ochoa"
Facultad de Ciencias
Campus de Cantoblanco
Universidad Autónoma de Madrid
28049 Madrid
Spain

D Barak
Department of Organic Chemistry
Israel Institute for Biological Research
Ness-Ziona 74100
Israel

P Bar-On
Department of Neurosciences
University of California
San Diego
La Jolla, CA 92093-0624
USA

Y Barhum MSc
Laboratory of Neuroscience
Felsenstein Medical Research Center and
    Department of Neurology
Rabin Medical Center
Beilinson Campus
Tel Aviv University
Sackler School of Medicine
Petah-Tikva 49100
Israel

KFS Bell
Departments of Pharmacology and Therapeutics
McGill University
McIntyre MS Building
3655 Promenade Sir William Osler
Montreal, Quebec
Canada H3G 1Y6

Y Ben-Shaul PhD
The Eric Roland Center of Neurodegenerative Diseases
and
Center for Computational Neuroscience
Department of Biological Chemistry and
    Department of Physiology
The Hebrew University of Jerusalem
Jerusalem 91904
Israel

H Bergman MD PhD
The Eric Roland Center of Neurodegenerative Disease
and
Department of Physiology
The Hebrew University of Jerusalem
Jerusalem 91904
Israel

M Bronfman
Centro FONDAP de Regulación Celular y Patología
    "Joaquín V. Luco"
MIFAB, Facultad de Ciencias Biológicas
Pontificia Universidad Católica de Chile
Chile

S Bulvik MD
Laniado Medical Center
Natanya 42150
Israel

A Burshtein MSc
Laboratory of Neuroscience
Felsenstein Medical Research Center and
    Department of Neurology
Rabin Medical Center
Beilinson Campus
Tel Aviv University
Sackler School of Medicine
Petah-Tikva 49100
Israel

R Cacabelos MD PhD DMSci
EuroEspes Biomedical Research Center
Institute for CNS Disorders
Department of Clinical Neuroscience
15166 Bergondo, La Coruña, and
Department of Biotechnology and Genomics
Camilo José Cela University
Madrid
Spain

F Checler PhD
Institut de Pharmacologie Moléculaire et Cellulaire
UMR6097 CNRS/UNSA
660 Route des Lucioles
06560 Valbonne
France

P Choi MD PhD
Department of Surgery
University of Washington
Seattle, WA 98195
USA

M Citron
Amgen Inc.
Department of Neuroscience
M/S 29-2-B, One Amgen Center Drive
Thousand Oaks, CA 91320
USA

MR Cookson PhD
Cell Biology and Gene Expression Unit
Laboratory of Neurogenetics
National Institute on Aging, NIH
Building 35, Room 1A116
MSC 3707, 35 Convent Drive
Bethesda MD 20892-3707
USA

M Cornelli
Cornelli Consulting
Corso Indipendenza, 1
20129 Milan
Italy

U Cornelli MD PhD
Department of Pathology & Pharmacology
Loyola University Chicago Medical Center
2160 S. First Avenue
Maywood, IL 60153
USA

L Corzo
EuroEspes Biomedical Research Center
Institute for CNS Disorders
15166 Bergondo, La Coruña, and
Department of Biotechnology and Genomics
Camilo José Cela University
Madrid
Spain

KA Crutcher
Department of Neurosurgery (MSB 4313)
231 Albert Sabin Way
University of Cincinnati College of Medicine
Cincinnati, OH 45267-0515
USA

AC Cuello MD
Departments of Pharmacology and Therapeutics
Anatomy and Cell Biology
Neurology and Neurosurgery
McGill University
McIntyre MS Building
3655 Promenade Sir William Osler
Montreal, Quebec
Canada H3G 1Y6

ST DeKosky MD
Departments of Neurology and Psychiatry, and
Alzheimer's Disease Research Center
University of Pittsburgh
Pittsburgh, PA 15213
USA

A del C Alonso PhD
Chemical Neuropathology Laboratory
Department of Neurochemistry
New York State Institute for Basic Research in
    Developmental Disabilities
1050 Forest Hill Road
Staten Island, NY 10314-6399
USA

A Delacourte PhD
INSERM Director
Unit INSERM 422
1, place de Verdun
59045 Lille Cedex
France

JC de la Torre MD PhD
Institute of Pathology
Case Western Reserve University
2085 Adelbert Road
Cleveland, OH 44106
USA

L De Ambrosi
Laboratori Derivati Organici
VM Barozzi 4
Milan 21022
Italy

DW Dickson MD
Neuropathology Laboratory
Mayo Clinic College of Medicine
Birdsall Medical Research Building
4500 San Pablo Road
Jacksonville, FL 32224
USA

I D'Souza
Geriatric Research Education and Clinical Center
Veterans Affairs Puget Sound Health Care System,
    Seattle Division
1660 S. Columbian Way, Seattle WA 98108, and
Divisions of Gerontology and Geriatric Medicine
Department of Medicine
University of Washington
Seattle, WA 98195
USA

B Dudas
Loyola University Chicago School of Medicine
2160 S. First Avenue
Maywood, IL 60153
USA

V Echeverria
Departments of Pharmacology and Therapeutics
McGill University
McIntyre MS Building
3655 Promenade Sir William Osler
Montreal, Quebec
Canada H3G 1Y6

P Eikelenboom
Department of Neurology and Academic Medical
    Center
University of Amsterdam, and
Department of Psychiatry
Vrije Universiteit Medical Center
Amsterdam
The Netherlands

E El-Akkad PhD
Chemical Neuropathology Laboratory
Department of Neurochemistry
New York State Institute for Basic Research in
    Developmental Disabilities
1050 Forest Hill Road
Staten Island, NY 10314-6399
USA

I Etcheverría PhD
Biotechnology Department
EBIOTEC
Santa Marta de Babío s/n
15166 Bergondo
La Coruña
Spain

M Fahnestock PhD
Department of Psychiatry and Behavioural
 Neurosciences
McMaster University
Hamilton, Ontario
Canada L8N 3Z5

GG Farias
Centro FONDAP de Regulación Celular y Patología
 "Joaquín V. Luco"
MIFAB, Facultad de Ciencias Biológicas
Pontificia Universidad Católica de Chile
Chile

J Fareed PhD
Department of Pathology and Pharmacology
Loyola University Chicago Medical Center
2160 S. First Avenue
Maywood, IL 60153
USA

MR Farlow MD
Department of Psychiatry and Neurology
Institute of Psychiatric Research
Indiana University School of Medicine
791 Union Drive, Rm PR-313
Indianapolis, IN 46202-4887
USA

L Fernández-Novoa MD PhD
EuroEspes Biomedical Research Center
Institute for CNS Disorders
15166 Bergondo, La Coruña, and
Department of Biotechnology and Genomics
Camilo José Cela University
Madrid
Spain

A Fisher
Israel Institute for Biological Research
Ness-Ziona 74100
Israel

LR Fodero PhD
Department of Pathology
University of Melbourne
Victoria 3010
Australia

M Frasier PhD
Eli Lilly and Company
Lilly Corporate Center
Building 48 Dock
Indianapolis, IN 46285-0533
USA

RA Fuentealba
Centro FONDAP de Regulación Celular y Patología
 "Joaquín V. Luco"
MIFAB, Facultad de Ciencias Biológicas
Pontificia Universidad Católica de Chile
Chile

P Gambetti MD
Division of Neuropathology
Institute of Pathology
School of Medicine
Case Western Reserve University
10900 Euclid Avenue
Cleveland, OH 44120
USA

N Giladi
Movement Disorders Unit
Tel-Aviv Sourasky Medical Center
6 Weizmann Street
Tel Aviv 64239, and
Sackler School of Medicine
Tel-Aviv University
Tel-Aviv
Israel

N Golts
Becton Dickinson
4665 North Avenue
Oceanside
San Diego, CA 92056-3590
USA

A Gómez-Ramos PhD
Centro de Biología Molecular "Severo Ochoa"
Facultad de Ciencias
Campus de Cantoblanco
Universidad Autónoma de Madrid
28049 Madrid
Spain

C-X Gong MD MS
Brain Metabolism Laboratory
Department of Neurochemistry
New York State Institute for Basic Research in
 Developmental Disabilities
1050 Forest Hill Road
Staten Island, NY 10314-6399
USA

NH Greig PhD
National Institute of Aging
National Institutes of Health
Baltimore, MD 21224
USA

I Grundke-Iqbal PhD
Neuroimmunology Laboratory
Department of Neurochemistry
New York State Institute for Basic Research in
    Developmental Disabilities
1050 Forest Hill Road
Staten Island, NY 10314-6399
USA

RA Halverson PhD
Department of Pharmacology
Loyola University Chicago Medical Center
2160 S. First Avenue
Maywood, IL 60153
USA

I Hanin PhD
Department of Pharmacology and Experimental
    Therapeutics
Loyola University Chicago Medical Center
2160 S. First Avenue
Maywood, IL 60153
USA

T Hänninen PhD
Department of Neurology
University and University Hospital of Kuopio
Building 5, 8th Floor
PO Box 1777
FIN 70211 Kuopio
Finland

N Haque PhD
Neuroimmunology Laboratory
Department of Neurochemistry
New York State Institute for Basic Research in
    Developmental Disabilities
1050 Forest Hill Road
Staten Island, NY 10314-6399
USA

M Hashimoto
Department of Neurosciences
University of California
San Diego
La Jolla, CA 92093-0624
USA

JM Hausdorff
Movement Disorders Unit
Tel-Aviv Sourasky Medical Center
Sackler School of Medicine
Tel-Aviv University
Tel-Aviv, Israel, and
Division on Aging
Harvard Medical School
Boston, Massachusetts
USA

M Hejna
Department of Pathology
Loyola University Chicago Medical Center
2160 S. First Avenue
Maywood, IL 60153
USA

J Henao
EuroEspes Biomedical Research Center
Institute for CNS Disorders
15166 Bergondo, La Coruña, and
Department of Biotechnology and Genomics
Camilo José Cela University
Madrid
Spain

F Hernández PhD
Centro de Biología Molecular "Severo Ochoa"
Facultad de Ciencias
Campus de Cantoblanco
Universidad Autónoma de Madrid
28049 Madrid
Spain

J Hitomi
Department of Anatomy and Neuroscience
Osaka University Graduate School of Medicine
2-2, Yamadaoka, Suita
Osaka 565-0871
Japan

JJM Hoozemans
Department of Psychiatry
Vrije Universiteit Medical Center
Amsterdam
The Netherlands

K Imahori PhD
Mitsubishi Kasei Institute of Life Sciences
Machida
Japan

K Imaizumi
Division of Structural Cell Biology
Nara Institute of Science and Technology
8916-5, Takayama, Ikoma
Nara 630-0101
Japan

NC Inestrosa
FONDAP Biomedical Center P
Universidad Católica de Chile
Alameda 340, Santiago
Chile

K Iqbal PhD
Department of Neurochemistry
Chemical Neuropathology Laboratory
New York State Institute for Basic Research in
   Developmental Disabilities
1050 Forest Hill Road
Staten Island, NY 10314-6399
USA

O Iqbal MD
Department of Pathology
Loyola University Chicago Medical Center
2160 S. First Avenue
Maywood, IL 60153
USA

C Isaza
EuroEspes Biomedical Research Center
Institute for CNS Disorders
15166 Bergondo, La Coruña, and
Department of Biotechnology and Genomics
Camilo José Cela University
Madrid
Spain

K Ishiguro PhD
Mitsubishi Kasei Institute of Life Sciences
Machida
Japan

N Itoh MD PhD
Department of Neurology
Mie University School of Medicine
Tsu 514-8507
Japan

KA Jellinger MD
Department of Neuropathology
Institute of Clinical Neurobiology
Kenyongasse 18
A-1070 Vienna
Austria

D Kanayama
Department of Psychiatry and Behavioral Science
Osaka University Graduate School of Medicine
2-2, Yamadaoka, Suita
Osaka 565-0871
Japan

S-C Kang MS
Institute of Pathology
School of Medicine
Case Western Reserve University
10900 Euclid Avenue
Cleveland, OH 44120
USA

D Kaplan
Department of Biochemistry and Molecular Genetics
Israel Institute for Biological Research
Ness-Ziona 74100
Israel

T Katayama
Department of Anatomy and Neuroscience
Osaka University Graduate School of Medicine
2-2, Yamadaoka, Suita
Osaka 565-0871
Japan

S Khatoon PhD
Chemical Neuropathology Laboratory
Department of Neurochemistry
New York State Institute for Basic Research in
   Developmental Disabilities
1050 Forest Hill Road
Staten Island, NY 10314-6399
USA

H-C Kim PhD
Neurotoxicology Program
College of Pharmacy
Kangwon National University
Chunchon 200-701
South Korea

M Kivipelto MD PhD
Neurotec
Karolinska Institute
Huddinge Hospital
SE-171 76 Stockholm
Sweden

JH Kordower PhD
Department of Neurological Sciences
Rush University Medical Center
1735 W. Harrison Street, Suite 300
Chicago, IL 60612
USA

B Kraemer
Geriatric Research Education and Clinical Center
Veterans Affairs Puget Sound Health Care System
Seattle Division, 1660 S. Columbian Way
Seattle, WA 98108, and
Divisions of Gerontology and Geriatric Medicine
Department of Medicine
University of Washington
Seattle, WA 98195
USA

C Kronman
Department of Biochemistry and Molecular Genetics
Israel Institute for Biological Research
Ness-Ziona 74100
Israel

Y Kubota MD PhD
EuroEspes Biomedical Research Center
Institute for CNS Disorders
15166 Bergondo, La Coruña, and
Department of Biotechnology and Genomics
Camilo José Cela University
Madrid
Spain

T Kudo MD Phd
Psychiatry and Behavioral Science
Osaka University Graduate School of Medicine
2-2, Yamadaoka, Suita
Osaka 565-0871
Japan

S Kuzuhara MD PhD
Department of Neurology
Mie University School of Medicine
Tsu 514-8507
Japan

FM LaFerla PhD
Department of Neurobiology and Behavior
University of California, Irvine
1109 Gillespie Neuroscience Research Facility
Irvine, CA 92697-4545
USA

DK Lahiri PhD
Department of Psychiatry and Neurology
Institute of Psychiatric Research
Indiana University School of Medicine
791 Union Drive, Rm PR-313
Indianapolis, IN 46202-4887
USA

J Lee MD PhD
Department of Pathology & Pharmacology
Loyola University Chicago Medical Center
2160 S. First Avenue
Maywood, IL 60153
USA

O Levi MSc
Department of Neurobiochemistry
The George S. Wise Faculty of Life Sciences
Tel Aviv University
Tel Aviv 69978
Israel

YS Levy MScPharm
Laboratory of Neuroscience
Felsenstein Medical Research Center and
    Department of Neurology
Rabin Medical Center
Beilinson Campus
Tel Aviv University
Sackler School of Medicine
Petah-Tikva 49100
Israel

L Li
Max-Planck-Unit for Structural Molecular Biology
Notkestrasse 85
22607 Hamburg
Germany

R Li MS
Institute of Pathology
School of Medicine
Case Western Reserve University
10900 Euclid Avenue
Cleveland, OH 44120
USA

J Lochhead PhD
Sun Health Research Insititute
10515 W. Santa Fe Drive
Sun City, AZ 85351
USA

VRM Lombardi PhD
Biotechnology Department
EBIOTEC
Santa Marta de Babío s/n
15166 Bergondo
La Coruña
Spain

E Lopez
Departments of Pharmacology and Therapeutics
McGill University
McIntyre MS Building
3655 Promenade Sir William Osler
Montreal, Quebec
Canada H3G 1Y6

S Lorens
Department of Pharmacology
Loyola University Chicago Medical Center
2160 S. First Avenue
Maywood, IL 60153
USA

JJ Lucas PhD
Centro de Biología Molecular "Severo Ochoa"
Facultad de Ciencias
Campus de Cantoblanco
Universidad Autónoma de Madrid
28049 Madrid
Spain

Q Ma PhD
Department of Pharmacology
Loyola University Chicago Medical Center
2160 S. First Avenue
Maywood, IL 60153
USA

E Mandelkow
Max-Planck-Unit for Structural Molecular Biology
Notkestrasse 85
22607 Hamburg
Germany

E-M Mandelkow
Max-Planck-Unit for Structural Molecular Biology
Notkestrasse 85
22607 Hamburg
Germany

T Martin DVM
Sun Health Research Institute
10515 W. Santa Fe Drive
Sun City, AZ 85351
USA

E Masliah MD
Departments of Neurosciences and Pathology
University of California
San Diego
La Jolla, CA 92093-0624
USA

E Melamed MD
Laboratory of Neuroscience
Felsenstein Medical Research Center and
    Department of Neurology
Rabin Medical Center
Beilinson Campus
Tel Aviv University
Sackler School of Medicine
Petah-Tikva 49100
Israel

DM Michaelson PhD
Department of Neurobiochemistry
The George S. Wise Faculty of Life Sciences
Tel Aviv University
Tel Aviv 69978
Israel

EJ Mufson PhD
Department of Neurological Sciences
Rush University Medical Center
1735 W. Harrison Street, Suite 300
Chicago, IL 60612
USA

NA Muma PhD
Department of Pharmacology
Loyola University Chicago Medical Center
2160 S. First Avenue
Maywood, IL 60153
USA

T Nabeshima PhD
Department of Neuropsychopharmacology and
    Hospital Pharmacy
Nagoya University Graduate School of Medicine
Nagoya 466-8560
Japan

K Nakashima MD PhD
Department of Neurology
Institute of Neurological Sciences, Faculty of Medicine
Tottori University
Yonago 683-8503
Japan

S Oddo
Department of Neurobiology and Behavior
University of California, Irvine
1216 Gillespie Neuroscience Building
Irvine, CA 92697
USA

D Offen PhD
Laboratory of Neuroscience
Felsenstein Medical Research Center and
  Department of Neurology
Rabin Medical Center
Beilinson Campus
Tel Aviv University
Sackler School of Medicine
Petah-Tikva 49100
Israel

M Okochi
Department of Psychiatry and Behavioral Science
Osaka University Graduate School of Medicine
2-2, Yamadaoka, Suita
Osaka 565-0871
Japan

H Oono PhD
Mitsubishi Kasei Institute of Life Sciences
Machida
Japan

A Ordentlich
Department of Biochemistry and Molecular Genetics
Israel Institute for Biological Research
Ness-Ziona 74100
Israel

T Pan PhD
Institute of Pathology
School of Medicine
Case Western Reserve University
10900 Euclid Avenue
Cleveland, OH 44120
USA

M Pappolla MD
Department of Neurosciences
Louisiana State University
Baton Rouge, LA 70803
USA

C Pennanen MD
Department of Neurology
University and University Hospital of Kuopio
Building 5, 8th Floor
PO Box 1777
FIN 70211 Kuopio
Finland

M Pérez PhD
Centro de Biología Molecular "Severo Ochoa"
Facultad de Ciencias
Campus de Cantoblanco
Universidad Autónoma de Madrid
28049 Madrid
Spain

S Petanceska PhD
Center for Dementia Research
Nathan S. Kline Institute for Psychiatric Research
New York University
New York, NY 10962
USA

V Pichel
EuroEspes Biomedical Research Center
Institute for CNS Disorders
15166 Bergondo, La Coruña, and
Department of Biotechnology and Genomics
Camilo José Cela University
Madrid
Spain

R Quirion PhD
Department of Psychiatry
McGill University and Douglas Hospital Research
  Center
Montreal, Quebec
Canada H4H 1R3

LM Refolo PhD
Department of Neurodegeneration
National Institute for Neurological Disorders and
  Stroke
NSC Room 2223
6001 Executive Boulevard
Rockville, MD 20852
USA

H Reichmann
Klinik und Poliklinik für Neurologie
Universitätsklinikum Carl Gustav Carus
Technische Universität Dresden
Germany

A Ribeiro-da-Silva
Departments of Pharmacology and Therapeutics
Anatomy and Cell Biology
McGill University
McIntyre MS Building
3655 Promenade Sir William Osler
Montreal, Quebec
Canada H3G 1Y6

P Riederer
Clinical Neurochemistry
Department of Psychiatry and Psychotherapy
University of Würzburg
Füchsleinstrasse 15
97080 Würzburg
Germany

E Rockenstein
Department of Neurosciences
University of California
San Diego
La Jolla, CA 92093-0624
USA

JT Rogers PhD
Massachusetts General Hospital
Genetics and Aging Research Unit
Department of Psychiatry
Bldg 114, 16th Street
Charleston, MA 02129
USA

M Rose
Loyola University Chicago School of Medicine
2160 S. First Avenue
Maywood, IL 60153
USA

JM Rozemuller
Department of Pathology
Academic Medical Center
University of Amsterdam
The Netherlands

J Sáez-Valero PhD
Instituto de Neurociencias
Universidad Miguel Hernández
San Juan de Alicante
Spain

H Sasaki MD PhD
Department of Geriatrics
Tohoku University School of Medicine
Sendai 980-8578
Japan

GD Schellenberg
Geriatric Research Education and Clinical Center
Veterans Affairs Puget Sound Health Care System
Seattle Division
1660 S. Columbian Way, Seattle WA 98108, and
Divisions of Gerontology and Geriatric Medicine
Department of Medicine
University of Washington, Seattle, WA 98195, and
Departments of Neurology and Pharmacology
University of Washington
Seattle, WA 98195
USA

J Scheu
Centro FONDAP de Regulación Celular y Patología
    "Joaquín V. Luco"
MIFAB, Facultad de Ciencias Biológicas
Pontificia Universidad Católica de Chile
Chile

S Seoane MSci
Molecular Biology Department
EBIOTEC
Santa Marta de Babío s/n
15166 Bergondo
La Coruña
Spain

A Shafferman
Department of Biochemistry and Molecular Genetics
Israel Institute for Biological Research
Ness-Ziona 74100
Israel

PL Sheridan
Division on Aging
Harvard Medical School, Boston, Massachusetts, and
Behavioral Neurology Division
Department of Neurology
Beth Israel Deaconess Medical Center
Boston, Massachusetts
USA

DH Small PhD
Department of Biochemistry and Molecular Biology
Monash University
Clayton
Victoria 3800
Australia

H Snyder PhD
Feinberg School of Medicine
Northwestern University
Department of Pediatrics
Children's Memorial Hospital
2300 Children's Plaza Mox 209
Chicago, IL 60614
USA

H Soininen MD PhD
Department of Neurology
University and University Hospital of Kuopio
Building 5, 8th Floor
PO Box 1777
FIN 70211 Kuopio
Finland

H Soreq PhD
The Eric Roland Center of Neurodegenerative Disease
and
Department of Biological Chemistry
The Hebrew University of Jerusalem
Jerusalem 91904
Israel

DL Sparks PhD
Sun Health Research Institute
10515 W. Santa Fe Drive
Sun City, AZ 85351
USA

K Sugaya PhD
Department of Molecular Biology and Microbiology
Biomolecular Science Center
Burnett College of Biomedical Sciences
University of Central Florida
4000 Central Florida Blvd
BMS Building, Rm 223
Orlando, FL 32816-2364
USA

M-S Sy PhD
Institute of Pathology and Department of
  Neuroscience
School of Medicine
Case Western Reserve University
10900 Euclid Avenue
Cleveland, OH 44120
USA

M Szyf
Departments of Pharmacology and Therapeutics
McGill University
McIntyre MS Building
3655 Promenade Sir William Osler
Montreal, Quebec
Canada H3G 1Y6

M Takeda
Department of Psychiatry and Behavioral Science
Osaka University Graduate School of Medicine
2-2, Yamadaoka, Suita
Osaka 565-0871
Japan

H Tanimukai MD PhD
Chemical Neuropathology Laboratory
Department of Neurochemistry
New York State Institute for Basic Research in
  Developmental Disabilities
1050 Forest Hill Road
Staten Island, NY 10314-6399
USA

M Taniguchi PhD
Section of Environment and Health Science
Department of Biological Regulation, School of Health
  Science
Faculty of Medicine
Tottori University
Nishimachi 86
Yonago 683-8503
Japan

M Tohyama
Department of Anatomy and Neuroscience
Osaka University Graduate School of Medicine
2-2, Yamadaoka, Suita
Osaka 565-0871
Japan

I Tsujio MD PhD
Chemical Neuropathology Laboratory
Department of Neurochemistry
New York State Institute for Basic Research in
  Developmental Disabilities
1050 Forest Hill Road
Staten Island, NY 10314-6399
USA

S Tuomainen MSci
Department of Neurology
University and University Hospital of Kuopio
Building 5, 8th Floor
PO Box 1777
FIN 70211 Kuopio
Finland

H Uchikado MD PhD
Department of Psychiatry
Yokohama City University
22-2 Seto Kanazawa-ku
Yokohama
Japan

K Urakami MD PhD
Section of Environment and Health Science
Department of Biological Regulation
School of Health Science, Faculty of Medicine
Tottori University
Nishimachi 86
Yonago 683-8503
Japan

MS Urra
Centro FONDAP de Regulación Celular y Patología
  "Joaquín V. Luco"
MIFAB, Facultad de Ciencias Biológicas
Pontificia Universidad Católica de Chile
Chile

WA van Gool
Deptment of Neurology and Academic Medical Center
University of Amsterdam
The Netherlands

R Veerhuis
Department of Psychiatry
Vrije Universiteit Medical Center
Amsterdam
The Netherlands

B Velan
Department of Biochemistry and Molecular Genetics
Israel Institute for Biological Research
Ness-Ziona 74100
Israel

M von Bergen
Max-Planck-Unit for Structural Molecular Biology
Notkestrasse 85
22607 Hamburg
Germany

K Wada-Isoe MD PhD
Department of Neurology
Institute of Neurological Sciences, Faculty of Medicine
Tottori University
Yonago 683-8503
Japan

Y Wakutani MD PhD
Department of Neurology
Institute of Neurological Sciences, Faculty of Medicine
Tottori University
Yonago 683-8503
Japan

M Walzer
Department of Pharmacology
Loyola University Chicago Medical Center
2160 S. First Avenue
Maywood, IL 60153
USA

M Weinstock PhD
Department of Pharmacology
Hebrew University Medical Center
Jerusalem
Israel

B Wolozin MD PhD
Department of Pharmacology
Boston University School of Medicine
715 Albany St., Rm 614
Boston, MA 02118-2526
USA

B-S Wong PhD
Institute of Pathology
School of Medicine
Case Western Reserve University
10900 Euclid Avenue
Cleveland, OH 44120
USA

K Yamada PhD
Laboratory of Neuropsychopharmacology
Division of Life Sciences
Graduate School of National Science and Technology
Kanazawa University
Kanazawa 920-1192
Japan

K Yanagisawa MD
National Institute for Longevity Sciences
National Center for Geriatrics and Gerontology
Gengo 36-3 Morioka
OBU, Aichi 474-8522
Japan

MBH Youdim
Department of Pharmacology
Eve Topf and NPF Centers for Neurodegenerative
    Diseases
Faculty of Medicine
Haifa
Israel

W-H Zheng PhD
Department of Psychiatry
McGill University and Douglas Hospital Research
    Center
Montreal
Quebec
Canada H4H 1R3

Preface

Set amidst the splendor of Seville and the magnificence of Spain, and elevated by the regal presence of Her Majesty, Queen Sophia of Spain, we celebrated The 6th International Congress on Alzheimer's and Parkinson's Diseases during May 8–12, 2003. Her Majesty served as Honorary President of the congress, and chaired the opening session.

This event proved to be most successful. With approximately 1200 scientific participants in attendance, Invited Speaker sessions, Oral presentation sessions, and Poster sessions, the four-and-a-half day meeting provided much scientific stimulation and opportunities for discussion, exchange of ideas, and development of new collaborations.

This book includes chapters contributed by selected invited speakers at the congress.

The generosity of corporate sponsors enabled us to enjoy a meaningful and comprehensive congress. Our appreciation goes to Amersham Health; Ceretec; Datscan; Elan; GlaxoSmithKline; Hunter Fleming; The Institute for the Study of Aging (ISOA); Janssen-Cilag; Merck; and Merz.

In particular, we, the organizers, would like to extend our deepest appreciation to Her Majesty, Queen Sophia. The success of this congress and its attendance (which far surpassed our expectations) is due to the Queen's interest and active participation in this meeting. We were honored by the extent of Her Majesty's knowledge, and humbled by her encouragement. We would also like to acknowledge the participation of Spain's government officials, Her Excellency Ana Pastor, Minister of Health, Government of Spain; His Excellency Manuel Chaves, President of the Autonomous Government of Andalusia; and His Excellency Alfredo Sanchez Monteseirin, Mayor of the city of Seville, in the opening ceremonies.

On behalf of the scientists and researchers in the AD/PD field, we dedicate these proceedings to Her Majesty, Queen Sophia of Spain.

Israel Hanin PhD
Ramón Cacabelos MD PhD DMSci
Abraham Fisher PhD

Chapter 1

Mechanisms of degeneration in Parkinson's disease

B Wolozin, M Frasier, H Snyder, P Choi, N Golts

INTRODUCTION

Parkinson's disease (PD) is a progressive neurodegenerative disease that is the most prevalent movement disorder in the elderly. The symptoms of the disease are tremor, brady-kinesia, muscular rigidity and loss of balance. These symptoms result primarily from the degeneration of dopaminergic neurons in the substantia nigra. The neuropathological hallmark of the disease is the Lewy body, which is an intracellular proteinaceous inclusion that accumulates in the remaining neurons of the substantia nigra.

Both genetic and environmental factors appear to contribute to the etiology of PD. Epidemiological studies show that PD is more prevalent among rural farming communities and among factory workers exposed to heavy metals.[1–5] Pesticides, herbicides and fungicides all appear to contribute to PD, and pesticides, such as rotenone, model some aspects of PD in rodent models.[3]

Studies of twins with PD suggest a genetic contribution to the etiology of PD.[6] Mutations in several genes have been associated with PD. One protein, termed α-synuclein, exhibits an autosomal dominant mode of inheritance.[7,8] α-Synuclein is particularly interesting, because it

appears to be the principal component of Lewy bodies.[9,10] The autosomal dominant mode of inheritance suggests that the mutation causes a gain of function for α-synuclein. As will be described below, research from a number of laboratories suggests that the particular 'function' that is gained by the mutation in α-synuclein is an increased propensity to aggregate, which leads to Lewy body formation.

The other genes that have been shown to be associated with PD all exhibit a recessive mode of inheritance, which suggests a loss of function. Mutations in *parkin*, *DJ-1* and *NURR1* are all associated with recessive parkinsonisms that resemble some aspects of sporadic PD, but often not the entire pathological spectrum.[11–13] For instance, mutations in *parkin* are associated with autosomal recessive juvenile parkinsonism, which is a parkinsonism that presents in the teenage years, leads to motor deficits and degeneration of the substantia nigra, but lacks Lewy bodies.

PROTEIN AGGREGATION: A CENTRAL HYPOTHESIS

Protein aggregation is thought to play a critical role in the pathophysiology of many late-onset neurodegenerative diseases, because each of the diseases is characterized by a protein that accumulates to form an inclusion, and in each case the protein that accumulates either has a strong tendency to aggregate, or disease-related mutations in the protein tend to increase its tendency to aggregate. β-Amyloid accumulates in Alzheimer's disease, and the disease-related mutations in amyloid precursor protein and presenilins mostly lead to increased production of a β-amyloid that is 42 rather than 40 amino acids long and has a much greater tendency to aggregate. Similarly, mutations in polyglutamine disorders, such as Huntington's disease, lead to production of polyglutamine expansions that aggregate readily, and mutations in fronto-temporal dementias of chromosome 17 are caused by mutations in tau protein that increase the tendency of tau to aggregate.

The mutations in α-synuclein that are associated with PD follow a similar pattern. Two mutations are associated with PD: the A53T and the A30P mutations. Each of these mutations increases the tendency of α-synuclein to aggregate. The A53T mutation increases the tendency of α-synuclein to fibrillize, and the A30P mutation increases the tendency of α-synuclein to nucleate.[14–18]

Protein aggregation proceeds through a two-step process that starts with nucleation and proceeds to fibrillization (Figure 1.1). The process of protein aggregation can be understood by considering the process of crystallization. Crystallization exhibits a strong lag phase during which nucleation occurs. Nucleation is the rate-limiting step in crystallization. Once nucleation occurs and crystal niduses are generated, crystal formation occurs rapidly. Protein aggregation exhibits similar phenomena. Protein aggregation begins slowly and exhibits a strong lag phase. During the lag phase, small protofibrils form. Once sufficient numbers of protofibrils have formed, the fibrils

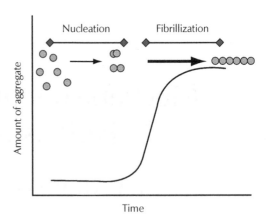

Figure 1.1 The biphasic aggregation of α-synuclein begins with a lag phase during which time nucleation occurs, generating protofibrils. This process is quite slow. Following formation of sufficient protofibrils, fibrillization occurs rapidly

begin to coalesce to form large fibrils, and the rate of protein aggregation increases greatly (Figure 1.1).

The biphasic process of protein aggregation has important implications. Factors that affect the rate of either step will increase the rate of protein aggregation. One factor that has already been mentioned is mutation. Another factor is concentration. Studies *in vitro*, in cell culture and *in vivo*, show that increasing the concentration of α-synuclein increases the rate of its aggregation.[14–22] Exogenous agents that increase the tendency of α-synuclein to bind to itself also increases the tendency to aggregate. Dopamine, for instance, increases the tendency of α-synuclein to form protofibrils, and increases the rate of α-synuclein aggregation. Iron also increases the tendency of α-synuclein to fibrillate and also increases the tendency of α-synuclein to aggregate. Finally, free radicals tend to cause α-synuclein to dimerize, and also increase the tendency of α-synuclein to fibrillate. Hence, agents such as arachidonic acid, hydrogen peroxide and other oxidants increase the rate of α-synuclein fibrillization.[16,23,24]

Taken together, these factors explain much of the aggregation behavior of α-synuclein. For instance, the tendency of α-synuclein to aggregate in dopaminergic neurons of the substantia nigra might result in part from the abundance of dopamine in the substantia nigra and the tendency of the substantia nigra to accumulate iron with age. Similarly, diseases in which iron accumulates, such as iron accumulation disease, type I (Hallovorden Spatz disease), show extensive α-synuclein aggregation.[25] The biphasic aggregation process also needs to be considered when designing assays to monitor α-synuclein aggregation. Some monitoring methods, such as the thioflavin T or turbidity assays, primarily detect the formation of large fibrils of α-synuclein. Other assays such as enzyme-linked immunosorbent assay (ELISA) capture assays primarily detect the formation of

protofibrils. Each assay yields particular kinetic results that depend on the accumulation of the particular aggregation intermediate being studied.[26]

INHIBITORS OF AGGREGATION

The ability to recapitulate the aggregation process *in vivo* enables detection of agents that can inhibit the aggregation process. For instance, while iron promotes α-synuclein aggregation, magnesium inhibits the process. Magnesium dramatically inhibits both spontaneous and iron-induced α-synuclein aggregation *in vitro*.[27] Magnesium also inhibits iron-induced α-synuclein aggregation in neurons grown in cell culture (Figure 1.2). To demonstrate this, we took primary cultures of cortical neurons and exposed them to 0.1 mmol/l $FeCl_2$ in the presence of 0–3 mmol/l $MgCl_2$ during 24-h incubation. We then counted the number of

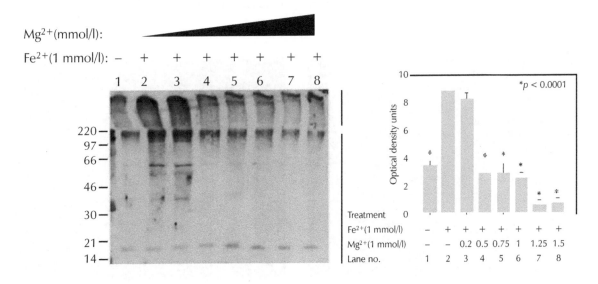

Figure 1.2 Magnesium inhibits the aggregation of α-synuclein in primary cortical neurons. Primary cortical neuronal cultures were exposed to 1 mmol/l $FeCl_2 \pm 0$–1.5 mmol/l $MgCl_2$ for 72 h and then the number of processes over 10 μm in length was quantified

neurons with processes longer than 100 μm. As shown in Figure 1.2, magnesium almost completely inhibited the aggregation of α-synuclein. These results suggest that one might be able to be use magnesium to inhibit α-synuclein aggregation *in vivo*, and that endogenous levels of magnesium *in vivo* might modify the tendency of α-synuclein to aggregate.

ANIMAL MODELS: PROTEIN AGGREGATION *IN VIVO*

By combining over-expression with aggregation-increasing mutations, investigators have been able to model some aspects of the process of α-synuclein aggregation *in vivo*. Our studies of α-synuclein aggregation *in vivo* have utilized a transgenic mouse overexpressing A30P α-synuclein driven by a Thy1 promoter that was developed by Philipp Kahle and Christian Haass and their co-investigators.[22] Prior studies showed that this mouse model develops a progressive loss of motor function beginning with tremor, which progresses to bradykinesia, then postural instability and ultimately death. The motor decline is accompanied by the accumulation of inclusions in the brain stem that contain aggregated α-synuclein and, to a lesser extent, ubiquitin (Figure 1.3).

The accumulation of inclusions that contain aggregated α-synuclein and ubiquitin in the transgenic A30P α-synuclein mouse partially recapitulates the pathology of PD. However, the anatomical distribution of the inclusions does not reflect that of PD, because the inclusions accumulate in the brain stem rather than the substantia nigra. The similarities and differences between the pathology of the transgenic mouse and PD subjects suggests that the A30P α-synuclein transgenic mouse might provide a useful model of α-synuclein aggregation but does not provide a model relevant to understanding the mechanisms of degeneration specific to dopaminergic neurons.

Using the A30P α-synuclein transgenic mouse, we have begun to explore the

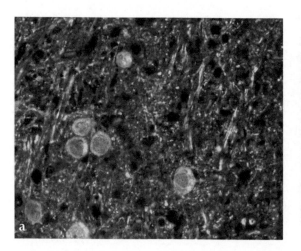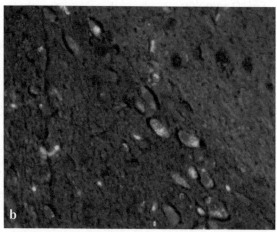

Figure 1.3 The accumulation of α-synuclein and ubiquitin inclusions in the brains of A30P α-synuclein mice partially recapitulates the pathology of Parkinson's disease. (a) Staining of α-synuclein in the brain stem of a symptomatic transgenic A30P mouse; (b) staining of α-synuclein in the brain stem of a non-transgenic age-matched mouse

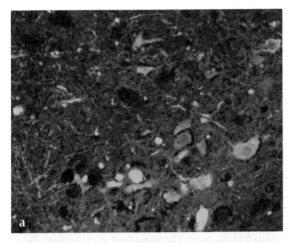

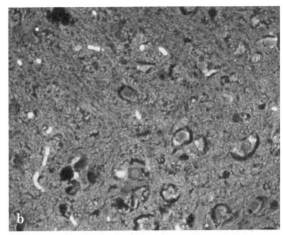

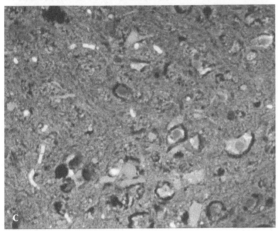

Figure 1.4 Phosphorylated tau epitopes appear in the brain stem of symptomatic A30P α-synuclein transgenic mice. Neurons that stain positive with antibodies to PHF1 appear in symptomatic A30P α-synuclein transgenic mice and co-localize with α-synuclein reactivity. (a) α-Synuclein staining; (b) PHF1 staining; (c) combination of (a) and (b)

pathophysiology of α-synuclein aggregation *in vivo*. One of the key questions that we examined first is whether aggregation of α-synuclein stimulates other pathological changes. Increasing data suggest that fibrillization of α-synuclein frequently occurs along with fibrillization of tau protein.[28,29] This observation prompted us to examine whether tau was affected by the presence of aggregated α-synuclein. To investigate this question, we performed immunocytochemistry with the antibodies PHF1 and AT8, both of which recognize phosphorylated epitopes characteristically observed in neuro-

fibrillary tangles and pre-tangles. We observed that neurons in the ventral brain stem of symptomatic A30P α-synuclein mice stained with both PHF1 and AT8 (Figure 1.4). Approximately 40% of these neurons also contained small foci of α-synuclein staining. Interestingly, the neurons that exhibited the greatest amount of α-synuclein staining occurred in dorsal nuclei of the brain stem. Very little PHF1 or AT8 reactivity was seen in the brain stems from asymptomatic transgenic A30P α-synuclein mice or non-transgenic mice. We also stained the brains with thioflavin to determine whether the abnormally phosphorylated tau was present as a tangle or a pretangle. The neurons that were positive for PHF1 and AT8 did not stain with thioflavin.

The selective appearance of abnormal phosphorylated epitopes in tau protein in symptomatic transgenic A30P α-synuclein mice suggests that aggregation of α-synuclein stimulates pathological changes in tau protein. This could explain why tau pathology occurs alongside α-synuclein pathology in human diseases. The absence of thioflavin staining in the PHF1- and AT8-positive neurons indicates that the tau was present as pre-tangles rather than as tangles. The pre-tangle nature of the phosphorylated tau is to be expected, because mouse tau protein does not aggregate nearly as quickly as human tau protein. Thus, phosphorylated mouse tau is unlikely to progress to the tangles. The identification of these correlated changes allows us to begin to determine what types of stress kinases are activated by aggregated α-synuclein.

PARKIN ACCUMULATES IN LEWY BODIES IN PARKINSON'S DISEASE BRAINS BUT NOT IN THE A30P α-SYNUCLEIN MOUSE

Prior work has suggested that parkin is present in Lewy bodies in brains of subjects with PD. We were curious to determine whether parkin might also occur in the inclusions that accumulate in A30P α-synuclein mice. Brains from symptomatic A30P α-synuclein mice were stained with antibody either to α-synuclein or to parkin. None of the neurons that accumulated α-synuclein stained positive for parkin. This suggests that α-synuclein aggregation can accumulate without a concomitant accumulation of parkin.

CONCLUSION

The application of molecular genetics to the study of PD has led to the identification of a number of genes that participate in the pathophysiology of PD. α-Synuclein has garnered particular interest because it is the only genetic mutation associated with a dominant form of the illness that has been identified to date, and because α-synuclein accumulates in Lewy bodies.[7,9,10] Studies in vitro and in vivo have shown that α-synuclein tends to aggregate, and that mutations in α-synuclein that are associated with PD increase the tendency of α-synuclein to aggregate.[15,16,22] Using these α-synuclein models we have shown that factors such as iron and dopamine increase the tendency of α-synuclein to aggregate, while magnesium inhibits α-synuclein aggregation.[16] The studies of α-synuclein aggregation in vivo using A30P α-synuclein mice show that α-synuclein accumulates in neurons of the brain stem and that this accumulation also elicits the accumulation of ubiquitin reactivity, but not parkin reactivity. Interestingly, aggregation of α-synuclein also stimulates abnormal phosphorylation of tau protein, which is apparent using the PHF1 and AT8 antibodies. Since the phosphorylation events associated with PHF1 and AT8 reactivity are one of the preliminary steps associated with tangle formation, these results suggest that aggregation of α-synuclein moves tau protein towards tangle pathology. These results emphasize the interrelated nature of the different pathologies that occur in neurodegenerative diseases in human illnesses.

There remains an important mechanistic gap between studies of environmental factors implicated in PD, and genetic factors implicated in PD. Studies with rotenone suggest that prolonged application stimulates selective degeneration of the substantia nigra and formation of α-synuclein positive inclusions.[30,31]

In contrast, overexpressing α-synuclein in a transgenic mouse stimulates α-synuclein aggregation but not in the substantia nigra.[19-22] The identification of proteins such as α-synuclein that are specifically implicated in the neurodegeneration associated with PD provides an important target for pharmaceutical intervention. However, the disparity between the pathology elicited by α-synuclein overexpression and the pathology of PD presents an important challenge for applying this new knowledge to identification of novel therapeutic approaches for the treatment of PD.

ACKNOWLEDGEMENTS

This work was supported by grants from NIH (NIA, NINDS) and USAMRC.

REFERENCES

1. Langston J. Epidemiology versus genetics in Parkinson's disease: progress in resolving an age-old debate. Ann Neurol 1998; 44: S45–52

2. Semchuk KM, Love EJ, Lee RG. Parkinson's disease and exposure to rural environmental factors: a population based case–control study. Can J Neurol Sci 1991; 18: 279–86

3. Liou HH, Tsai MC, Chen CJ, et al. Environmental risk factors and Parkinson's disease: a case–control study in Taiwan. Neurology 1997; 48: 1583–8

4. Gorell J, Rybicki B, Cole-Johnson C, Peterson E. Occupational metal exposures and the risk of Parkinson's disease. Neuroepidemiology 1999; 18: 303–8

5. Rybicki BA, Johnson CC, Uman J, Gorell JM. Parkinson's disease mortality and the industrial use of heavy metals in Michigan. Mov Disord 1993; 8: 87–92

6. Tanner CR, Ottman R, Goldman S, et al. Parkinson disease in twins: an etiologic study. J Am Med Assoc 1999; 281: 341–6

7. Polymeropoulos MH, Lavedan C, Leroy E, et al. Mutation in the alpha-synuclein gene identified in families with Parkinson's disease. Science 1997; 276: 2045–7

8. Kruger R, Kuhn W, Muller T, et al. Ala30Pro mutation in the gene encoding α-synuclein in Parkinson's disease. Nat Genet 1998; 18: 106–8

9. Spillantini M, Schmidt M, Lee VM, et al. α-Synuclein in Lewy bodies. Nature 1997; 388: 839–40

10. Spillantini MG, Crowther RA, Jakes R, et al. α-Synuclein in filamentous inclusions of Lewy bodies from Parkinson's disease and dementia with lewy bodies. Proc Natl Acad Sci USA 1998; 95: 6469–73

11. Kitada T, Asakawa S, Hattori N, et al. Mutations in the parkin gene cause autosomal recessive juvenile parkinsonism. Nature 1998; 392: 605–8

12. Bonifati V, Rizzu P, van Baren MJ, et al. Mutations in the DJ-1 gene associated with autosomal recessive early-onset parkinsonism. Science 2003; 299: 256–9

13. Le WD, Xu P, Jankovic J, et al. Mutations in NR4A2 associated with familial Parkinson disease. Nat Genet 2003; 33: 85–9

14. Conway K, Harper J, Lansbury P. Accelerated in vitro fibril formation by a mutant alpha-synuclein linked to early-onset Parkinson disease. Nature Med 1998; 4: 1318–20

15. Conway KA, Lee SJ, Rochet JC, et al. Acceleration of oligomerization, not

fibrillization, is a shared property of both alpha-synuclein mutations linked to early-onset Parkinson's disease: implications for pathogenesis and therapy. Proc Natl Acad Sci USA 2000; 97: 571–6

16. Ostrerova-Golts NL, Petrucelli J, Hardy J, et al. The A53T α-synuclein mutation increases iron-dependent aggregation and toxicity. J Neuroscience 2000; 20: 6048–54

17. Hashimoto M, Hsu L, Sisk A, et al. Human recombinant NACP/α-synuclein is aggregated and fibrillated in vitro: relevance for Lewy body disease. Brain Res 1998; 799: 301–6

18. Hashimoto M, Hsu LJ, Xia Y, et al. Oxidative stress induces amyloid-like aggregate formation of NACP/α-synuclein in vitro. NeuroReport 1999; 10: 717–21

19. Masliah E, Rockenstein E, Veinbergs I, et al. Dopaminergic loss and inclusion body formation in alpha-synuclein mice: implications for neurodegenerative disorders. Science 2000; 287: 1265–9

20. Giasson BI, Duda JE, Quinn SM, et al. Neuronal alpha-synucleinopathy with severe movement disorder in mice expressing A53T human alpha-synuclein. Neuron 2002; 34: 521–33

21. Lee M, Stirling W, Xu Y, et al. Human α-synuclein-harboring familial Parkinson's disease-linked Ala-53 to Thr mutation causes neurodegenerative disease with α-synuclein aggregation in transgenic mice. Proc Natl Acad Sci USA 2002; 99: 8968–73

22. Kahle PJ, Neumann M, Ozmen L, et al. Selective insolubility of alpha-synuclein in human Lewy body diseases is recapitulated in a transgenic mouse model. Am J Pathol 2001; 159: 2215–25

23. Perrin RJ, Woods WS, Clayton DF, George JM. Exposure to long chain polyunsaturated fatty acids triggers rapid multimerization of synucleins. J Biol Chem 2001; 276: 41958–62

24. Perrin, RJ, Woods WS, Clayton DF, George JM. Interaction of human α-synuclein and Parkinson's disease variants with phospholipids:structural analysis using site-directed mutagenesis. J Biol Chem 2000; 275: 34393–8

25. Galvin JE, Giasson B, Hurtig HI, et al. Neurodegeneration with brain iron accumulation, type 1 is characterized by alpha-, beta-, and gamma-synuclein neuropathology. Am J Pathol 2000; 157: 361–8

26. El-Agnaf O, Jakes R, Curran M, Wallace A. Effects of the mutations Ala30 to Pro and Ala53 to Thr on the physical and morphological properties of α-synuclein protein implicated in Parkinson's disease. FEBS Lett 1998; 440: 67–70

27. Golts N, Snyder H, Frasier M, et al. Magnesium inhibits spontaneous and iron-induced aggregation of alpha-synuclein. J Biol Chem 2002; 277: 16116–23

28. Ishizawa T, Mattila P, Davies P, et al. Colocalization of tau and alpha-synuclein epitopes in Lewy bodies. J Neuropathol Exp Neurol 2003; 62: 389–97

29. Giasson BI, Forman MS, Higuchi M, et al. Initiation and synergistic fibrillization of tau and alpha-synuclein. Science 2003; 300: 636–40

30. Betarbet R, Sherer TB, MacKenzie G, et al. Chronic systemic pesticide exposure reproduces features of Parkinson's disease. Nat Neurosci 2000; 3: 1301–6

31. Sherer TB, Betarbet R, Stout AK, et al. An in vitro model of Parkinson's disease: linking mitochondrial impairment to altered alpha-synuclein metabolism and oxidative damage. J Neurosci 2002; 22: 7006–15

Chapter 2

Underlying biochemical and molecular mechanisms of dyskinesia

H Reichmann, P Riederer

PATHOBIOCHEMICAL ASPECTS OF DYSKINESIA

Clinical features of dyskinesia

Most patients with Parkinson's disease experience dyskinesia and motor fluctuations during the course of their disease. There are several reports that have indicated that long-term use of levodopa, particularly with doses higher than 600 mg/day, leads to motor complications such as wearing off (end of dose), the on–off phenomenon, freezing, peak-dose dyskinesia, biphasic dyskinesia and dystonia. Kostic and colleagues[1] have shown that up to 90% of young-onset patients who use levodopa present with dyskinesia after 5 years, whilst 50% of old-onset patients also develop dyskinesia after this period. These findings strengthen the view that young-onset patients should preferentially be treated with dopamine agonists to avoid dyskinesia. Dyskinesias are involuntary movements that are related to levodopa administration. Cederbaum *et al*.[2] demonstrated that, within the first 5 years of levodopa treatment, 45% of parkinsonian patients developed dyskinesia. After 10 years this figure increased to 66% and after 15 years to 88%. In some young patients the so-called priming phenomenon occurs in which dyskinesia starts spontaneously, even years after a short period of levodopa intake. In the DATATOP study 21–31% of patients had dyskinesia even after only 20.5 months of levodopa therapy.[3] Therefore, we advocate using levodopa as late as possible, with a dose as low as possible but as high as necessary.[4]

Dyskinesias normally start on the most affected side of the patient and include chorea, dystonia, athetosis, ballismus, myoclonus and akathisia. These symptoms help to differentiate between peak-dose dyskinesia, which most often involves choreiform movements, and biphasic dyskinesia (onset and end-of dose), and end-of dose dyskinesia, which normally presents with dystonic movements. In early phases of Parkinson's disease, endogenous dopamine production is not high enough to reach a necessary baseline for continuous dopamine receptor stimulation. This problem is easily overcome by adding oral levodopa. In later stages the endogenous synthesis of dopamine decreases even more, owing to the continual dying of dopamine neurons in the substantia nigra. Here it becomes difficult to administer levodopa in such a way that continuous receptor stimulation is guaranteed. It is under these circumstances that peak-dose dyskinesias[5,6] occur when the levodopa level is very high. As mentioned above, peak-dose dyskinesias consist of choreiform movements of the head, trunk and limbs and sometimes even of the respiratory muscles.[7] Biphasic dyskinesias (dyskinesia–improvement–dyskinesia)[8] occur both when the threshold is surpassed following oral administration of levodopa (onset) and when levels fall beneath the threshold after dopamine degradation. Dystonia seems to be particularly related to a fall in plasma or presumably brain dopamine levels. In both instances patients experience dyskinesias.

While dystonia is rather painful, owing to the extensive involuntary flexion or extension of toes or other body parts, it is sometimes surprising how little patients are bothered by choreiform movements which may sometimes be very irritating to their relatives. While choreic movements are normally most pronounced in the upper part of the body, dystonia affects the distal extremities. Dystonia may herald the beginning of dyskinesias and, shortly thereafter, is followed by choreiform dyskinesia. Dystonia most often occurs in the morning or during the night when not enough levodopa or dopamine agonist were administered during the night. Patients mostly report painful foot cramps and painful toe distraction. It is important to distinguish between dystonia in off-periods, which is due to levodopa levels that are too low, or in on-periods, when it is due to levodopa levels that are too high. Myoclonus is also levodopa related and occurs both during the day or at night.[9,10]

The severity of dyskinesia seems to be dose dependent;[11] thus patients with high dosages of levodopa present with more severe choreiform dyskinesia than patients with lower levodopa dosages. For this reason we will discuss later that lowering the levodopa dosage is an important tool in the treatment of dyskinesia. Subtle

observation of patients will reveal that akathisia is also quite common in parkinsonian patients.[12]

For many years it has been debated whether dyskinesia is a result of the progression of the disease or of the intake of levodopa.[13–15] Nowadays, it is generally accepted that levodopa is mostly responsible for the dyskinesia. There are, however, other anti-parkinsonian drugs that may induce dyskinesia. Anticholinergics also lead to bucco-oro-lingual dyskinesia, as known from tardive dyskinesias. However, even dopamine agonists, which together with amantadine are in our view the best suited drugs to overcome dyskinesia, lead to dyskinesias in a very small percentage of cases.[16]

Treatment of dyskinesia

Treatment of peak-dose dyskinesia

Optimum treatment of dyskinesia depends upon obtaining good information from the patient and his/her caregivers. It is of importance to differentiate between peak-dose-related dyskinesias and those which occur when levodopa levels are low. It is helpful to ask the patient to use a diary and mark in this booklet the intake of medication, on- and off-periods and occurrence of dyskinesia. If this is impossible, short-term observation on the ward may be necessary. Peak-dose dyskinesia occurs normally 60 min after intake of levodopa, and can be diagnosed by levodopa analysis in the blood. In this situation it is mandatory to decrease the dosage of levodopa even if mobility also decreases. Patients will usually be less happy with this, since they prefer to be hyperkinetic than to be hypokinetic, in contrast to their caregivers, who find it difficult to deal with long-lasting dyskinesias. In some instances lowering of levodopa dosage or the administration of lower but more frequent doses of levodopa may be enough to improve dyskinesia. Another option would be the consumption of small portions of dissolved levodopa throughout the day. This drink must be made fresh each day. We were not happy with the use of controlled-release levodopa in such a situation, because absorption in the gut is greatly hampered in these patients and some patients report worsening of dyskinesias. Basically, the use of controlled-release levodopa could be advantageous in peak-dose dyskinesias but not in biphasic-dyskinesia.

Catechol-O-methyltransferase inhibitors may allow a reduction of levodopa and thus a more phasic stimulation of dopamine receptors and a concomitant reduction of dyskinesia. It is important to inform the patient that initially, while levodopa is not yet reduced, dyskinesias may worsen. There are new results on the possible use of COMT inhibitors and slow-release levodopa which increase the time 'on' and decrease the duration of dyskinesia (Stocchi, personal communication). If co-morbidity of the patients is not a contra-indication, the best approach would be to decrease levodopa and to compensate with dopamine agonists. In some highly selected patients high-dose dopamine agonist therapy may be appropriate to achieve maximal lowering of levodopa.[17-19] If a sufficient compensation with dopamine agonists is impossible, the use of amantadine is recommended.[20-22] Rajput's study included 19 patients with hyperkinesias, of whom 13 showed choreiform peak-dose dyskinesias. Fourteen out of 19 patients showed an improvement of dyskinesia after 2 weeks and seven also showed an improvement of parkinsonian symptoms. Verhagen-Metmann and colleagues achieved a reduction of peak-dose dyskinesias of 60%. A follow-up study (1 year later) supported this finding, since a 56% reduction of dyskinesia and a considerable improvement of on-time was reported. If medication does not achieve a sufficient improvement of dyskinesia, deep brain stimulation may be an option. In our view deep brain stimulation of the subthalamic nucleus is the most appropriate method.[23,24]

Treatment of biphasic dyskinesias

Therapy of biphasic dyskinesia is often rather difficult and can sometimes even be unsuccessful. Most patients have the so-called D-I-D pattern (dyskinesia–improvement–dyskinesia). As mentioned above, patients experience dyskinesia as long as the levodopa level is not high enough. Thus, to keep this phase short, it is important to increase the levodopa level rapidly. When patients have reached their peak they function well, and when levodopa decreases again they have their second phase of dyskinesia. In contrast to peak-dose dyskinesia, this type of dyskinesia often involves the lower extremities, and the period when the levodopa levels decrease is normally longer and more troublesome for the patient than the first dyskinetic phase when he/she turns 'on'. Our first approach is the use of more frequent and higher doses of levodopa to reach the plateau rapidly and keep the patient in the 'on' state. The use of a soluble fast-release levodopa led to improvement in some patients. Since low plasma doses of levodopa cause the first dyskinetic period, it is not advisable to use controlled-release levodopa or COMT inhibitors which cause too slow an increase in levodopa levels. To the best of our knowledge there are no studies on the effectiveness of dopamine agonists or amantadine in this situation, although we have used both drugs with good results for patients with biphasic dyskinesias. Finally, there is one study that has indicated the use of clozapine for dyskinesia.[25]

Treatment of dystonic dyskinesia

As mentioned for biphasic dyskinesia it is also mandatory if patients report dystonia to obtain a precise history of the relationship of the dyskinesia to levodopa intake. Dystonia occurs most often in the morning, is rather painful and presents with cramping of the toes and feet. A beneficial treatment of this early-morning dystonia is the use of soluble fast-release levodopa or subcutaneous application of apomorphine. Alternatively, the nightly administration of slow-release levodopa may be necessary. Another alternative would be the use of a dopamine agonist. Hypothetically, the use of botulinum injection should be helpful but is not very practical. Peak-dose dystonia can be treated by decreasing levodopa dose and/or applying dopamine agonists. End of dose dystonia may be improved by the use of a COMT inhibitor or the use of a long-acting dopamine agonist.

Underlying biochemical and molecular mechanisms of dyskinesia

Although the causal mechanisms underlying dyskinesia(s) are not known, current evidence from biochemical and molecular experimental approaches have raised reasonable hypotheses which are suited for testing under clinical conditions. These hypotheses are mainly, but not exclusively, based on biochemical/molecular alterations within the dopaminergic nigrostriatal systems. As motor fluctuations and dyskinesia(s) are not a prerequisite of physiological aging and have not been observed in long-term L-dopa-treated patients who were diagnosed originally with Parkinson's disease but finally did not suffer from a degenerative disorder, it is reasonable to assume that degeneration of the nigrostriatal system is a dominant prerequisite for developing dyskinesia. Degeneration in the striatum may then lead to hyperkinesia via final overactivity of the dopamine receptor D1-driven direct loop system, while final overactivity of the D2-receptor-driven indirect pathway causes hypoactivity. L-Dopa-induced choreiform dyskinesias (LID) in Parkinson's disease are based on risk factors which include young age, female gender, high L-dopa doses and long duration of L-dopa treatment.

Electrophysiological studies in MPTP (N-methyl-4-phenyl-1,2,3,6-tetrahydropyridine)-lesioned monkeys demonstrate that chronic L-dopa treatment causes reduced activities in the GPm (globus pallidus medialis) but not in GPl (globus pallidus lateralis).[26] Therefore, one may assume that the direct D1-driven motor loop is responsible for the development of dyskinesias. *In situ* hybridization studies showed increases in enkephalin concentration but reduced substance P mRNA in the striatum.[27] More recently the precursor gene of enkephalins, prepro-enkephalin (PPE), has been found to be increased at the mRNA level in the putamen of Parkinson's disease with LID.[28] These data agree with dopamine being inhibitory on enkephalinergic neurons, while relief of this inhibition induces increased expression of PPE. Although there is a relationship between the increase of PPE and the severity of motor impairment in MPTP monkeys, other studies using the MPTP model have challenged this causal link (reviewed by Calon *et al.*[28]). Based on work by Oh *et al.*[29] it has been suggested that intermittent, unphysiological stimulation of striatal dopamine receptors by L-dopa triggers phosphorylation of glutamatergic NMDA (N-methyl-D-aspartate) receptors and leads to facilitation of postsynaptic glutamatergic neurotransmission. This glutamatergic overactivity might contribute to the development of dyskinesia.[29] There are, however, many critical issues based on postmortem analyses, anatomical, functional and clinical arguments, which appear to make the current concept of the organization of the basal ganglia obsolete (reviewed by Gerlach et al.,[4] Parent and Cicchetti,[30] and Marsden and Obeso[31]).

Because of these uncertainties, clinical concepts concentrate on the action of L-dopa and dopaminergic receptor agonists on D1- and D2-receptors. Especially being considered are the half-life of drug action and receptor efficacy due to drug affinity (Tables 2.1 and 2.2).

It has been hypothesized that medication with drugs showing long half-life (in general

dopamine receptor agonists), thereby guaranteeing continuous receptor stimulation, should not cause motor fluctuations and dyskinesia, while short-acting substances such as L-dopa would lead to pulsatile receptor stimulation, resulting in this type of adverse reaction. This concept seems to be well accepted in clinical practice.

From a theoretical point of view, however, these data do not seem to explain the whole problem. Recent experimental evidence suggests that there is equipotent efficacy in MPTP-lesioned monkeys between L-dopa/carbidopa (12.5 mg/kg p.o. twice daily), apomorphine

Table 2.1 Half-life, affinities for D1- and D2-receptors, and daily doses of L-dopa and dopamine receptor agonists. Adapted in part from reference 39

| | Half-life (h) | D1 [³H]SCH23390 K_i (nmol/l) | D2 [³H]Racloprid K_i (nmol/l) | Typical daily dose as adjunct to L-dopa therapy | |
				Dose (mg)	No. of doses
L-Dopa/dopamine	<1	2729	117 000	50 to >250	3
Bromocriptine	3–8	119.6	2.9	15–40	3
Cabergoline	65–110	1462	0.61	4–5	1
α-Dihydroergocryptine	15	35.4	7.25	60–120	2–3
Lisuride	2–3	56.7	0.95	1.5–4	3
Pergolide	7–27	447	10.3	0.75–4	3
Pramipexole	8–12	>100 000	79 500	1.5–4.5	3
Ropinirole	3–6	>100 000	98 700	7–16	3

Table 2.2 Gross comparison of principal pharmacological action of L-dopa/dopamine and dopamine receptor agonists on intact and lesioned nigrostriatal dopaminergic neurons

	Intact neuron	Lesioned neuron
L-Dopa	low affinity	low affinity
	tonic release	pulsed release
	continuous receptor stimulation	pulsed receptor stimulation
	no motor fluctuations	dyskinesia
Dopamine receptor agonists	high affinity	high affinity
	continuous receptor stimulation	continuous receptor stimulation
	no motor fluctuations	no motor fluctuations

(0.15 mg/kg p.o. once daily) and pergolide (0.4 mg/kg s.c. twice daily).[32]

Interestingly, L-dopa (mean per 28-days' follow-up) showed significant and great potential for inducing (total) dyskinesias compared to apomorphine and pergolide, the latter showing (total) dyskinesias to a significantly lesser extent. Also, apomorphine and pergolide did not demonstrate significant differences in expressing dyskinesias despite great variances in half-life and duration of action. On the other hand, there was statistical significance between the effects of L-dopa and apomorphine, drugs with a similar and short half-life. These data by Maratos *et al.*[32] clearly demonstrate the difficulties when only the half-life of anti-parkinsonian drugs are considered important in explaining the occurrence of L-dopa induced dyskinesias.

In addition, at early stages of Parkinson's disease one would suggest that L-dopa-induced dyskinesias would be less frequent, owing to the availability of more intact dopaminergic neurons, while in later stages pulsatile receptor stimulation should provoke dyskinesias to a greater extent. However, this is not confirmed by clinical observations. In fact, young patients elicit dyskinesias much earlier and to a greater severity than patients who develop the disease later in life.

Still keeping the concept of continuous receptor stimulation, we would rather assume that drugs' receptor affinity plays a much more important role to explain the occurrence of motor fluctuations/dyskinesia at the receptor signaling site: L-dopa/dopamine and dopamine receptor agonists might lead to different and long-lasting changes in the expression of certain but still unknown genes. This hypothesis would explain differences in the occurrence of dyskinesia, differences in the priming efficacy of L-dopa (high) and dopaminergic receptor agonists (low);[33] and the surprisingly effective clinical action of dopaminergic receptor agonists with short half-life.

We have not yet discussed the importance of cAMP stimulating D1- and cAMP inhibiting G-protein-dependent D2-dopaminergic receptors in developing dykinesias. It has been reported that D1- and D2-receptor agonists such as apomorphine and pergolide elicit higher levels of dyskinesia than do pure D2-receptor agonists. However, as pointed out above, they show less of this effect following chronic L-dopa treatment. These data imply that D1-receptor activation increases the risk for dyskinesia(s).

Furthermore, L-dopa induces ectopic expression of the D3-receptor on D1/dynorphin/substance P-expressing neurons. Intermittent D1-receptor stimulation reverses the denervation-induced down-regulation of dynorphin and substance P. Therefore, L-dopa, via D3-receptors, would dissociate the response of dynorphin and substance P to the D1-agonist, leading to a high dynorphin/substance P ratio. An excess inhibitory action in the globus pallidus internus and reduction in the discharge rates of its neurons would be the consequence. Dyskinesias would be the behavioral correlate.[34–36] Others hypothesize from a set of observations indicating plastic changes in striatal function produced by the combination of substantial striatal dopamine denervation and L-dopa treatment. The key factor in the emergence of this behavioral sensitization is suggested to be continuity of dopamine receptor occupancy. The interpretation of the sensitization phenomenon relates to the magnitude of the nigrostriatal lesion. The incidence of dyskinesia, however, is not correlated with the duration of treatment.

In addition, non-physiological pulsatile dopamine receptor stimulation changes the dopamine–glutamate interaction, leads to glutamate-receptor subtype phosphorylation (therefore enhancing the efficacy of those receptors), and consequently alters the output signal from medium spiny neurons in the putamen.[37] In agreement with such data, Bedard (personal communication) reported an increased glutamate concentration in monkeys with L-dopa-induced dyskinesias. Continuous stimulation of the subthalamic nucleus (STN) induces long-term plastic changes in the dopaminergic system with slow and partial desensitization.[38] The question remains open whether STN stimulations may directly facilitate the improvement of L-dopa-induced dyskinesias.

CONCLUSIONS

From the available data it is hypothesized that drugs with: preference for D2-receptors and high affinity for D2-receptors will have low incidence for dyskinesias. In this case the half-life of a drug does not seem to have a decisive role. In contrast, drugs with: preferred actions on D1-receptors, low affinity for dopamine receptors and short half-life seem to facilitate dyskinesias.

Duration of treatment is of less importance. The extent of nigrostriatal degeneration, suggested to play a major role in the development of dyskinesias, is a factor to be further elucidated in this regard.

In addition, basic research is needed to elucidate the mechanisms by which other drugs, such as dopamine receptor antagonists, anticonvulsants (carbamazepine, phenytoin) and benzodiazepines, antihistaminic drugs, metoclopramide, digoxin, flunarizin, cimetidine and methadone, facilitate dyskinesias.

REFERENCES

1. Kostic V, Przedborski S, Flaster E, Sternic N. Early development of levodopa-induced dyskinesias and response fluctuations in young-onset Parkinson's disease. Neurology 1991; 41: 202–5

2. Cederbaum JM, Gandy SE, McDowell FH. 'Early' initiation of levodopa treatment does not promote the development of motor response fluctuations, dyskinesias, or dementia in Parkinson's disease. Neurology 1991; 41: 622–9

3. Parkinson Study Group. Impact of deprenyl and tocopherol treatment on Parkinson's disease in DATATOP patients requiring levodopa. Ann Neurol 1996; 39: 37–45

4. Gerlach M, Reichmann H, Riederer P. Die Parkinson Krankheit. Vienna: Springer, 2003

5. Nutt JG. Levodopa induced dyskinesia: review, observations and speculations. Neurology 1990; 40: 340–5

6. Luquin MR, Scipioni O, Vaamonde J, et al. Levodopa-induced dyskinesia in Parkinson's disease: clinical and pharmacological classification. Mov Disord 1992; 7: 117–24

7. Jankovic J, Nour F. Respiratory dyskinesia in Parkinson's disease. Neurology 1986; 36: 303–4

8. Muenter MD, Sharpless NS, Tyce GM, Darley FL. Patterns of dystonia ('I-D-I' and 'D-I-D') in response to L-dopa therapy for Parkinson's disease. Mayo Clin Proc 1977; 52: 163–74

9. Klawans HL, Goetz C, Bergen D. Levodopa-induced myoclonus. Arch Neurol 1975; 32: 231–4

10. Klawans HL, Tanner CM, McDermott J. Myoclonus and parkinsonism. Clin Neuropharmacol 1986; 9: 202–5

11. Poewe WH, Lees AJ, Stern GM. Low-dose L-dopa therapy in Parkinson's disease: a 6-year follow-up study. Neurology 1986; 36: 1528–30

12. Comella CL, Goetz CG. Akathisia in Parkinson's disease. Mov Disord 1994; 9: 545–9

13. Diamond SG, Markham CH, Hoehn MM, et al. Multicenter study of Parkinson mortality with early versus later dopa treatment. Ann Neurol 1987; 22: 8–12

14. Fahn S, Bressman SB. Should levodopa therapy for parkinsonism be started early or late? Evidence against early treatment. Can J Neurol Sci 1984; 11: 2000–6

15. Rajput AH, Stern W, Laverty WH. Chronic low-dose levodopa therapy in Parkinson's disease: an argument for delaying levodopa therapy. Neurology 1984; 34: 991–7

16. Rascol O, Brooks D, Korczyn AD, et al. for the 056 Study Group. A five-year study of the incidence of dyskinesia in patients with early Parkinson's disease who were treated with ropinirole or levodopa. N Engl J Med 2000; 342: 1484–91

17. Facca A, Sanchez-Ramos J. High-dose pergolide monotherapy in the treatment of severe levodopa-induced dyskinesias. Mov Disord 1996; 11: 327–9

18. Müngersdorf M, Sommer U, Sommer M, Reichmann H. High-dose therapy with ropinirole in patients with Parkinson's disease. J Neural Transm 2001; 108: 1309–17

19. Cristina S, Zangaglia R, Mancini F, et al. High-dose ropinirole in advanced Parkinson's disease with severe dyskinesia. Clin Neuropharmacol 2003; 26: 146–50

20. Rajput A, Wallkai M, Rajput AH. 18 month prospective study of amantadine (Amd) for Dopa (LD) induced dyskinesias (DK) in idiopathic Parkinson's disease. Can Neurol Sci 1997; 24: S23

21. Verhagen-Metmann L, Del Dotto P, van-den-Munckhof P, et al. Amantadine as treatment for dyskinesias and motor fluctuations in Parkinson's disease. Neurology 1998; 50: 1323–6

22. Verhagen-Metmann L, Del Dotto P, LePoole K, et al. Amantadine for levodopa-induced dyskinesias – a 1-year follow-up study. Arch Neurol 1999; 56: 1383–6

23. Limousin P, Krack P, Pollack P, et al. Electrical stimulation of the subthalamic nucleus in advanced Parkinson's disease. N Engl J Med 1998; 339: 1105–11

24. Krack P, Pollack P, Limousin P, et al. From 'off' period dystonia to peak-dose chorea: the clinical spectrum of varying subthalamic nucleus activity. Brain 1999; 122: 1133–46

25. Pierelli F, Adipietro A, Soldati G, et al. Low dosage clozapine effects on L-dopa induced dyskinesias in parkinsonian patients. Acta Neurol Scand 1998; 97: 295–9

26. Fox SH, Brotchie JM. New treatments for movement disorders? Trends Pharmacol Sci 1996; 17: 339–42

27. Jolkkonen J, Jenner P, Marsden CD. L-DOPA reverses altered gene expression of substance P but not enkephalin in the caudate-putamen of common marmosets treated with MPTP. Brain Res Mol Brain Res 1995; 32: 297–307

28. Calon F, Morissette M, Rajput AH, et al. Changes of GABA receptors and dopamine turnover in the postmortem brains of Parkinsonians with levodopa-induced motor complications. Mov Dis 2003; 18: 241–53

29. Oh JD, Russell D, Vaughan CL, Chase TN. Enhanced tyrosine phosphorylation of striatal NMDA receptor subunits: effect of dopaminergic denervation and L-DOPA administration. Brain 1998; 813: 150–9

30. Parent A, Cicchetti F. The current model of basal ganglia organization under scrutiny. Mov Disord 1998, 13: 199–202

31. Marsden CD, Obeso JA. The functions of the basal ganglia and the paradox of stereotaxic surgery in Parkinson's disease. Brain 1994; 117: 887–97

32. Maratos EC, Jackson MJ, Pearce RKB, et al. Both short- and long-acting D-1/D-2 dopamine agonists induce less dyskinesia than L-DOPA in the MPTP-lesioned common marmoset (Callithrix jacchus). Exp Neurol 2003; 179, 90–102

33. Andersson M, Hilbertson A, Cenci MA, Striatal fosB expression is causally linked with L-DOPA-induced abnormal involuntary movements and the associated upregulation of striatal prodynorphin mRNA in rat model of Parkinson's disease. Neurobiol Dis 1999; 6: 461–74

34. Bezard E, Ferry A, Mach U, et al. Attenuation of levodopa-induced dyskinesia by normalizing dopamine D3 receptor function. Nature Med 2003; 9: 762–7

35. Wooten GF. Agonists vs levodopa in PD. Neurology 2003; 60: 360–2

36. Smith LA, Jackson MJ, Hansard MJ, et al. Effect of pulsatile administration of Levodopa on dyskinesia induction in drug-naive MPTP-treated common marmosets: effect of dose, frequency of administration, and brain exposure. Mov Dis 2003; 18: 487–95

37. Chase TN, Konitsiotis S, Oh JD. Striatal molecular mechanisms and motor dysfunction in Parkinson's disease. Adv Neurol 2001; 86: 355–60

38. Moro E, Esselink RJ, Benabid AL, Pollak P. Response to levodopa in parkinsonian patients with bilateral subthalamic nucleus stimulation. Brain 2002; 125: 2408–17

39. Foley P, Gerlach M, Double KL, Riederer P. Dopamine receptor agonists in the therapy of Parkinson's disease. J Neural Transm 2004; 111: 1375–446

Chapter 3

Molecular neuropathology of parkinsonism

DW Dickson

INTRODUCTION

Parkinson's disease (PD) is primarily a clinical diagnosis with a phenotype characterized by bradykinesia, rigidity, tremor and postural instability. Non-motor manifestations, such as anosmia and autonomic dysfunction, are also common in PD. Another clinical feature used by some investigators to confirm the diagnosis of PD is sustained clinical response to dopamine replacement therapy.[1] While the usual pathological substrate of PD is Lewy body disease (LBD), other pathological entities such as progressive supranuclear palsy (PSP) and multiple system atrophy (MSA) less often clinically resemble PD.[2] The latter disorders usually have other features that are not common in PD such as eye movement abnormalities and cerebellar signs.

At present, postmortem neuropathological studies of the brain are the only way to differentiate among the various causes of parkinsonism. It should also be acknowledged that pathological criteria for PD have not been validated using modern neuropathological methods for detecting Lewy bodies (LBs) and that the clinical phenotype of LBD is more diverse than that of PD, including dementia, psychosis, autonomic dysfunction and sleep disorders. Moreover, there is as yet no way to predict with certainty the clinical phenotype of LBD given the pathological findings.

GENETICS OF PARKINSONISM

The discovery that mutations in the α-synuclein gene (*SNCA*) can cause familial PD[3] and that α-synuclein is the major structural component of LBs[4] has opened a new avenue in the investigation of parkinsonism. At present, 11 genetic assignments have been proposed for familial PD (Table 3.1).[5] PARK1 is autosomal dominant early-onset PD due to mutations in *SNCA*.[3] PARK2 and PARK7 are autosomal recessive early-onset PD due to mutations in *parkin*[6] and *DJ-1*,[7] respectively. Genes for the other familial PD assignments remain unknown or controversial. Mutations in the tau gene (*MAPT*) have been discovered in some forms of frontotemporal dementia,[8] and some of these kindreds have prominent parkinsonism,[9] most often with features similar to PSP or corticobasal degeneration (CBD). The accepted term for this disorder is FTDP-17.[10] For this reason, *MAPT* is sometimes included among the genes responsible for parkinsonism. Some forms of spinocerebellar ataxia (SCA), particularly

Table 3.1 Genetic assignments for familial Parkinson's disease

Chromosome	Gene	Name	Neuropathology
17q12-22	MAPT (tau)	FTDP-17	NFT and tau-positive glial lesions
4q21	SNCA (α-synuclein)	PARK1	LBs
6q25.2-27	parkin	PARK2	non-specific nigral degeneration (tau-positive lesions; LBs in some cases)
2p13	unknown	PARK3	LBs
4q21 (initially linked to 4p15)	SNCA[43]	PARK4	LBs
4p14-15	UCHL-1	PARK5	not described (giant axonal dystrophy in mouse UCHL1 mutants)
1q35-36	PINK1[42]	PARK6	not described
1p36	DJ-1	PARK7	not described (LBs in heterozygous individuals)
12p11.2-q13.1	unknown	PARK8	variable pathology (non-specific nigral degeneration; LBs; NFT[44])
1p36	unknown	PARK9	not described (pallidal-pyramidal degeneration on imaging)
1p32	unknown	PARK10	not described
2q36-37	unknown	PARK11	not described

NFT, neurofibrillary tangles; LBs, Lewy bodies

SCA2 and SCA3,[11] may also have prominent parkinsonism and might also be added to the list of PD genes.

MOLECULAR CLASSIFICATION OF PARKINSON'S DISEASE

Immunochemical, biochemical and genetic studies have provided a basis for a molecular classification of parkinsonism. The major parkinsonian disorders fall into two groups: those characterized by synuclein abnormalities ('synucleinopathies') and those characterized by tau abnormalities ('tauopathies').[12] Among the former are LBD and MSA, while the latter include PSP, CBD and FTDP-17. Neuro-pathological studies are sparse or absent in most of the familial PD assignments. Even the most common of the familial PD, autosomal recessive juvenile-onset PD (ARJP) due to parkin mutations, has been the subject of only a limited number of autopsy studies.[13] The available autopsy studies of ARJP have shown substantia nigra degeneration with no specific histopathological lesions, sparse tau-related lesions or LBs, making it difficult to assign ARJP to one of the molecular categories, at present. The pathology of DJ-1-related PD is unknown. Two other assignments (PARK3 and PARK4) are also synucleinopathies, in that LBs have been described in autopsies from some kindred linked to these loci.[14,15]

SYNUCLEINOPATHIES

The most common of the synucleinopathies is LBD. LBs are granulofilamentous lesions composed of synuclein within the perikarya of neurons. Similar lesions are also found within neuronal processes, also known as Lewy neurites (LNs). While originally described in the hippocampus[16] and later the amygdala,[17] LNs are now more widespread than originally suspected and may be the most abundant type of pathological lesion in a given region of brain affected by the disease. The contribution of neuritic degeneration to the clinical phenotype is increasingly recognized.[18] The lesions detected in sporadic LBD are essentially identical to those found in genetically determined forms of LBD.

MSA is a sporadic synucleinopathy in which there is neuronal loss and demyelination in the striatonigral system and the olivoponto-cerebellar systems.[19] The hallmark histopathological lesion is the glial cytoplasmic inclusion (GCI), which is a cytoplasmic inclusion within oligodendrocytes in the white matter in affected regions.[20] While most of the synuclein pathology in MSA is within glia, in many cases synuclein-immunoreactive neuronal cytoplasmic inclusions and neuritic lesions are also present.[21] While these lesions resemble LBs and LNs, the anatomical distribution of the pathology is distinct from LBD. Interestingly, synuclein-immunoreactive glial lesions have also been reported in LBD,[22] especially in early-onset familial forms,[15] suggesting that MSA and LBD are part of a pathological spectrum. Biochemical studies of brain homogenates from MSA and LBD also support this contention in that abnormal forms of synuclein are detected in detergent- and formic acid-extractable fractions in both MSA and LBD.[23] Moreover, high molecular weight forms that may represent post-translationally modified or aggregated forms of synuclein are detected in both.

The different selectively neuronal vulnerability in LBD and MSA is striking, with the major overlap being in the nigrostriatal system. The forebrain, especially olfactory and limbic areas, has far more pathology in LBD than in MSA. The pattern of selective vulnerability of LBD has been the focus of several recent studies. Of particular note is the attempt to develop a staging system for LBD in PD by Braak and co-workers.[24] In this staging system nigral pathology occurs at mid-stage disease, whereas involvement of the medulla and pontine tegmentum occur earlier (Table 3.2). The anterior olfactory nucleus is also affected early in the course. In the endstage, LBs involve cortical areas, and at this stage many patients with PD are expected to have significant cognitive problems. The pathology at this stage is similar to that found in diffuse LBD, an increasingly recognized late-life dementing disorder.[25] Several studies have suggested that the most common cause of later-developing dementia in patients who initially had typical PD is in fact diffuse LBD.[26,27]

Despite the heuristic value of this proposed staging system, it requires validation. A large cross-sectional study by Parkkinen and co-workers[28] of 904 brains studied with synuclein immunohistochemistry largely concurred with the Braak staging scheme; however, they also described six cases in which LBs were found only in the substantia nigra without involvement of the medulla. Another area in which the staging scheme breaks down is the presence of LBs in the setting of advanced Alzheimer's disease (AD). It is increasingly recognized that many cases of AD have LBs[29] and that the most common location for LBs in advanced AD is the amygdala.[30] We have termed this AD with amygdala LBs (ALB).[31] In a cross-sectional study of 345 consecutive cases of AD in the Mayo Clinic Jacksonville neuropathology files, LBs were found in 94 cases in multiple brain stem,

Table 3.2 Braak staging of Lewy body Parkinson's disease

Stage 1
Medulla tegmentum: dorsal motor nucleus of vagus–glossopharyngeal complex

Stage 2
Pontine tegmentum: locus ceruleus

Stage 3
Substantia nigra

Stage 4
Basal forebrain and medial temporal cortex

Stage 5
Higher-order-association cortices (especially temporal and frontal lobes)

Stage 6
Primary cortices

---

diencephalic and forebrain regions, but in the remaining 251 AD cases no brain stem LBs were detected. The amygdala was screened with synuclein immunohistochemistry in this group and 38 (15%) had LBs. On re-examination the brain stem had only isolated and sparse LNs in eight cases, but the other cases did not have brain stem LBs. Thus, LBs in advanced AD begin *de novo* in the amygdala without progressing through the several brain stem stages that have been described for PD. Further studies are warranted to determine whether there are other patterns of LB acquisition in different diseases in which LBs are occasionally found.

TAUOPATHIES AND THE ROLE OF TAU IN PARKINSON'S DISEASE

Besides FTDP-17, tau is implicated in the molecular neuropathology of several other parkinsonian disorders. The most common is PSP, but others include CBD, post-encephalitic parkinsonism, Guam parkinsonism–dementia complex and dementia pugilistica.[32] All of these disorders have neuronal loss in the substantia nigra, and some of the residual neurons have

neurofibrillary tangles (NFTs). NFTs are intra-neuronal filamentous inclusions composed of tau protein, a microtubule-associated protein encoded by a gene on chromosome 17. The tau gene (*MAPT*) has a number of polymorphisms that are inherited as two major haplotypes – H1 and H2.[33] The *MAPT* gene is alternatively transcribed to generate at least six isoforms. Alternative splicing of exon 10 generates tau with either three or four 31–32 homologous ('repeat', R) sequences – thus 3R and 4R tau.[34] The nature of the tau differs among the various tauopathies associated with parkinsonism.[35] Depending upon the *MAPT* mutation, the tau protein that accumulates in FTDP-17 is 3R and 4R, only 3R or only 4R. In AD, Guam parkinsonism–demenita complex, postencephalitic parkinsonism and dementia pugilistica tau in NFTs is composed of 3R and 4R tau. In PSP and CBD, 4R is the predominant species.

The 4R tauopathies are associated with a high frequency of the *MAPT* H1/H1 genotype, suggesting that the H1 haplotype may confer risk for PSP and CBD.[36] Interestingly, several studies have also suggested that the H1 haplotype may be more frequent in PD.[37,38] The mechanism for this association is uncertain, given that the major pathology of PD is the LB. Moreover, in a recent study of LBD cases in the Mayo Clinic Jacksonville brain bank, the frequency of the H1/H1 genotype in LBD was no greater than in controls, while there was a significant increase in the H1/H1 genotype in PSP and CBD (unpublished observation). Interpretation of these results needs to be made with caution, since the majority of the LBD brains in the Mayo Clinic Jacksonville brain bank are derived from patients with dementia syndromes rather than parkinsonism.

Of possible relevance to this observation is the fact that tau immunoreactivity is occasionally reported in LBs.[39,40] In a study of tau immunoreactivity in LBs using a panel of tau antibodies recognizing epitopes that span the entire length of the tau molecule, tau immunoreactivity was detected in 5–40% of LBs, with the highest frequency detected in neurons known to be vulnerable to both NFTs and LBs and with tau antibodies that recognized phosphorylated epitopes.[40] Excluding the possibility of co-occurrence of NFTs in neurons with LBs and possible cross-reactivity of phosphoepitopes, there still remains a small proportion of LBs with tau immunoreactivity. In most cases this immunoreactivity is detected at the periphery of the LB, which suggests that tau may be co-deposited in the late stages of LB formation. This is at variance with the hypo-

thesis that synuclein may serve as a seed for tau polymerization, as shown recently in reconstitution experiments *in vitro*.[41]

Summary

The number of molecules important to the pathogenesis of PD continues to grow with the advent of molecular biological approaches to brain tissue and genetic studies of familial PD. The molecules of current interest are linked to ubiquitin-mediated proteolysis (*parkin* and *UCHL1*), synaptic plasticity (*SNCA*) and oxidant stress. The role of tau remains controversial, but several points are clear: synuclein is often detected in neurons that are also vulnerable to NFT, for example in the amygdala; tau is present in some LBs; and the *MAPT* H1/H1 genotype is increased in clinical series of PD, but not in pathological series of LBD. The latter is of particular interest, since it raises the possibility that there may be genetically distinct forms of LBD (one presenting with parkinsonism and associated with H1 and one presenting with other phenotypes, such as dementia, and not associated with H1). Additional molecular genetic studies on autopsy-confirmed cases are necessary, since multiple pathological processes with different molecular mechanisms can present with parkinsonism.

REFERENCES

1. Hughes AJ, Daniel SE, Ben-Shlomo Y, Lees AJ. The accuracy of diagnosis of parkinsonian syndromes in a specialist movement disorder service. Brain 2002; 25: 861–70

2. Bower JH, Dickson DW, Taylor L, et al. Clinical correlates of the pathology underlying parkinsonism: a population perspective. Mov Disord 2002; 17: 910–16

3. Polymeropoulos MH, Lavedan C, Leroy E, et al. Mutation in the alpha-synuclein gene identified in families with Parkinson's disease. Science 1997; 276: 2045–7

4. Spillantini MG, Schmidt ML, Lee VM, et al. Alpha-synuclein in Lewy bodies. Nature 1997; 388: 839–40

5. Gwinn-Hardy K. Genetics of parkinsonism. Mov Disord 2002; 17: 645–56

6. Kitada T, Asakawa S, Hattori N, et al. Mutations in the parkin gene cause autosomal recessive juvenile parkinsonism. Nature 1998; 392: 605–8

7. Bonifati V, Rizzu P, van Baren MJ, et al. Mutations in the DJ-1 gene associated with autosomal recessive early-onset parkinsonism. Science 2003; 299: 256–9

8. Hutton M, Lendon CL, Rizzu P, et al. Association of missense and 5′-splice-site mutations in tau with the inherited dementia (FTDP-17). Nature 1998; 393: 702–5

9. Wszolek ZK, Tsuboi Y, Farrer M, et al. Hereditary tauopathies and parkinsonism. Adv Neurol 2003; 91: 153–63

10. Foster NL, Wilhelmsen K, Sima AAF, et al. Frontotemporal dementia and parkinsonism linked to chromosome 17: a consensus conference. Ann Neurol 1997; 41: 706–15

11. Payami H, Nutt J, Gancher S, et al. SCA2 may present as levodopa-responsive parkinsonism. Mov Disord 2003; 18: 425–9

12. Hardy J, Gwinn-Hardy K. Genetic classification of primary neurodegenerative disease. Science 1998; 282: 1075–9

13. Hayashi S, Wakabayashi K, Ishikawa A, et al. An autopsy case of autosomal-recessive juvenile parkinsonism with a homozygous exon 4 deletion in the parkin gene. Mov Disord 2000; 15: 884–8

14. Wszolek ZK, Gwinn-Hardy K, Wszolek EK, et al. Neuropathology of two members of a German-American kindred (Family C) with late onset parkinsonism. Acta Neuropathol 2002; 103: 344–50

15. Gwinn-Hardy K, Mehta ND, Farrer M, et al. Distinctive neuropathology revealed by α-synuclein antibodies in hereditary parkinsonism and dementia linked to chromosome 4p. Acta Neuropathol 2000; 99: 663–72

16. Dickson DW, Ruan D, Crystal H, et al. Hippocampal degeneration differentiates diffuse Lewy body disease (DLBD) from Alzheimer's disease: light and electron microscopic immunocytochemistry of CA2-3 neurites specific to DLBD. Neurology 1991; 41: 1402–9

17. Braak H, Braak E, Yilmazer D, et al. Amygdala pathology in Parkinson's disease. Acta Neuropathol 1994; 88: 493–500

18. Churchyard A, Lees AJ. The relationship between dementia and direct involvement of the hippocampus and amygdala in Parkinson's disease. Neurology 1997; 49: 1570–6

19. Lantos PL. The definition of multiple system atrophy: a review of recent developments. J Neuropathol Exp Neurol 1998; 57: 1099–111

20. Papp MI, Kahn JE, Lantos PL. Glial cytoplasmic inclusions in the CNS of patients with multiple system atrophy (striatonigral degeneration, olivopontocerebellar atrophy and Shy–Drager syndrome). J Neurol Sci 1989; 94: 79–100

21. Arima K, Ueda K, Sunohara N, et al. NACP/α-synuclein immunoreactivity in fibrillary components of neuronal and oligodendroglial cytoplasmic inclusions in the pontine nuclei in multiple system atrophy. Acta Neuropathol 1998; 96: 439–44

22. Takahashi H, Wakabayashi K. The cellular pathology of Parkinson's disease. Neuropathology 2001; 21: 315–22

23. Dickson DW, Liu W-K, Hardy J, et al. Widespread alterations of alpha-synuclein in multiple system atrophy. Am J Pathol 1999; 155: 1241–51

24. Braak H, Del Tredici K, Rub U, et al. Staging of brain pathology related to sporadic Parkinson's disease. Neurobiol Aging 2003; 24: 197–211

25. Kosaka K. Diffuse Lewy body disease in Japan. J Neurol 1990; 237: 197–204

26. Hurtig HI, Trojanowski JQ, Galvin J, et al. Alpha-synuclein cortical Lewy bodies correlate with dementia in Parkinson's disease. Neurology 2000; 54: 1916–21

27. Apaydin H, Ahlskog JE, Parisi JE, et al. Parkinson disease neuropathology: later-developing dementia and loss of the levodopa response. Arch Neurol 2002; 59: 102–12

28. Parkkinen L, Soininen H, Alafuzoff I. Regional distribution of alpha-synuclein pathology in unimpaired aging and Alzheimer disease. J Neuropathol Exp Neurol 2003; 62: 363–7

29. Hamilton RL. Lewy bodies in Alzheimer's disease: a neuropathological review of 145 cases using alpha-synuclein immunohistochemistry. Brain Pathol 2000; 10: 378–84

30. Lippa CF, Schmidt ML, Lee VM, Trojanowski JQ. Alpha-synuclein in familial Alzheimer disease: epitope mapping parallels dementia with Lewy bodies and Parkinson disease. Arch Neurol 2001; 58: 1817–20

31. DeLucia MW, Cookson N, Dickson DW. Synuclein-immunoreactive Lewy bodies are detected in the amygdala in less than 20% of Alzheimer (AD) cases. J Neuropathol Exp Neurol 2002; 61: 454

32. Dickson DW. Neuropathology of Parkinsonian disorders. In Jankovic JJ, Tolosa E, eds. Parkinson's Disease and Movement Disorders, 4th edn. Philadelphia: Lippincott Williams & Wilkins, 2002: 256–69

33. Baker M, Litvan I, Houlden H, et al. Association of an extended haplotype in the tau gene with progressive supranuclear palsy. Hum Mol Gen 1999; 8: 711–15

34. Andreadis A, Brown WM, Kosik KS. Structure and novel exons of the human tau gene. Biochemistry 1992; 31: 10626–33

35. Spillantini MG, Goedert M. Tau protein pathology in neurodegenerative diseases. Trends Neurosci 1998; 21: 428–33

36. Di Maria E, Tabaton M, Vigo T, et al. Corticobasal degeneration shares a common genetic background with progressive supranuclear palsy. Ann Neurol 2000; 47: 374–7

37. Martin ER, Scott WK, Nance MA, et al. Association of single-nucleotide polymorphisms of the tau gene with late-onset Parkinson disease. J Am Med Assoc 2001; 286: 2245–50

38. Farrer M, Skipper L, Berg M, et al. The tau H1 haplotype is associated with Parkinson's disease in the Norwegian population, Neurosci Lett 2002; 322: 83–6

39. Duda JE, Giasson BI, Mabon ME, et al. Concurrence of alpha-synuclein and tau brain pathology in the Contursi kindred, Acta Neuropathol 2002; 104: 7–11

40. Ishizawa T, Mattila P, Davies P, et al. Colocalization of tau and alpha-synuclein epitopes in Lewy bodies. J Neuropathol Exp Neurol 2003; 62: 389–97

41. Giasson BI, Forman MS, Higuchi M, et al. Initiation and synergistic fibrillization of tau and alpha-synuclein. Science 2003; 300: 636–40

42. Valente EM, Abou-Sleiman PM, Caputo V, et al. Hereditary early-onset Parkinson's disease caused by mutations in PINK1. Science 2004; 304: 1158–60

43. Singleton AB, Farrer M, Johnson J, et al. alpha-Synuclein locus triplication causes Parkinson's disease. Science 2003; 302: 841

44. Wszolek ZK, Pfeiffer RF, Tsuboi Y, et al. Autosomal dominant parkinsonism associated with variable synuclein and tau pathology. Neurology 2004; 62: 1619–22

Familial parkinsonian mutations affect the ability of catecholaminergic neurons to withstand proteasome inhibition

MR Cookson

INTRODUCTION

Identification of genes that cause familial parkinsonism may allow us to identify some of the pathways that lead to nigral degeneration in Parkinson's disease (PD) and related disorders. One gene in particular, parkin, implicates dysfunction in the ubiquitin–roteasome pathway as a causal route to nigral cell loss as the gene encodes a critical enzyme in this system. Recessive mutations in parkin sensitize cells to proteasome dysfunction and dominant mutations in α-synuclein have similar effects. How we might begin to address some of these questions will be discussed in this chapter.

PARKINSON'S DISEASE, CELL LOSS AND LEWY PATHOLOGY

The two pathological hallmarks of PD are a complex patchwork of neuronal cell loss including dopaminergic neurons in the substantia nigra pars compacta and the formation of protein aggregates that are collectively recognized as Lewy pathology.[1] In the rare familial forms of PD, mutations in α-synuclein or parkin both invariably cause nigral cell loss (for a review of the genetics of PD see

reference 2). Lewy bodies and Lewy neurites are prominent in cases with α-synuclein mutations but generally lacking in cases with parkin mutations, although some unusual parkin mutations are associated with Lewy-like pathology.[3] Therefore, mutations in either of these genes produce an overlapping but non-identical pathology. They also differ in the course of the disease (faster for α-synuclein mutations, more benign for parkin), age of onset (earlier for parkin mutations) and in some of the clinical parameters.[4] These observations show that there is overlap between these two Mendelian forms of PD, but there is distinctness as well.

This concept of overlap and distinctness applies to the comparison with genetic and sporadic forms of PD. It was shown several years ago that the wild-type form of α-synuclein is a substantial component of Lewy pathology.[5] In postmortem brain, α-synuclein forms extensive fibrils and is deposited into the insoluble fraction. Although there is argument about whether mature fibrils[6] or oligomeric precursors (protofibrils) mediate toxicity,[7] most commentators agree that the aggregation of α-synuclein is an important prerequisite for neuronal damage. More recently, genetic variability in expression of both α-synuclein[8] and parkin[9] have been shown to influence risk for developing idiopathic PD. This chapter will discuss how examining the mechanistic overlaps between different genes that cause the same disease might help us understand the underlying pathophysiological pathway that drives neurodegeneration. We also hope that there is sufficient overlap between sporadic and familial syndromes to gain eventual understanding of the nature of neuronal damage in all these situations. This may aid the development of rational interventions that address the underlying degenerative process in PD.

The ubiquitin–proteasome system and familial parkinsonism

There have been many proposals for causal biochemical events that might cause cell death in PD. Many of these, including mitochondrial function and oxidative stress, are dealt with in other chapters in this book. An additional hypothesis that has gained some currency recently is that subsets of neurons are vulnerable to a failure in proteasome-mediated protein turnover.[10,11] The proteasome system is a major route for protein degradation, especially for short-lived or misfolded/damaged proteins. Most proteins that are degraded by the proteasome require the addition of chains of a small modifier protein, ubiquitin. Ubiquitin is activated in a two-step process, and then added to target proteins by a series of enzymes referred to as 'E3' protein–ubiquitin ligases.[12,13]

There are a number of pieces of evidence that broadly support the idea that failure in the ubiquitin–proteasome system underlies aspects of neurological damage in sporadic PD. Proteasome activity is lower in the substantia nigra of brain from PD patients[14,15] (although not in other brain regions,[16] nor in diffuse Lewy body disease[17]). Application of proteasome inhibitors, in vivo or in vitro, result in selective toxicity towards catecholaminergic neurons. Although ubiquitin marks some Lewy bodies, whether this supports the idea of proteasome dysfunction or not in PD is unclear. For example, ubiquitylation of α-synuclein seems to be a consequence rather than cause of fibril formation[18] and therefore may occur rather late in the disease.

Strong evidence for the idea that proteasome dysfunction underlies familial PD comes from the identification of parkin as one of the group of E3 protein–ubiquitin ligases. Parkin has a number of substrates (reviewed by Cookson[19]) and several groups have suggested that accumulation of substrates for parkin's ubiquitylation activity leads to neuronal damage. Whether there is one critical substrate or a multitude, perhaps having additive effects, is not known. Pael-R (parkin-associated endothelin receptor-like receptor) is a substrate associated with the endoplasmic reticulum, and its expression is sufficient to drive toxicity in vitro and in transgenic flies.[20] Other substrates for parkin include a number that might have similar effects, such as cyclinE, which might trigger apoptosis directly.[21] Perhaps as a result of having multiple substrates, parkin can protect against a number of different cellular triggers for damage.

Additional important support for the proteasome hypothesis comes from the observation by several independent laboratories that mutant α-synuclein also increases sensitivity to proteasome inhibitors by decreasing net proteasome function.[22–24] The mechanism is not completely clear at this time, although a direct effect of aggregated α-synuclein on purified proteasomes in vitro has been reported.[25] Other proteins that aggregate have similar effects (see below). Linking these observations into selective vulnerability, we have recently shown that expression of mutant α-synucleins results in toxicity towards catecholaminergic neurons in primary midbrain cultures.[24] Parkin both decreases sensitivity to proteasome inhibitors in cell lines and is capable of rescuing the toxic effects of mutant α-synuclein in primary neurons. This has been confirmed in an *in vitro* model. The mechanism is not through parkin regulating bulk levels of α-synuclein, as might be expected if parkin were an E3-ligase for α-synuclein itself. A parsimonious but unproven explanation is that, as α-synuclein aggregates, it indirectly affects the turnover of critical proteasome substrates that accumulate and damage the cell. Parkin may maintain lower steady-state levels of these proteins, if it is a key E3 ligase modulating steady-state levels. However, it is clear that there is a great deal of work to be done on the relationship between these two gene products.

TESTING THE PROTEASOME HYPOTHESIS

One of the difficulties with placing the proteasome at the center of the PD pathogenic cascade is that this seems to be a shared event with other neurological disorders. For example, the expanded forms of poly-glutamine proteins,[26] or mutant forms of Cu/Zn superoxide dismutase associated with amyotrophic lateral sclerosis (ALS),[27] also inhibit the proteasome. Other groups of neurons show differential vulnerability, importantly including spinal cord motor neurons affected in ALS.[27] Therefore, PD is not the only disorder where the proteasome is inhibited. However, the phenotype of parkin mutations is reasonably specific to a PD-like disorder, and so there must be some

degree of specificity for dopaminergic neurons. It is possible that there are additional common links between these two proteins; for example, mitochondrial function can be impaired by α-synuclein[22] and its impairment can be protected against by parkin.[28]

What is clear is that parkin and α-synuclein are linked by common effects on a specific pathway associated with selective cell death in catecholaminergic neurons. What is the molecular basis for the differential sensitivity of neuronal groups to α-synuclein-mediated damage? α-Synuclein has multiple effects on the dopamine systems, including affecting expression of the genes involved in dopamine synthesis.[29] Moreover, α-synuclein oligomers can be stabilized by catecholamines.[30] However, as the patterns of selective vulnerability in PD are more complex than simple loss of only dopaminergic cells, there are clearly other contributing factors to the patterns of cell damage.

How might we test some of these different ideas about centrality in PD and the roles of α-synuclein and parkin? Another definitive gene for PD, *DJ-1*, has recently been cloned.[31] At the time of this writing, the relationship to α-synuclein is unknown and there are a number of possible links.[32] What we do know is that the reported mutations induce a simple loss-of-function in DJ-1 leading, in one case, to protein instability.[33] A reasonable conjecture is that DJ-1 is, like parkin, a protein that protects against the damaging effects of α-synuclein accumulation. This provides a unique opportunity to understand the pathophysiological pathway underlying this condition and to test the hypothesis that proteasome function is critical in PD.

REFERENCES

1. Braak H, Braak E. Pathoanatomy of Parkinson's disease. J Neurol 2000; 247 (Suppl 2): 3–10

2. Hardy J, Cookson MR, Singleton A. Genes and parkinsonism. Lancet Neurol 2003; 2: 221–8

3. Farrer M, Chan P, Chen R, et al. Lewy bodies and parkinsonism in families with parkin mutations. Ann Neurol 2001; 50: 293–300

4. Gwinn-Hardy K. Genetics of parkinsonism. Mov Disord 2002; 17: 645–56

5. Spillantini MG, Schmidt ML, Lee VM, et al. Alpha-synuclein in Lewy bodies. Nature 1997; 388: 839–40

6. Giasson BI, Lee VM. Are ubiquitination pathways central to Parkinson's disease? Cell 2003; 114: 1–8

7. Volles MJ, Lansbury PT Jr. Zeroing in on the pathogenic form of alpha-synuclein and its mechanism of neurotoxicity in Parkinson's disease. Biochemistry 2003; 42: 7871–8

8. Farrer M, Maraganore DM, Lockhart P, et al. alpha-Synuclein gene haplotypes are associated with Parkinson's disease. Hum Mol Genet 2001; 10: 1847–51

9. West AB, Maraganore D, Crook J, et al. Functional association of the parkin gene promoter with idiopathic Parkinson's disease. Hum Mol Genet 2002; 11: 2787–92

10. McNaught KS, Olanow CW, Halliwell B, et al. Failure of the ubiquitin-proteasome system in Parkinson's disease. Nat Rev Neurosci 2001; 2: 589–94

11. McNaught KS, Olanow CW. Proteolytic stress: a unifying concept for the etiopathogenesis of Parkinson's disease. Ann Neurol 2003; 53 (Suppl 3): S73–84; discussion S84–6

12. Pickart CM. Mechanisms underlying ubiquitination. Annu Rev Biochem 2001; 70: 503–33

13. Hershko A, Ciechanover A. The ubiquitin system. Annu Rev Biochem 1998; 67: 425–79

14. McNaught KS, Jenner P. Proteasomal function is impaired in substantia nigra in Parkinson's disease. Neurosci Lett 2001; 297: 191–4

15. McNaught KS, Belizaire R, Jenner P, et al. Selective loss of 20S proteasome alpha-subunits in the substantia nigra pars compacta in Parkinson's disease. Neurosci Lett 2002; 326: 155–8

16. Furukawa Y, Vigouroux S, Wong H, et al. Brain proteasomal function in sporadic Parkinson's disease and related disorders. Ann Neurol 2002; 51: 779–82

17. Tofaris GK, Razzaq A, Ghetti B, et al. Ubiquitination of alpha-synuclein in Lewy bodies is a pathological event not associated with impairment of proteasome function. J Biol Chem 2003; 278: 44405–11

18. Sampathu DM, Giasson BI, Pawlyk AC, et al. Ubiquitination of alpha-synuclein is not required for formation of pathological inclusions in alpha-synucleinopathies. Am J Pathol 2003; 163: 91–100

19. Cookson MR. Parkin's substrates and the pathways leading to neuronal damage. Neuromol Med 2003; 3: 1–13

20. Yang Y, Nishimura I, Imai Y, et al. Parkin suppresses dopaminergic neuron-selective neurotoxicity induced by Pael-R in Drosophila. Neuron 2003; 37: 911–24

21. Staropoli JF, McDermott C, Martinat C, et al. Parkin is a component of an SCF-like ubiquitin ligase complex and protects postmitotic neurons from kainate excitotoxicity. Neuron 2003; 37: 735–49

22. Tanaka Y, Engelender S, Igarashi S, et al. Inducible expression of mutant alpha-synuclein decreases proteasome activity and

increases sensitivity to mitochondria-dependent apoptosis. Hum Mol Genet 2001; 10: 919–26

23. Stefanis L, Larsen KE, Rideout HJ, et al. Expression of A53T mutant but not wild-type α-synuclein in PC12 cells induces alterations of the ubiquitin-dependent degradation system, loss of dopamine release, and autophagic cell death. J Neurosci 2001; 21: 9549–60

24. Petrucelli L, O'Farrell C, Lockhart PJ, et al. Parkin protects against the toxicity associated with mutant alpha-synuclein: proteasome dysfunction selectively affects catechola-minergic neurons. Neuron 2002; 36: 1007–19

25. Snyder H, Mensah K, Theisler C, et al. Aggregated and monomeric alpha-synuclein bind to the S6′ proteasomal protein and inhibit proteasomal function. J Biol Chem 2003; 278: 11753–9

26. Bence NF, Sampat RM, Kopito RR. Impairment of the ubiquitin-proteasome system by protein aggregation. Science 2001; 292: 1552–5

27. Urushitani M, Kurisu J, Tsukita K, Takahashi R. Proteasomal inhibition by misfolded mutant superoxide dismutase 1 induces selective motor neuron death in familial amyotrophic lateral sclerosis. J Neurochem 2002; 83: 1030–42

28. Darios F, Corti O, Lucking CB, et al. Parkin prevents mitochondrial swelling and cytochrome c release in mitochondria-dependent cell death. Hum Mol Genet 2003; 12: 517–26

29. Baptista MJ, O'Farrell C, Daya S, et al. Co-ordinate transcriptional regulation of dopamine synthesis genes by alpha-synuclein in human neuroblastoma cell lines. J Neurochem 2003; 85: 957–68

30. Conway KA, Rochet JC, Bieganski RM, Lansbury PT Jr. Kinetic stabilization of the alpha-synuclein protofibril by a dopamine-alpha-synuclein adduct. Science 2001; 294: 1346–9

31. Bonifati V, Rizzu P, van Baren MJ, et al. Mutations in the DJ-1 gene associated with autosomal recessive early-onset parkinsonism. Science 2003; 299: 256–9

32. Cookson MR. Pathways to parkinsonism. Neuron 2003; 37: 7–10

33. Miller DW, Ahmad R, Hague S, et al. L166P mutant DJ-1, causative for recessive Parkinson's disease, is degraded through the ubiquitin-proteasome system. J Biol Chem 2003; 278: 36588–95

Chapter 5

Acetylcholinesterase, cholinergic signaling and Parkinson's disease

Y Ben-Shaul, H Bergman, H Soreq

INTRODUCTION

Parkinson's disease (PD) is the leading neurodegenerative disorder with primary effects on motion control. The classic symptoms of PD include tremor, muscle rigidity, postural abnormalities and slowness of volitional movements. Cognitive and mood disorders are also common, usually at more advanced stages of the disease.[1,2] Although both genetic and environmental factors may account for instances of so-called sporadic (idiopathic) PD,[3] the etiology of the disease is only partially understood.

PD pathology involves damage to multiple neuronal circuits, including the dopaminergic, noradrenergic, serotonergic and cholinergic projection systems.[1] Nonetheless, the most crucial deficit underlying PD is depletion of dopamine in the striatum (the input stage of the basal ganglia, BG) due to loss of midbrain dopaminergic cells. This has been most convincingly demonstrated by the efficacy of the dopamine precursor L-dopa, as well as other dopaminergic agonists, in alleviating the symptoms of PD.[4] However, the cellular and molecular events which lead to parkinsonism are still debatable,[5] and it is still unclear how loss of dopaminergic (and other) neurons leads to the characteristic symptoms of PD.[6,7]

The cholinergic system is closely involved with normal BG function and hence with its pathology.[8] While it has been suggested that a relatively simple balance between acetylcholine (ACh) and dopamine is essential for normal BG function, the involvement of the cholinergic system in PD is multifaceted. Thus, whereas cholinergic antagonists can alleviate motor symptoms,[9] presumably by restoring the ACh/dopamine balance within the striatum, cortical cholinergic deficiencies may underlie the cognitive impairments in PD.[10]

The enzyme acetylcholinesterase (AChE) is most obviously related to PD through its role in terminating cholinergic transmission by hydrolyzing ACh.[11] However, it is now accepted that AChE has additional, non-catalytic roles in both cholinergic and non-cholinergic neurons.[12] Moreover, AChE is subject to complex transcriptional and splicing modulations in response to various insults to the central nervous system (CNS),[13] some of which may be directly relevant to PD etiology. While over-expressed AChE normally serves to attenuate the possible outcomes of such insults,[14] under severe and/or long-term damage the response may be disproportionate and can therefore lead to deleterious outcomes.[15]

The aim of this chapter is to highlight the putative links between PD pathology and symptoms and changes in cholinergic signaling which involve modified properties and levels of AChE. As will be detailed below, AChE may shape PD symptoms and progress at multiple levels, some of which can lead to opposing effects. A deeper understanding of the relationship between PD, AChE and the various insults which modulate its expression may suggest both preventive measures and novel therapies targeted to the function of specific AChE forms in treating the symptoms and attenuating the progress of PD.

THE CHOLINERGIC SYSTEM IN PARKINSON'S DISEASE

The understanding that cholinergic function is involved in PD emerged during the mid-19th century after observing the beneficial effects of cholinergic antagonists on PD symptoms. Indeed, for almost a century, muscarinic anti-cholinergics (e.g. atropine, scopolamine) were the only available treatment for PD.[9] However, following the introduction of L-dopa, a dopamine precursor that can cross the blood–brain barrier, the use of anti-cholinergics has declined. This was mainly due to the supremacy of L-dopa as a treatment, as well as to increasing awareness of the deleterious cognitive side-effects of anti-cholinergic therapy.[9] The observation that either restitution of striatal dopamine or antagonism of ACh could alleviate PD symptoms led to the 'ACh/dopamine balance hypothesis of striatal function'.[16] According to this hypothesis, ACh and dopamine exert opposing effects on striatal circuitry; consequently, a proper balance between these neurotransmitters is essential for normal function. Supporting this hypothesis, it was subsequently shown that the centrally acting AChE inhibitor physostigmine

exacerbated, whereas muscarinic antagonists alleviated PD symptoms.[17]

Further evidence for the role of the cholinergic system in PD, though not directly for the ACh/DA balance hypothesis, is that muscarinic and nicotinic binding sites, as well as levels of the ACh synthesizing enzyme choline acetyltransferase (ChAT), are altered in the brains of PD patients.[18–20] In addition, post-mortem studies of PD brains reveal substantial loss of basal forebrain[1] and pedunculopontine cholinergic neurons.[21] Loss of basal forebrain cholinergic neurons and the consequent depletion of cortical ACh is now thought by some researchers to underlie the cognitive deficits in PD.[22] Indeed, AChE inhibitors have proved to be effective for treatment of cognitive deficits in PD, highlighting the multifaceted role of the cholinergic system in this disease.[23]

Major efforts have been directed to the elucidation of the physiological mechanisms underlying the ACh/dopamine balance hypothesis of BG function. The most dramatic interplay between the cholinergic and dopaminergic systems is apparent in the striatum, which contains the highest density of both dopaminergic and cholinergic markers in the entire brain.[24] The anatomical distributions of cholinergic and dopaminergic terminals in the striatum overlap extensively and their co-ordinated activity seems essential for proper BG function. Striatal dopaminergic innervation consists of dense and widespread terminals formed by afferent axons from midbrain dopaminergic neurons, whereas striatal ACh originates primarily from local cholinergic interneurons.[25] Although these cholinergic interneurons represent no more than 5% of the striatal population, they innervate it extensively. Similar to the dopaminergic innervation, these interneurons target mainly dendrites and dendritic spines of the inhibitory (GABAergic) medium spiny neurons. These neurons constitute the majority of striatal neurons and are the only projection neurons in this structure.[26]

A possible mechanism underlying the ACh/dopamine balance may act via the effects of these neurotransmitters on the spiny projection neurons. These neurons express metabotropic dopaminergic receptors of both the D1 and the D2 families.[27] Activation of D1 family receptors (i.e. D1 and D5) leads to increased intracellular cyclic AMP (cAMP) concentrations, whereas receptors from the D2 family mediate a decrease in cAMP.[28] As with dopaminergic receptors, metabotropic cholinergic muscarinic receptors are also classified into two groups: M1-like receptors (M1, M3, M5) and M2-like receptors (M2, M4), each group activating a distinct intracellular pathway.[24] Striatal projection neurons express mainly the M1 and M4 muscarinic receptors, and M4 receptors generally co-localize with dopaminergic D1 receptors.[29] Since M4 receptors act to decrease cAMP concentration, and D1 receptors act to increase it, this suggests that the ACh/dopamine balance is at least partially mediated by the opposing effects of these neurotransmitters on the striatal projection neurons.

However, in addition to the specific example described above, there is a range of additional points of interaction between the dopaminergic and cholinergic systems in the BG. For example, dopamine and ACh can also affect each other's release in the striatum, ACh can influence midbrain dopaminergic neurons, and both ACh and dopamine can modulate the activity of projection neurons and interneurons within the BG.[24] Moreover, in addition to dopamine and ACh muscarinic receptors, striatal and midbrain neurons also express various ACh nicotinic receptors.[30] The distinct effects mediated by each of these receptors, together with their compound and often overlapping distribution on specific neuronal components, highlight the intricacy of the interactions between the cholinergic and dopaminergic systems. Thus, detailed investigation of the midbrain and striatal systems suggests that the cholinergic–dopaminergic interaction is complex rather than simply antagonistic. The picture is further complicated by the finding that the effect of a given neurotransmitter at a given site may crucially depend on the time course of administration, prolonged administration often leading to desensitization.[31]

Finally, a causal role for AChE in mediating dopaminergic–cholinergic interactions in the substantia nigra has been documented in several studies by Greenfield and co-workers. Specifically, it has been shown that, in the rat, nigral release of AChE is enhanced by extracellular levels of dopamine, as well as by locomotion, presumably as a result of nigral activation.[32,33] On the other hand, AChE was reported to inhibit nigral cell discharge both *in vitro* and *in vivo*, via mechanisms independent of its hydrolytic function.[34] As described below, in addition to the obvious effects of AChE release on cholinergic transmission, AChE has been shown to exert a specific trophic action on the developing substania nigra.[34]

POSSIBLE GENETIC AND ENVIRONMENTAL FACTORS IN PARKINSON'S DISEASE

The events leading to neurodegeneration in PD are still debated. The emerging picture is that PD results from a combination of genetic and environmental factors, which may well interact with each other. Analysis of familial cases of PD has led to the discovery of eight genetic markers obeying Mendelian inheritance patterns (named PARK1–8).[35] Of these, three have been characterized and shown to involve proteins associated with the ubiquitin protease pathway (UPP) or with its degradation substrates. Specific polymorphisms in these genes probably result in failure of the UPP to degrade defective proteins. Failure of the UPP may be related to one common marker (though not obligatory and not sufficient) of PD, i.e. Lewy bodies, neuronal intracytoplasmic inclusions of filamentous and granular material.[36]

Other genetic and functional studies have demonstrated an association between enzymes related to the metabolism of reactive oxygen species (ROS) and PD. Dopaminergic neurons are especially vulnerable to oxidative stress, owing to their high dopamine content, which by itself can spontaneously form ROS.[37] It seems that failure of the UPP and accumulation of ROS mutually enhance each other, so that a positive vicious feedback cycle leading to accelerated neurodegeneration may ensue.[38] Nevertheless, it is still not clear which are the ultimate cellular events leading to cell damage. Recently, it was shown that inflammation, probably in response to the initial cellular damage, can play an active role in the pathogenesis of PD.[39] Thus, microglial, and to a lesser extent astroglial elements, once activated, may express sustained activity leading to further cell damage. Various studies showing direct and causal involvement in animal models of PD of these inflammatory cells and of pro-inflammatory cytokines support this hypothesis.[39–42]

Currently, only a minority of PD cases can be attributed to specific genetic causes.[35] Identification of additional genetic markers is likely, however, to reveal that cases of so-called sporadic (or idiopathic) PD are in fact associated with one or more genetic origins. Nonetheless, it is also known that various environmental factors play a key role in PD etiology.[43,44] Thus, prolonged exposure to pesticides, and specifically organophosphate compounds that inhibit AChE, is positively correlated with PD.[45–49] Such long-term exposure may act by different mechanisms than those of acute organophosphate

exposure, which has also been shown to induce parkinsonism, albeit transient in certain cases.[50] In fact, biochemically debilitating polymorphisms in several genes involved in metabolizing toxic compounds are associated with severe responses to organophosphates and specifically with susceptibility to PD.[51–55]

Intriguingly, it seems that certain personality types are associated with increased PD risk. Specifically, low scores on novelty seeking and high scores on harm avoidance (associated with anxious, pessimistic and shy personalities) are implicated in PD.[56–58] Extending these findings, it was recently suggested that psychological stress, by triggering neurodegeneration-promoting processes, also constitutes a risk factor in PD.[59] Acute psychological and physical traumatic events (including closed head injuries) have also been implicated in PD.[60,61] A related finding is that the symptoms of PD (and primarily tremor) are exacerbated following stress.[62] Together, these findings suggest a link between stress, anxiety and PD.

DISTINCT ROLES FOR ALTERNATIVELY SPLICED ACETYLCHOLINESTERASE VARIANTS

Although the link between AChE function and cholinergic transmission is apparently straightforward, its connection to the abovementioned environmental risk factors for PD is less obvious. However, as described below, it turns out that changes in the expression patterns of AChE are associated with each and all of the risk factors mentioned above, namely, exposure to organophosphates (and other AChE inhibitors), closed head injury, psychological stress and specific personality traits.

To explain the significance of these changes in gene expression and their suggested link with neurodegeneration, we will briefly review some of the properties of AChE. In mammals, AChE exists primarily as one of three 3′ alternatively spliced variants.[63] The predominant form in the nervous system is AChE-S (S for 'synaptic') which is associated with neuromuscular and CNS synapses through the structural subunit PRiMA.[64] This variant usually forms membrane-bound tetramers, but can exist in a number of other configurations as well, including dimers and monomers. Another variant is the C-terminal hydrophilic AChE-R which is normally expressed in low levels in the adult nervous system (R is for 'read-through' as, in this variant, the mRNA transcript is read through the fourth pseudo-intron).[65] The third variant, AChE-E (E for 'erythrocytic') is found as glycophosphatydilinositol-linked dimers on erythrocytic membranes, but is unlikely to play a specialized role in nervous system function.

The alternatively spliced forms of nervous tissue AChE (the S and R forms) share the same catalytic core, yet differ in their C terminal regions.[65] These terminal regions are responsible for the quaternary structure and localization patterns of the different variants, and confer additional, currently investigated non-hydrolytic roles, at least to some of the variants.[66] Of these functions, some are probably associated with the core domain of the AChE protein. This domain shares structure and function properties[67] with neuroligins, the β-neurexin partner proteins which participate in neuritogenesis and synapse formation.[68] Variant-specific roles should principally stem from the C-terminal peptides that are unique to each variant.[12] The neuroligin homology hence predicts that AChE is involved in cell differentiation, process extension and dendritic modeling. In fact, it has been specifically shown that AChE can enhance neurite growth of cultured frog neurons[69] and chick neurons[70,71] and of rodent midbrain dopaminergic neurons in organotypic cultures.[72] These growth-enhancing functions are likely to differ for the AChE-S and AChE-R variants and are not restricted to neural tissue.[65,69]

Although AChE-R is normally present at very low levels, its neuronal prevalence increases dramatically following various insults, including exposure to organophosphates and other AChE inhibitors,[13] psychological stress,[73] and closed head injury.[74] Up-regulation of AChE transcription and a shift to the AChE-R splice variant were thus implicated as being an inherent component of mammalian stress responses.[14] Consistent with this is the location of a glucocorticoid response element upstream of the AChE gene.[75] Additionally, changes in AChE expression are often accompanied by co-ordinated reductions in expression of ChAT and the vesicular acetylcholine transporter (VAChT).[13] Acting in concert, these modulations constitute a feedback response attenuating the cholinergic hyperexcitation resulting from stress insults.[14]

SIGNIFICANCE OF STRESS-INDUCED SHIFTS IN ALTERNATIVE SPLICING

We have described above how up-regulation of AChE-R expression follows various psychological and physical insults, implying a protective role for this splice variant. What, then, are the possible merits of AChE-R over the normally predominant synaptic form, AChE-S, in the CNS?

First, we consider a purely hydrolytic function of AChE. Since AChE-R, unlike AChE-S, is soluble, it is well suited to scavenge organophosphates and other toxins which may otherwise inhibit the crucial hydrolytic role of AChE-S. Indeed, the other cholinesterase in the mammalian brain, butyrylcholinesterase (BuChE) probably has a similar scavenging function, attesting to the importance of this role.[76] A second hydrolysis-related function, also associated with the solubility of AChE-R, involves the recently discovered role of ACh in regulating the inflammatory response. Specifically, it has been shown that ACh attenuates inflammation, and the term 'cholinergic reflex' was coined to describe this phenomenon.[77] The soluble AChE-R, which can reduce ACh levels throughout the brain, is well suited to relieve the ACh blockade of pro-inflammatory responses in regions distal from synaptic sites. Appropriate levels of AChE-R, by enhancing the inflammatory response (which may be associated with at least some of the insults mentioned above) may well be adaptive at moderate levels.[78] A third merit of AChE-R is related to the growth-promoting effects of AChE. Both the AChE-S and the AChE-R forms include a neuroligin-homologous domain.[65] Nevertheless, AChE-R does not exhibit membrane anchoring as does AChE-S, implying that distinct processes are mediated by each of these variants. Thus, AChE-S has been shown to facilitate process extension from PC12 cells, and this function shows apparent redundancy with that of neuroligin.[67] Presumably, this is mediated by the heterosynaptic interaction between neuroligin-like domains and β-neurexin.[79] It is tempting to speculate that, by virtue of localizing a neurotransmitter-hydrolytic function and a growth-promoting function on the same molecule, AChE-S may mediate a synaptic learning rule. Thus, modulation of the expression of the synaptic AChE variant at cholinergic synapses may reflect the fluctuations in activity in these synapses under normal conditions, and therefore may play a role in regulating the strength of synaptic contacts.[80] On the other hand, cholinergic hyperexcitation, as induced, for example, by stress, may lead through alternative splicing to the increased expression of the soluble AChE-R variant, potentially leading to disruption of synaptic contacts and hence synaptic remodeling. Synaptic modeling is probably advantageous

under stress-induced, abnormal functioning of the cholinergic system. Moreover, by binding to β-neurexin, AChE-R may even disrupt cell-to-cell contacts in glutamatergic synapses.[81] Fourth, AChE-R promotes intracellular processes independently of its hydrolytic role and specific to its unique C-terminus. Among these functions are interaction with intracellular signaling cascades,[82] and enhancement of fear conditioning and hippocampal long-term potentiation.[83] These functions may be related both to adaptive stress-induced changes in synaptic transmission and to additional intracellular processes in non-neuron brain cells.[82,84,85] Behaviorally, excess of transgenic AChE-S is associated with secondary accumulation of AChE-R.[86] This induces progressive cognitive alterations which can be viewed as impairments,[87] but may also be interpreted as adaptive cautiousness following the inherited cholinergic imbalance. The causal involvement of AChE-R in these changes is demonstrated by the capacity of antisense oligonucleotides targeting this variant to reverse many of these cognitive alterations.[74,86]

Direct evidence for the protective role of AChE-R, compared to AChE-S, comes from studies in mice and humans expressing AChE at abnormally high levels. A mouse model overexpressing the very similar human AChE-S form shows increased markers of neurodegeneration when compared to normal mice or mice expressing the human AChE-R.[87–89] Humans with a transcription-activating mutation in the AChE upstream region are especially sensitive to organophosphate exposure, suggesting that normal up-regulation and changes in splicing patterns are essential for efficient handling of organophosphates.[90]

Considering all the abovementioned aspects, controlled up-regulation of AChE-R may be adaptive in response to common and relatively mild stressors. However, extreme insults such as closed head injury or events leading to the initiation of neurodegenerative processes may induce exaggerated expression, leading to deleterious outcomes. Each of the functions of AChE-R, when overdriven, is expected to be maladaptive. Thus, excessive hydrolysis may impair cholinergic transmission, which can lead to diminished cognitive function,[22] and to excessive inflammation. The latter is especially relevant in PD, for which one of the key initiator events may be an unregulated inflammatory response.[39] Disproportionate disruption of cell-to-cell contacts and initiation of intracellular cascades triggered by AChE-R may also be deleterious. Exaggerated long-term potentiation may lead to neuronal hyperexcitation and hence to consequent neuronal death by glutamate-induced toxicity.[91] Finally, concerning the trophic roles of AChE on substania nigra neurons, it has been suggested that the trophic effect at moderate doses[72] can turn into a toxic effect at higher doses.[34] The beneficial and deleterious effects of the functions of AChE-R at moderate and high doses respectively are summarized in Figure 5.1.

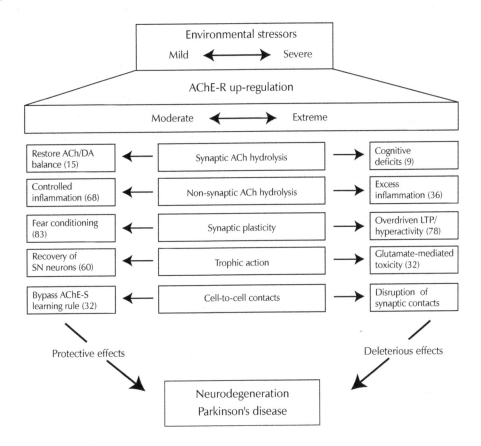

Figure 5.1 Putative roles of acetylcholinesterase read-through variant (AChE-R) in the etiology of Parkinson's disease. Various psychological and physical stressors lead to up-regulation of AChE-R. Mild stressors will lead to correspondingly moderate and hence adaptive up-regulation. However, following extreme stressors or an accumulation of mild stressors, levels of AChE-R may reach a stage in which they are no longer protective. Rather, they may cause cumulative and progressive damage. Numbers in brackets denote references which favor the specific functions. DA, dopamine; AChE-S, synaptic variant; LTP, long-term potentiation; SN, substantia nigra

POTENTIAL IMPLICATIONS FOR TREATING PARKINSON'S DISEASE

This short overview shows that understanding the precise roles played by the cholinergic system and AChE in PD await further research. On the one hand, cholinergic antagonists have been used to alleviate motor symptoms, while on the other hand, inhibitors of AChE (leading to cholinergic overactivity) can improve cognitive impairment in PD. In fact, perhaps it will prove best to inhibit cholinergic functions in some regions (e.g. substantia nigra pars compacta and striatum with respect to motor function) yet to increase cholinergic function in regions that are normally innervated by the degenerating basal forebrain cholinergic neurons (e.g. cortex, hippocampus, amygdala). A major theme of this chapter is that, in addition to its role in cholinergic transmission, AChE is probably involved in the pathogenesis of PD via additional, non-hydrolytic functions.

Our hypothesis concerning the role of AChE in PD remains to be tested experimentally, initially in animal models. We predict that events causing AChE overexpression, whether inhibition of AChE hydrolytic activity, psychological stress, closed head injury, or transgenically induced overexpression of AChE, will increase the susceptibility to parkinsonism. If this turns out to be true, manipulations leading to decreased expression of specific AChE variants should be considered as potential protective treatments against PD.

ACKNOWLEDGEMENTS

This research was supported by grants from the US Army Medical Research and Materiel Command (DAMD 17-99-1-9547 (to H.S.)), the Eric Roland Center for Neurodegenerative Diseases and the Interdisciplinary Center for Neuronal Computation of the Hebrew University (ICNC; to H.S. and H.B.). Y.B.S. was a recipient of an ICNC post-doctoral fellowship.

REFERENCES

1. Lang AE, Lozano AM. Parkinson's disease. First of two parts. N Engl J Med 1998; 339: 1044–53

2. Lang AE, Lozano AM. Parkinson's disease. Second of two parts. N Engl J Med 1998; 339: 1130–43

3. Dauer W, Przedborski S. Parkinson's disease: mechanisms and models. Neuron 2003; 39: 889–909

4. Martin WR, Wieler M. Treatment of Parkinson's disease. Can J Neurol Sci 2003; 30 (Suppl 1): S27–33

5. Huang Z, de la Fuente-Fernandez R, Stoessl AJ. Etiology of Parkinson's disease. Can J Neurol Sci 2003; 30 (Suppl 1): S10–18

6. Bar-Gad I, Bergman H. Stepping out of the box: information processing in the neural networks of the basal ganglia. Curr Opin Neurobiol 2001; 11: 689–95

7. Wichmann T, DeLong MR. Functional neuroanatomy of the basal ganglia in Parkinson's disease. Adv Neurol 2003; 91: 9–18

8. Calabresi P, Centonze D, Gubellini P, et al. Acetylcholine-mediated modulation of striatal function. Trends Neurosci 2000; 23: 120–6

9. Lang AE, Lees AJ. Anticholinergic therapies in the treatment of Parkinson's disease. Mov Disord 2002; 17 (Suppl 4): S7–12

10. Perry E, Walker M, Grace J, Perry R. Acetylcholine in mind: a neurotransmitter correlate of consciousness? Trends Neurosci 1999; 22: 273–80

11. Massoulie J. The origin of the molecular diversity and functional anchoring of cholinesterases. Neurosignals 2002; 11: 130–43

12. Soreq H, Seidman S. Acetylcholinesterase – new roles for an old actor. Nat Rev Neurosci 2001; 2: 294–302

13. Kaufer D, Friedman A, Seidman S, Soreq H. Acute stress facilitates long-lasting changes in cholinergic gene expression. Nature 1998; 393: 373–7

14. Kaufer D, Friedman A, Seidman S, Soreq H. Anticholinesterases induce multigenic transcriptional feedback response suppressing cholinergic neurotransmission. Chem Biol Interact 1999; 119–120: 349–60

15. Kaufer D, Soreq H. Tracking cholinergic pathways from psychological and chemical stressors to variable neurodeterioration paradigms. Curr Opin Neurol 1999; 12: 739–43

16. Barbeau A. The pathogenesis of Parkinson's disease: a new hypothesis. Can Med Assoc J 1962; 87: 802–7

17. Duvoisin RC. Cholinergic–anticholinergic antagonism in parkinsonism. Arch Neurol 1967; 17: 124–36

18. Asahina M, Suhara T, Shinotoh H, et al. Brain muscarinic receptors in progressive supranuclear palsy and Parkinson's disease: a positron emission tomographic study. J Neurol Neurosurg Psychiatry 1998; 65: 155–63

19. Mattila PM, Roytta M, Lonnberg P, et al. Choline acetytransferase activity and striatal dopamine receptors in Parkinson's disease in relation to cognitive impairment. Acta Neuropathol (Berl) 2001; 102: 160–6

20. Guan ZZ, Nordberg A, Mousavi M, et al. Selective changes in the levels of nicotinic acetylcholine receptor protein and of corresponding mRNA species in the brains of patients with Parkinson's disease. Brain Res 2002; 956: 358–66

21. Jellinger K. The pedunculopontine nucleus in Parkinson's disease, progressive supranuclear palsy and Alzheimer's disease. J Neurol Neurosurg Psychiatry 1988; 51: 540–3

22. Dubois B, Pillon B. Cognitive deficits in Parkinson's disease. J Neurol 1997; 244: 2–8

23. Werber EA, Rabey JM. The beneficial effect of cholinesterase inhibitors on patients suffering from Parkinson's disease and dementia. J Neural Transm 2001; 108: 1319–25

24. Zhou FM, Wilson C, Dani JA. Muscarinic and nicotinic cholinergic mechanisms in the mesostriatal dopamine systems. Neuroscientist 2003; 9: 23–36

25. Kawaguchi Y, Wilson CJ, Augood SJ, Emson PC. Striatal interneurones: chemical, physiological and morphological characterization. Trends Neurosci 1995; 18: 527–35

26. Parent A, Hazrati LN. Functional anatomy of the basal ganglia. I. The cortico-basal ganglia-thalamo-cortical loop. Brain Res Brain Res Rev 1995; 20: 91–127

27. Nicola SM, Surmeier J, Malenka RC. Dopaminergic modulation of neuronal excitability in the striatum and nucleus accumbens. Annu Rev Neurosci 2000; 23: 185–215

28. Sealfon SC, Olanow CW. Dopamine receptors: from structure to behavior. Trends Neurosci 2000; 23 (Suppl 10): S34–40

29. Ince E, Ciliax BJ, Levey AI. Differential expression of D1 and D2 dopamine and m4 muscarinic acetylcholine receptor proteins in identified striatonigral neurons. Synapse 1997; 27: 357–66

30. Zhou FM, Wilson CJ, Dani JA. Cholinergic interneuron characteristics and nicotinic properties in the striatum. J Neurobiol 2002; 53: 590–605

31. Zhou FM, Liang Y, Dani JA. Endogenous nicotinic cholinergic activity regulates dopamine release in the striatum. Nat Neurosci 2001; 4: 1224–9

32. Dally JJ, Schaefer M, Greenfield SA. The spontaneous release of acetylcholinesterase in rat substantia nigra is altered by local changes in extracellular levels of dopamine. Neurochem Int 1996; 29: 629–35

33. Heiland B, Greenfield SA. Rat locomotion and release of acetylcholinesterase. Pharmacol Biochem Behav 1999; 62: 81–7

34. Greenfield SA. Non-cholinergic actions of acetylcholinesterase in the substantia nigra. In Doctor BP, Quinn DM, Rotundo RL, Taylor P, eds. Structure and Function of Cholinesterases and Related Proteins. New York: Plenum Press, 1998: 557–62

35. Foltynie T, Sawcer S, Brayne C, Barker RA. The genetic basis of Parkinson's disease. J Neurol Neurosurg Psychiatry 2002; 73: 363–70

36. Maries E, Dass B, Collier TJ, et al. The role of alpha-synuclein in Parkinson's disease: insights from animal models. Nat Rev Neurosci 2003; 4: 727–38

37. Zhang Y, Dawson VL, Dawson TM. Oxidative stress and genetics in the pathogenesis of Parkinson's disease. Neurobiol Dis 2000; 7: 240–50

38. McNaught KS, Olanow CW, Halliwell B, et al. Failure of the ubiquitin-proteasome system in Parkinson's disease. Nat Rev Neurosci 2001; 2: 589–94

39. Orr CF, Rowe DB, Halliday GM. An inflammatory review of Parkinson's disease. Prog Neurobiol 2002; 68: 325–40

40. Vila M, Jackson-Lewis V, Guegan C, et al. The role of glial cells in Parkinson's disease. Curr Opin Neurol 2001; 14: 483–9

41. Wu DC, Jackson-Lewis V, Vila M, et al. Blockade of microglial activation is neuroprotective in the 1-methyl-4-phenyl-1,2,3,6-tetrahydropyridine mouse model of Parkinson disease. J Neurosci 2002; 22: 1763–71

42. Wu DC, Tieu K, Cohen O, et al. Glial cell response: a pathogenic factor in Parkinson's disease. J Neurovirol 2002; 8: 551–8

43. Foltynie T, Brayne C, Barker RA. The heterogeneity of idiopathic Parkinson's disease. J Neurol 2002; 249: 138–45

44. Sherer TB, Betarbet R, Greenamyre JT. Environment, mitochondria, and Parkinson's disease. Neuroscientist 2002; 8: 192–7

45. Baldi I, Cantagrel A, Lebailly P, et al. Association between Parkinson's disease and exposure to pesticides in southwestern France. Neuroepidemiology 2003; 22: 305–10

46. Liu B, Gao HM, Hong JS. Parkinson's disease and exposure to infectious agents and pesticides and the occurrence of brain injuries: role of neuroinflammation. Environ Health Perspect 2003; 111: 1065–73

47. Uversky VN, Li J, Fink AL. Pesticides directly accelerate the rate of alpha-synuclein fibril formation: a possible factor in Parkinson's disease. FEBS Lett 2001; 500: 105–8

48. Jenner P. Parkinson's disease, pesticides and mitochondrial dysfunction. Trends Neurosci 2001; 24: 245–7

49. Giasson BI, Lee VM. A new link between pesticides and Parkinson's disease. Nat Neurosci 2000; 3: 1227–8

50. Shahar E, Andraws J. Extra-pyramidal parkinsonism complicating organophosphate insecticide poisoning. Eur J Paediatr Neurol 2001; 5: 261–4

51. Kelada SN, Costa-Mallen P, Checkoway H, et al. Paraoxonase 1 promoter and coding region polymorphisms in Parkinson's disease. J Neurol Neurosurg Psychiatry 2003; 74: 546–7

52. Taylor MC, Le Couteur DG, Mellick GD, Board PG. Paraoxonase polymorphisms, pesticide exposure and Parkinson's disease in a Caucasian population. J Neural Transm 2000; 107: 979–83

53. Kondo I, Yamamoto M. Genetic polymorphism of paraoxonase 1 (PON1) and susceptibility to Parkinson's disease. Brain Res 1998; 806: 271–3

54. Bharath S, Hsu M, Kaur D, et al. Glutathione, iron and Parkinson's disease. Biochem Pharmacol 2002; 64: 1037–48

55. Menegon A, Board PG, Blackburn AC, et al. Parkinson's disease, pesticides, and glutathione transferase polymorphisms. Lancet 1998; 352: 1344–6

56. Ogawa T. Personality characteristics of Parkinson's disease. Percept Mot Skills 1981; 52: 375–8

57. Kaasinen V, Nurmi E, Bergman J, et al. Personality traits and brain dopaminergic function in Parkinson's disease. Proc Natl Acad Sci USA 2001; 98: 13272–7

58. Menza M. The personality associated with Parkinson's disease. Curr Psychiatry Rep 2000; 2: 421–6

59. Smith AD, Castro SL, Zigmond MJ. Stress-induced Parkinson's disease: a working hypothesis. Physiol Behav 2002; 77: 527–31

60. Taylor CA, Saint-Hilaire MH, Cupples LA, et al. Environmental, medical, and family history risk factors for Parkinson's disease: a New England-based case control study. Am J Med Genet 1999; 88: 742–9

61. Lees AJ. Trauma and Parkinson disease. Rev Neurol (Paris) 1997; 153: 541–6

62. Schwab RS, Zieper I. Effects of mood, motivation, stress and alertness on the performance in Parkinson's disease. Psychiatr Neurol (Basel) 1965; 150: 345–57

63. Massoulie J. Molecular forms and anchoring of acetylcholinesterase. In Cholinesterases and Cholinesterase Inhibitors. London: Martin Dunitz, 2000: 81–101

64. Perrier AL, Massoulie J, Krejci E. PRiMA: the membrane anchor of acetylcholinesterase in the brain. Neuron 2002; 33: 275–85

65. Grisaru D, Sternfeld M, Eldor A, et al. Structural roles of acetylcholinesterase variants in biology and pathology. Eur J Biochem 1999; 264: 672–86

66. Massoulie J, Anselmet A, Bon S, et al. Acetylcholinesterase: C-terminal domains, molecular forms and functional localization. J Physiol Paris 1998; 92: 183–90

67. Grifman M, Galyam N, Seidman S, Soreq H. Functional redundancy of acetylcholinesterase and neuroligin in mammalian neuritogenesis. Proc Natl Acad Sci USA 1998; 95: 13935–40

68. Brose N. Synaptic cell adhesion proteins and synaptogenesis in the mammalian central nervous system. Naturwissenschaften 1999; 86: 516–24

69. Sternfeld M, Ming G, Song H, et al. Acetylcholinesterase enhances neurite growth and synapse development through alternative contributions of its hydrolytic capacity, core protein, and variable C termini. J Neurosci 1998; 18: 1240–9

70. Layer PG, Willbold E. Cholinesterases in avian neurogenesis. Int Rev Cytol 1994; 151: 139–81

71. Bigbee JW, Sharma KV, Chan EL, Bogler O. Evidence for the direct role of acetylcholinesterase in neurite outgrowth in primary dorsal root ganglion neurons. Brain Res 2000; 861: 354–62

72. Holmes C, Jones SA, Budd TC, Greenfield SA. Non-cholinergic, trophic action of recombinant acetylcholinesterase on mid-brain dopaminergic neurons. J Neurosci Res 1997; 49: 207–18

73. Meshorer E, Erb C, Gazit R, et al. Alternative splicing and neuritic mRNA translocation under long-term neuronal hypersensitivity. Science 2002; 295: 508–12

74. Shohami E, Kaufer D, Chen Y, et al. Antisense prevention of neuronal damage following head injury in mice. J Mol Med 2000; 78: 228–36

75. Grant AD, Shapira M, Soreq H. Genomic dissection reveals locus response to stress for mammalian acetylcholinesterase. Cell Mol Neurobiol 2001; 21: 783–97

76. Soreq H, Glick D. Novel roles for cholinesterases in stress and inhibitor responses. In Giacobini E, ed. Cholinesterases and Cholinesterase Inhibitors. London: Martin Dunitz, 2000: 47–61

77. Tracey KJ. The inflammatory reflex. Nature 2002; 420: 853–9

78. Schwartz M, Moalem G, Leibowitz-Amit R, Cohen IR. Innate and adaptive immune

responses can be beneficial for CNS repair. Trends Neurosci 1999; 22: 295–9

79. Cantallops I, Cline HT. Synapse formation: if it looks like a duck and quacks like a duck. Curr Biol 2000; 10: R620–3

80. Nitsch RM, Rossner S, Albrecht C, et al. Muscarinic acetylcholine receptors activate the acetylcholinesterase gene promoter. J Physiol Paris 1998; 92: 257–64

81. Song JY, Ichtchenko K, Sudhof TC, Brose N. Neuroligin 1 is a postsynaptic cell-adhesion molecule of excitatory synapses. Proc Natl Acad Sci USA 1999; 96: 1100–5

82. Birikh KR, Sklan EH, Shoham S, Soreq H. Interaction of 'readthrough' acetyl-cholinesterase with RACK1 and PKCbeta II correlates with intensified fear-induced conflict behavior. Proc Natl Acad Sci USA 2003; 100: 283–8

83. Nijholt I, Farchi N, Kye M-J, et al. Alternative splicing modulation of hippocampal long-term potentiation and fear memory. Mol Psychol 2004; 9: 174–83

84. Perry C, Sklan EH, Birikh K, et al. Complex regulation of acetylcholinesterase gene expression in human brain tumors. Oncogene 2002; 21: 8428–41

85. Zhang XJ, Yang L, Zhao Q, et al. Induction of acetylcholinesterase expression during apopto-sis in various cell types. Cell Death Differ 2002; 9: 790–800

86. Cohen O, Erb C, Ginzberg D, et al. Neuronal overexpression of 'readthrough' acetyl-cholinesterase is associated with antisense-sup-pressible behavioral impairments. Mol Psychiatry 2002; 7: 874–85

87. Beeri R, Andres C, Lev-Lehman E, et al. Transgenic expression of human acetyl-cholinesterase induces progressive cognitive deterioration in mice. Curr Biol 1995; 5: 1063–71

88. Beeri R, Le Novere N, Mervis R, et al. Enhanced hemicholinium binding and attenuated dendrite branching in cognitively impaired acetylcholinesterase-transgenic mice. J Neurochem 1997; 69: 2441–51

89. Sternfeld M, Shoham S, Klein O, et al. Excess 'read-through' acetylcholinesterase attenuates but the 'synaptic' variant intensifies neurodeterioration correlates. Proc Natl Acad Sci USA 2000; 97: 8647–52

90. Shapira M, Tur-Kaspa I, Bosgraaf L, et al. A transcription-activating polymorphism in the AChE promoter associated with acute sensitivity to anti-acetylcholinesterases. Hum Mol Genet 2000; 9: 1273–81

91. Tapia R, Medina-Ceja L, Pena F. On the relationship between extracellular glutamate, hyperexcitation and neurodegeneration, in vivo. Neurochem Int 1999; 34: 23–31

Chapter 6

Bone marrow stem cells: possible source for cell therapy in Parkinson's disease

YS Levy, S Bulvik, A Burshtein, Y Barhum, E Melamed, D Offen

INTRODUCTION

Clinical trials with transplantation of human embryonic mesencephalic tissue into the caudate and putamen (striatum) of Parkinson's disease (PD) patients were initiated in 1987. About 350 patients have been operated upon since then.[1] At that time, it was not known whether neuronal replacement could be effective in the diseased human brain. The main objective of scientific efforts in the past 15 years have been to provide proof-of-principle that: the grafted dopamine neurons can survive and form connections in the PD patient's brain; the patient's brain can integrate and use the grafted neurons; and the grafts can induce a measurable clinical improvement.[2] Dopaminergic neurons isolated from human fetuses were transplanted to the striatum of PD patients, on one or both sides. The researchers who conducted the open trials in several medical centers reported on significant clinical benefits and demonstrated that the transplanted cells survived for years and produced dopamine.[1,2] However, practical and ethical issues such as the need for up to eight fetuses to provide sufficient numbers of dopaminergic neurons for one PD patient limited this specific treatment.[3–5] Recent reports on double-blind controlled trails of fetal nigral

transplantation raised serious questions on the safety and the efficacy of this procedure. They reported that improvement was not significant in most of the patients, while high percentages of the treated patients developed severe uncontrolled movements (tardive dyskinesia).[6,7] Moreover, Olanow's team found some evidence to suggest that an immunological reaction was destroying or disabling the tissue grafts.[7]

These observations add significantly to the other practical and ethical problematic issues concerning the use of up to eight human fetuses to provide sufficient numbers of dopaminergic neurons for one PD patient.[1,2,6,7] However, the challenge of cell replacement in PD is great, and finding the best cell source is a high priority. Advanced methods for isolating stem cells, the progenitors of all body tissues, have increased the expectation of these cells to provide an unlimited source that might be induced to differentiate into mature and functional dopaminergic cells.

BONE MARROW STROMAL CELLS

The use of cells originating from the same patient for autologous transplantation avoids the introduction of foreign material and reduces the possible rejection complications and the need for immunosuppression. This autologous transplantation strategy by-passes many ethical, technical and logistical issues. In recent years, there has been an increasing interest in adult bone marrow-derived stromal stem cells that support hematopoiesis. These mesenchymal stem cells differentiate into connective tissue, muscle, bone, cartilage and fat cells.[8–10] Evidence has accumulated that human, rat and mouse bone marrow stromal cells (BMSc) can also be induced to differentiate into neuron-like cells in culture.[11–18] Following induction, most (up to 80%) stromal cells may exhibit neuronal phenotypes. Moreover, it has been shown that the differentiated cells express neuronal protein markers such as neuron-specific enolase (NSE), neural nuclei protein (NeuN), neurofilament-M, and trkA. Other experiments with rodents demonstrated that transplanted bone marrow-derived cells might migrate into various brain regions and develop neuron-like features.[19–26] Furthermore, Mezey and co-investigators found Y-chromosomes in the human brains of females following transplantation of male bone marrow.[27] Donor cells were found in several brain regions, especially in the hippocampus and cerebral cortex. However, other researchers claim that bone-to-brain transdifferentiation may not be a general phenomenon but may reflect fusion with neurons or transient expression of many proteins, including neuronal markers.[28–32]

The evidence for differentiation of BMSc into dopaminergic neuron-like cells is limited. However, genes for human tyrosine hydroxylase (TH), the rate-limiting enzyme in dopamine biosynthesis, and GTP cyclohydrolase I (GC), the enzyme providing the tetrahydropterin (BH_4), cofactor for TH, were introduced into rat BMSc.[33,34] The engineered rat BMSc indeed synthesized and released 3,4,-dihydroxy-phenylalanine (L-dopa). When these rat BMSc were transplanted into the routinely used PD model, the striatum of 6-hydroxydopamine unilaterally lesioned rats, the synthesized L-dopa was converted into dopamine metabolites, and behavioral recovery was observed. However, the ameliorative effect of the modified BMSc transplantion was short-lived (up to 7 days), presumably owing to inactivation of transgenes introduced into the brain with retroviruses.

Woodbury and co-investigators developed a method for inducing rat BMSc to differentiate into neuron-like cells that express genes associated with neurotransmission.[13] Rat BMSc maintained in the induction medium for 10 days expressed tau in levels that correlated with the degree of neuronal morphological differentiation. β-Tubulin III, an intermediate filament characteristic of mature neurons, was present in virtually all cells. Analysis by reverse transcriptase-polymerase chain reaction (RT-PCR) indicated that synaptophysin mRNA, which is associated with synaptic vesicles and transmission, was not present in undifferentiated BMSc but was detected after 24 h of neuronal differentiation and continued to increase thereafter. The synaptophysin protein was detected in cell bodies as well as in varicose, putative transmitter-release sites along processes. Moreover, at 10 days of rat BMSc differentiation, a large population of the neuron-like cells expressed choline acetyl-transferase (ChAT), which catalyzes the synthesis of the excitatory transmitter acetylcholine. A smaller subpopulation of rat BMSc-derived neuron-like structures were reported to express TH. Nevertheless, Woodbury's group did not report on dopamine production or synthesis of other catecholamine neurotransmitters.

The search for a therapeutic potential of BMSc for the treatment of PD was stimulated by a publication from Li et al. in 2001.[20] Mouse

BMSc prelabeled with 5-bromo-2-deoxyuridine (BrdU) were grafted into the striatum of the 1-methyl-4-phenyl-1,2,3,6-tetrahydropyridine (MPTP) mouse model of Parkinson's disease. The grafted MPTP-treated mice exhibited a significant improvement on the rotarod test at 35 days after transplant, compared to non-grafted controls. Immunohistochemistry revealed BrdU-reactive cells in the striatum of the grafted MPTP-treated mice at least 4 weeks after transplantation. Double staining showed that only 0.8% of BrdU-reactive cells expressed TH. Although the injected mouse BMSc survived, expressed TH and promoted some functional recovery, much more work is required to understand the mechanism of recovery. It is not known whether the grafted cells increase production of dopamine or whether other processes, such as the secretion of neurotrophic factors by the marrow-derived cells, mediate the improvement in motor function.

Park and co-investigators introduced the glial cell line-derived neurotrophic factor (GDNF) gene into the mouse bone marrow cells, injected the cells intravenously and found GDNF-expressing cells within the brain parenchyma.[35] Furthermore, this *ex-vivo* gene transfer strategy, performed 6 weeks prior to exposure to the dopaminergic neurotoxin MPTP, provided protection of nigral neurons and their striatal terminals.

In our laboratory we have demonstrated that human BMSc might change their designations following induction in culture. The differentiation of human BMSc into neuron-like cells was associated with dramatic morphological changes. Before treatment, human BMSc displayed a flat, fibroblastic morphology (Figure 6.1a), whereas after 24 h of treatment the cells were rounded, exhibited highly retractile cell bodies and displayed prominent process-like extensions (Figure 6.1b). The neuron-like morphology of the cells was retained up to 26 days of culture (Figure 6.1c). The structural changes were accompanied by the expression of the tissue-specific neuronal marker, Neu-N, as indicated by nuclear immunostaining (Figure 6.1d). We also demonstrated, using RT-PCR methods, that the differentiated human BMSc expressed Nurr1, the transcription factor regulator of the midbrain dopamine neuron. Moreover, the dopamine-related genes; dopa-decarboxylase (DDC), D2 dopamine receptor (D2DR) and dopamine transporter (DAT) were increased during the induction of differentiation (Figure 6.2).

MULTIPOTENT ADULT PROGENITOR CELLS

Rare cells, termed the multipotent adult progenitor cell (MAPCs), were isolated from human and rat bone marrow mesenchymal stem cultures.[36–41] These cells can be expanded for more than 120 population doublings and differentiate into mesenchymal, endothelium[28,29] and endoderm lineages.[40] It was also shown that mouse MAPCs injected into the blastocyst contributed to most, if not all, somatic cell lineages including the brain, similar to embryonic stem (ES) cells.[41] Within the brain, region-specific appropriate differentiation occurred.[41]

Jiang and co-investigators cultured rodent MAPCs sequentially with basic fibroblast growth factor (bFGF) for 7 days, FGF-8 for 7 days and brain-derived neurotrophic factor (BDNF) for 7 days.[36] They demonstrated that the cells became polarized and expressed tau and microtubule-associated protein 2 (MAP2). Moreover, 30% of cells expressed markers of dopaminergic neurons, DDC and TH, 20% of serotonergic neurons and 50% were γ-aminobutyric acid (GABA)-ergic neurons. A particularly useful approach would be if the MAPCs

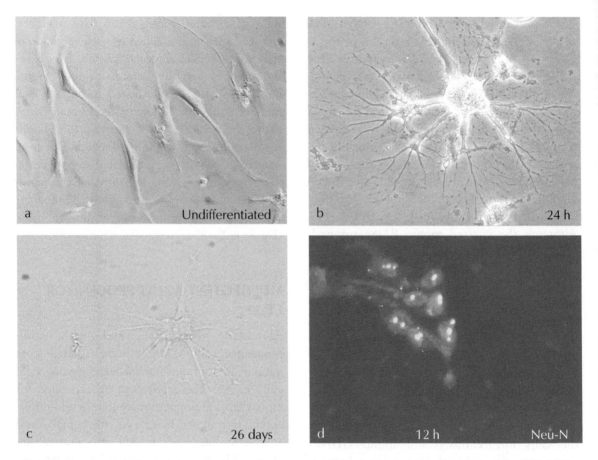

Figure 6.1 Formation of neural tissues by human bone marrow stromal cells (hBMSc). (a) hBMSc isolated from bone aspirate and grown as a sub-confluent monolayer. (b) Cultured hBMSc incubated in a combination of media supplements that induced significant morphological changes. During the first hours of exposure to induction medium, the cytoplasm in the adherent cells started to condense and retracted towards the nucleus, creating a spherical structure, and developed branches. (c) After 26 days of differentiation, hBMSc formed cells displaying a range of neuron-like morphologies. (d) Immunocytochemistry analysis confirms expression of neuronal nuclei (Neu-N) protein after 12 h of differentiation

could be administered systemically and could then find their way to the damaged central nervous system (CNS) region, where they would adopt the phenotype of the missing neuron. However, no significant engraftment of mouse MAPCs was seen in the brain after intravenous infusion, and rare donor cells found in the brain did not co-label with neuroectodermal markers.[36]

Recently, Jiang and co-investigators reported that, similar to mouse ES cells, mouse MAPCs could be induced to differentiate *in vitro* into cells with biochemical, anatomical and electrophysiological characteristics of midbrain neuronal cells.[42] Mouse MAPCs were cultured sequentially for 7 days with BFGF, FGF8 plus sonic hedgehog (SHH) and BDNF. They found that 23% of the cells were positive to nestin, a

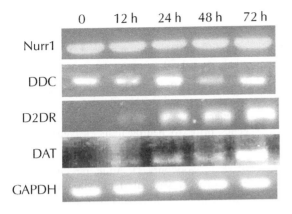

Figure 6.2 Differentiated human bone marrow stromal cells express genes associated with the dopaminergic lineage. mRNA isolated after 12–72 h of differentiation were analyzed by polymerase chain reaction with the primers of the genes found in dopaminergic neurons: nuclear receptor related 1 (Nurr1), dopa decarboxylase (DDC), D2 dopamine receptor (D2DR), dopamine transporter (DAT) and glyceraldehyde-3-phosphate dehydrogenase (GAPDH) a housekeeping gene used as a positive control

marker for neuronal progenitor, and expressed nuclear receptor related 1 (Nurr1), the key transcription factor for dopaminergic neuron development. Quantitative RT-PCR demonstrated that, on days 10 and 14, levels of GABA, TH and tryptophan hydroxylase (TPH) increased up to 120-fold. Immunophenotypic analysis on day 21 showed that 25% of cells expressed markers of dopaminergic neurons (DDC and TH), 18% expressed markers of serotonergic (TPH) neurons, and 52% expressed markers of GABAergic neurons. Double immunohistochemistry showed that GABA, TPH and TH were never detected in the same cell. They also demonstrated that mouse MAPC-derived neuron-like cells cultured in the presence of fetal brain astrocytes demonstrated much more mature neural morphology with more elaborate array axons.[42]

FUTURE STRATEGIES

In establishing stem cells as an alternative graft source, logistical, ethical and political issues need to be resolved. There is disagreement over the feasibility of 'adult' stem cells compared with ES cells. Adult stem cells might be capable of developing into only a limited number of cell types as compared to ES cells. However, ES cells could retain their mitotic ability after transplantation, which could give rise to tumors. Furthermore, ethical concerns surrounding the use of fetal tissues and ES cells will not apply to adult stem cells.[43] Thus, safety and efficacy issues on the use of stem cells include the following questions: Do they maintain long-term stable neuronal phenotypes crucial for rescuing the degenerating brain? Are transplanted stem cells functional as a dopaminergic neuron and thus able to provide beneficial effects?

It seems clear that there is an urgent need for more basic research if the field is to progress beyond the level of clinical phenomenology. There are three main challenges. First, it will be necessary to learn much more about neuronal development, in order to define cell types that can be cultured in sufficient quantities and that can adopt appropriate fates when transplanted to different sites *in vivo*. Second, it will be necessary to establish better animal models – perhaps including genetically modified primates – in order to perform more realistic tests of cognitive recovery after transplantation. Third, it will be important to develop methods for testing whether transplanted neurons can become functionally integrated into brain circuitry; in other words, whether they can contribute to the restoration of normal information processing in the damaged brain. This will require the identification and electrophysiological characterization of transplanted neurons *in vivo*.

REFERENCES

1. Lindvall O, Hagell P. Cell replacement therapy in human neurodegenerative disorders. Clin Neurosci Res 2002; 2: 86–92

2. Lindvall O. Stem cells for therapy in Parkinson's disease. Pharmacol Res 2003; 47: 279–87

3. Ungerstedt U, Arbuthnott GW. Quantitative recording of rotational behavior in rats after 6-hydroxy-dopamine lesions of the nigrostriatal dopamine system. Brain Res 1970; 24: 485–93

4. Bjorklund A, Stenevi U. Reconstruction of the nigrostriatal dopamine pathway by intra-cerebral nigral transplants. Brain Res 1979; 177: 555–60

5. Perlow MJ, Freed WJ, Hoffer BJ, et al. Brain grafts reduce motor abnormalities produced by destruction of nigrostriatal dopamine system. Science 1979; 204: 643–7

6. Freed CR, Greene PE, Breeze RE, et al. Transplantation of embryonic dopamine neurons for severe Parkinson's disease. N Engl J Med 2001; 344: 710–19

7. Olanow CW, Goetz CG, Kordower JH, et al. A double-blind controlled trial of bilateral fetal nigral transplantation in Parkinson's disease. Ann Neurol 2003; 54: 403–14

8. Prockop DJ. Marrow stromal cells as stem cells for nonhematopoietic tissues. Science 1997; 276: 71–4

9. Pittenger MF, Mackay AM, Beck SC, et al. Multilineage potential of adult human mesenchymal stem cells. Science 1999; 284: 143–7

10. Deans RJ, Moseley AB. Mesenchymal stem cells: biology and potential clinical uses. Exp Hematol 2000; 28: 875–84

11. Sanchez-Ramos J, Song S, Cardozo-Pelaez F, et al. Adult bone marrow stromal cells differentiate into neural cells in vitro. Exp Neurol 2000; 164: 247–56

12. Woodbury D, Schwarz EJ, Prockop DJ, Black IB. Adult rat and human bone marrow stromal cells differentiate into neurons. J Neurosci Res 2000; 61: 364–70

13. Woodbury D, Reynolds K, Black IB. Adult bone marrow stromal stem cells express germline, ectodermal, endodermal, and mesodermal genes prior to neurogenesis. J Neurosci Res 2002; 96: 908–17

14. Black I, Woodbury D. Adult rat and human bone marrow stromal stem cells differentiate into neurons. Blood Cells Mol Dis 2001; 27: 632–6

15. Deng W, Obrocka M, Fischer I, Prockop DJ. In-vitro differentiation of human marrow stromal cells into early progenitors of neural cells by conditions that increase intracellular cyclic AMP. Biochem Biophys Res Commun 2001; 282: 148–52

16. Kohyama J, Abe H, Shimazaki T, et al. Brain from bone: efficient 'meta-differentiation' of marrow stroma-derived mature osteoblasts to neurons with Noggin or a demethylating agent. Differentiation 2001; 68: 235–44

17. Brazelton TR, Rossi FMV, Keshet GI, Blau HM. From marrow to brain: expression of neuronal phenotypes in adult mice. Science 2000; 290: 1775–9

18. Mezey E, Chandross KJ, Harta G, et al. Turning blood into brain: cells bearing neuronal antigens generated in vivo from bone marrow. Science 2000; 290: 1779–82

19. Chen J, Li Y, Wang L, et al. Therapeutic benefit of intracerebral transplantation of bone marrow stromal cells after cerebral ischemia in rats. J Neurol Sci 2001; 189: 49–57

20. Li Y, Chen J, Wang L, et al. Intracerebral transplantation of bone marrow stromal cells in a 1-methyl-4-phenyl-1,2,3,6-tetrahydropyridine mouse model of Parkinson's disease. Neurosci Lett 2001; 316: 67–70

21. Li Y, Chen J, Chen XG, et al. Human marrow stromal cell therapy for stroke in rat: neurotrophins and functional recovery. Neurology 2002; 59: 514–23

22. Lu D, Li Y, Wang L, et al. Intra-arterial administration of marrow stromal cells in a rat model of traumatic brain injury. J Neurotrauma 2001; 18: 813–19

23. Lu D, Mahmood A, Wang L, et al. Adult bone marrow stromal cells administered intravenously to rats after traumatic brain injury migrate into brain and improve neurological outcome. Neuroreport 2001; 12: 559–63

24. Lu D, Li Y, Mahmood A, et al. Neural and marrow-derived stromal cell sphere transplantation in a rat model of traumatic brain injury. J Neurosurg 2002; 97: 935–40

25. Hess DC, Hill WD, Martin-Studdard A, et al. Bone marrow as a source of endothelial cells and NeuN-expressing cells after stroke. Stroke 2002; 33: 1362–8

26. Zhao LR, Duan WM, Reyes M, et al. Human bone marrow stem cells exhibit neural phenotypes and ameliorate neurological deficits after grafting into the ischemic brain of rats. Exp Neurol 2002; 174: 11–20

27. Mezey E, Key S, Vogelsang G, et al. Transplanted bone marrow generates new neurons in human brain. Proc Natl Acad Sci USA 2003; 100: 1364–9

28. Holden C, Vogel G. Plasticity: time for a reappraisal? Science 2002; 296: 2126–9

29. Lemischka I. A few thoughts about the plasticity of stem cell. Exp Hematol 2002; 30: 848–52

30. Wurmser AE, Gage FH. Cell fusion causes confusion. Nature 2002; 416: 485–7

31. Castro RF, Jackson KA, Goodell MA, et al. Failure of bone marrow cells to transdifferentiate into neural cells in vivo. Science 2002; 297: 1299

32. Terada N, Hamazaki T, Oka M, et al. Bone marrow adopt the phenotype of other cells by spontaneous cell fusion. Nature 2002; 416: 542–5

33. Schwarz EJ, Alexander GM, Prockop DJ, Azizi SA. Multipotential marrow stromal cells transduced to produce L-DOPA: engraftment in rat model of Parkinson disease. Hum Gene Ther 1999; 10: 2539–49

34. Schwarz EJ, Reger RL, Alexander GM, et al. Rat marrow stromal cells rapidly transduced with a self-inactivating retrovirus synthesize L-DOPA in vitro. Gene Ther 2001; 8: 1214–23

35. Park KW, Eglitis MA, Mouradian MM. Protection of nigral neurons by GDNF-engineered marrow cell transplantation. Neurosci Res 2001; 40: 315–23

36. Jiang Y, Jahagirdar BN, Reinhardt RL, et al. Pluripotency of mesenchymal stem cells derived from adult marrow. Nature 2002; 418: 41–9

37. Jiang Y, Vaessen B, Lenvik T, et al. Multipotent progenitor cells can be isolated from postnatal murine bone marrow, muscle, and brain. Exp Hematol 2002; 30: 896–904

38. Reyes M, Lund T, Lenvik T, et al. Purification and ex-vivo expansion of postnatal human marrow mesodermal progenitor cells. Blood 2001; 98: 2615–25

39. Reyes M, Dudek A, Jahagirdar B, et al. Origin of endothelial progenitors in human postnatal bone marrow. J Clin Invest 2002; 109: 337–46

40. Schwartz RE, Reyes M, Koodie L, et al. Multipotent adult progenitor cells from bone marrow differentiate into functional hepatocyte-like cells. J Clin Invest 2002; 109: 1291–302

41. Keene CD, Ortiz-Gonzalez XR, Jiang Y, et al. Neural differentiation and incorporation of bone marrow-derived multipotent adult progenitor cells after single cell transplantation into blastocyst stage mouse embryos. Cell Transplant 2003; 12: 201–13

42. Jiang Y, Henderson D, Blackstad M, et al. Neuroectodermal differentiation from mouse multipotent adult progenitor cells. Proc Natl Acad Sci USA 2003; 100 (Suppl 1) 11854–60

43. Borlongan CV, Sanberg PR. Neural transplantation for treatment of Parkinson's disease. Drug Discov Today 2002; 7: 674–82

Insulin-like growth factor I and intracellular signal transduction pathways in aging and dementia

W-H Zheng, R Quirion

INTRODUCTION

Insulin-like growth factor-I (IGF-I), also known as sulfation factor or somatomedin C, was originally isolated from human serum.[1,2] It is a 70-amino-acid peptide structurally very similar to insulin.[3] High levels of IGF-I are found in the plasma at concentrations of 20–80 nmol/l, and it mainly originates from the liver.[4,5] IGF-I is also present in most other tissues including the brain but at significantly lower concentrations.[4,5]

IGF-I plays a key role during normal development and in the maintenance of cellular integrity, including in the central nervous system (CNS).[6] It also has an important role in adulthood, especially under neurodegenerative conditions.[7] The expression of IGF-I and its receptors in the CNS is upregulated in response to injuries; this phenomenon probably relates to neuroprotection, as exogenous IGF-I protects the brain from hypoxic and ischemic injuries.[8–10] Moreover, IGF-I and IGF-I mRNA levels decrease during aging[11,12] while reduced efficacy of the IGF-I receptor signaling pathways has been reported in Alzheimer's disease (AD).[13,14] These findings, in addition to the well-established role of IGF-I in neuroprotection, neurogenesis, glucose metabolism, cerebral amyloidosis, tau phosphorylation and activity-dependent plasticity, suggest that the modulation of IGF-I receptor signaling by IGF-I itself or its mimetics could be an interesting therapeutic strategy in neurodegenerative disorders such as AD and stroke.[15–19]

IGF-I RECEPTOR SIGNALING

The biological functions of IGF-I are mediated by IGF-I receptors and modulated by IGF binding proteins.[20,21] The IGF-I receptor is a transmembrane tyrosine kinase receptor structurally very similar to the insulin receptor. It is a 1367-residue heterotetramer consisting of two α (115 kDa) and two β (94 kDa) subunits joined by disulfide bridges.[20] The interaction of this receptor with IGF-I induces its auto-phosphorylation and the activation of receptor tyrosine kinases, leading to tyrosine phosphorylation of its endogenous substrates such as the insulin receptor substrate (IRS)-1 to -4 proteins and SH2-plekstrin homology domain (Shc), followed by the downstream activation of various signaling pathways.[20–23]

The tyrosine phosphorylation of IRS-1/2 promotes the association with p85 phosphatidylinositol 3-kinase (PI3K), leading to the activation of the catalytic subunits of PI3K which, in turn, phosphorylate inositol lipids at the 3' position of the inositol ring to generate the 3-phosphoinositides PI(3)P, PI(3,4)P2 and PI(3,4,5)P3.[24] This event recruits Akt to the plasma membrane and its phosphorylation at residues Thr308 and Ser473 by PI(3,4,5) P3 dependent kinase (PDK)-1 and -2, respectively. The phosphorylation of these two residues fully activates Akt kinase, which then phosphorylates (in most cases here leading to inactivation of the target) its many substrates including glycogen synthase kinase-3 (GSK-3), the Bcl-2 family member Bad, caspase-9, nuclear factor-κB (NFκB) and the winged-helix family of transcription factors, FKHRL1, FKHR and AFX, as well as Mdm2/p53, nitric oxide synthase and calcium channels leading to various metabolic responses, cell survival and proliferation.[19,25–30] Other targets of PI3K include S6p70, some isoforms of protein kinase C (PKC), phospholipase Cγ, the small GTP-binding protein Rac, Bruton's tyrosine kinase and serum- and glucocorticoid-induced kinase (SGK).[25,30]

IGF-I and IGF-I receptors can also act via other signaling pathways. For example, the association of Shc proteins with the IGF-I receptor induces the phosphorylation of Shc on tyrosine residues that act as a docking site for the SH2 domain of GRB2. Binding of Grb2 to Shc, or IRS proteins, leads to the association of Grb2 with the guanine nucleotide exchange protein mSos, which then catalyzes the exchange of GTP to GDP on the small GTP-binding protein Ras, resulting in its activation and subsequently that of the MAPK pathway (also known as extracellular signal-related kinase or ERK) through the intermediary kinase c-Raf and MEK.[21,22,31] The activated mitogen-activated protein kinase (MAPK) phosphorylates its cytoplasmic and nuclear substrate proteins, including growth factor receptors, transcription factors and kinases, hence possibly

mediating various cellular responses of IGF-I and insulin[23,32]. Figure 7.1 is a diagram of the intracellular pathways involved in IGF-I receptor signaling.

Using various cell types including PC12 cells, hippocampal and cortical cultured neurons, we have systemically studied intracellular signaling pathways activated by IGF-I and its receptors in neuronal cells. IGF-I potently stimulates the Tyr phosphorylation of IGF-I receptors and IRS-1/2 and their association (IRS1/2>>IGF-IR) with PI3K leading to the activation of Akt kinases.[27,28] We also verified that Akt was able to phosphorylate Forkhead transcription factors directly.[27] This event leads to the inactivation of these transcription factors and plays an important role in neuronal survival properties of IGF-I and neurotrophins[27,29,30]. In contrast, the activation of the MAPK pathway by IGF-I or neurotrophins does not appear to play a significant role in the neuroprotective effects of these trophic factors in hippocampal neurons.[29,30] Activation of the PI3K/Rac pathway by IGF-I is apparently involved in neurite outgrowth.[33] Taken together, these results reveal the critical role of the PI3K/Akt pathway in mediating the neuroprotective effects of IGF-I in the CNS.

IGF-I RECEPTOR SIGNALING AND ALZHEIMER'S DISEASE

AD, the most common form of dementia in the elderly, is a progressive neurodegenerative disorder characterized by a gradual loss of memory and higher cognitive functions.[34,35] Intracellular neurofibrillary tangles, extracellular amyloid deposits and losses of neurons in selected regions of the brain are the most salient neuropathological features of this disease.[34] Mechanisms underlying the pathogenesis of AD are not fully clear. However, the

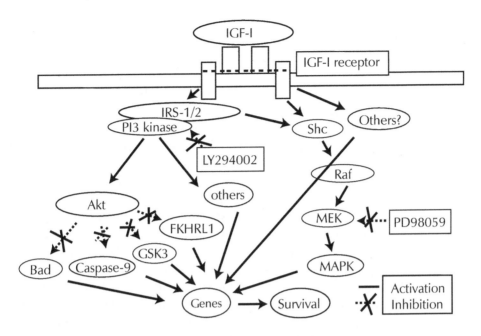

Figure 7.1 Intracellular signaling of IGF-I receptors in non-neuronal cells

accumulation of β-amyloid (Aβ) peptide or the abnormal processing of its precursor is believed to be a key player in this process.[19,34,36–38]

The precise relationship between the IGF-I receptor signaling cascades and AD mostly remains to be elucidated. The following sections will discuss some recent findings that should help in that regard.

IGF-I AND NEURONAL DEGENERATION IN ALZHEIMER'S DISEASE

IGF-I acts as a potent neuroprotective/neuro-rescuing factor of a broad range of neuronal and non-neuronal cells most probably by activating the PI3/Akt pathway.[16,19,29,30] Using cultured hippocampal neurons, we have shown that IGF-I not only protects hippocampal neurons against Aβ-induced toxicity, but can also 'rescue' neurons that have been pre-exposed to Aβ-peptides for an extended period of time.[16] This unique property of IGF-I is most likely to stem from its combined ability to maintain Ca^{2+} homeostasis, to protect against free radical damage, and to act as an anti-apoptotic factor via activation of the PI3K/Akt/FKHRL1 pathway.[19,29,30] IGF-I can also support the survival of basal forebrain cholinergic neurons and upregulate the expression of ChAT in these cells.[39] Additionally, we have shown that IGF-I and IGF-II can modulate the release of acetylcholine (ACh) from hippocampal and cortical brain slices,[40] two areas most severely affected in AD brains.[34] Taken together, these data suggest that alterations in IGF-I and its receptor signaling cascade could play a role in neuronal degeneration.

IGF-I AND CEREBRAL AMYLOIDOSIS

Apart from inhibiting Aβ neuronal toxicity, IGF-I was recently found to regulate Aβ load and clearance from the brain.[38,41] It is well established that plasma levels of IGF-I decrease with age, while those of Aβ have been reported to increase in the brains of rats and mice.[41] Interestingly, increasing serum levels of IGF-I in aged rats by subcutaneous, chronic infusions of IGF-I decreased Aβ levels in the brain of aged rats, compared to those found in young rats.[41] This finding is consistent with another result showing similar effects of IGF-I on endogenous Aβ levels in Tg2576 mice, a transgenic-mouse model of AD amyloidosis.[41] In this model, the administration of IGF-I significantly decreased the levels of Aβ and reduced Congo-red-positive fibrillar amyloid deposits in brain parenchyma of 1-year-old Tg2576 mice.[42] In contrast, increased cerebral levels of Aβ were seen in mutant mice with low circulating plasma levels of IGF-I. The mechanism involved here may be related to the ability of IGF-I to enhance the transport into the brain of Aβ carrier proteins such as albumin and transthyretin.[41]

IGF-I AND TAU PHOSPHORYLATION

The hyperphosphorylation of tau is a key component of neurofibrillary tangles present in the AD brain. IGF-I has been shown to reduce the phosphorylation of tau by activating the PI3K/Akt pathway which concurrently attenuates the activation of GSK3β, a kinase believed to be involved in the hyperphosphorylation of tau.[43] Moreover, a disruption of IGF-I receptor signaling increased tau phosphorylation in the brain of IRS-2 knockout mice.[38]

OTHER FINDINGS ABOUT IGF-I, AGING AND ALZHEIMER'S DISEASE

Some recent studies have provided evidence for possible alterations in IGF-I and IGF-I receptor signaling cascades in AD. Aging is a most important risk factor in AD. Circulating and brain levels of IGF-I are significantly reduced in aging and this may influence cognitive processes.[11–12,44] Moreover, a small, but significant increase in the level of [^{125}I]IGF-I binding sites was found in the prefrontal cortex of the AD brain, most probably as a compensatory adjustment to decreased amounts of IGF-I.[45] Additionally, a subset of reactive astrocytes and Aβ-containing neuritic plaques were shown to express IGF-I-like immunoreativity in the AD brain.[19,46] Finally, some recent data have suggested that the Tyr phosphorylation of the IGF-I receptor, the activity of Akt and the phosphorylation of CREB are all significantly decreased in the AD brain.[13,14] These data, together with evidence that IGF-I can facilitate working memory in aged rats[47,48] suggest the potential therapeutic relevance of modulating the IGF-I receptor signaling cascade using IGF-I itself or preferably small-molecule mimetics.

IGF-I-LIKE MIMETICS IN NEURODEGENERATIVE DISORDERS

A number of recent studies have shown that, following its peripheral administration, IGF-I can cross, to some extent, the blood–brain barrier, induce neurogenesis and protect neurons against toxic insults.[49–53] However, the development of IGF-I mimetics, particularly non-peptidyl mimetics, is required to ensure better brain penetration and improve stability.[54] These mimetics could be direct ligands of the IGF-I receptor, activators of receptor kinases, or compounds capable of either stimulating survival pathways induced by IGF-I or releasing IGF-I from its complex with various IGF-I binding proteins (IGFBP).

Progress toward the development of small ligands of IGF-I receptor has benefited from crystallographic studies and the phage display library. Several small peptides binding to IGF-I receptors were found using the phage display library and recombinant IGF-I receptor.[55] These small, peptide mimetics have affinities of 30–200 nmol/l, and have been classified into three groups on the basis of consensus sequences, competitive binding with IGF-I and activity studies. One group of peptides acts as agonists while the other two behave as antagonists. These peptides bind to hot spots on the IGF-I receptor (site 1 and site 2).[55] Both agonist and antagonist peptides bind to site 1, while only the antagonists bind to site 2.[55]

Regarding non-peptide mimetics, progress has particularly been made in the characterization of activators of insulin receptor kinase. Zhang et al. identified L-783,281, a small non-peptidyl agonist of the insulin receptor, which can induce the phosphorylation of the insulin receptor β subunit and IRS-I, as well as the activation of Akt without affecting IGF-I receptor signaling in transfected Chinese hamster ovary (CHO) cells.[54] In vivo, L-783,281 facilitated glucose transport in rat primary adipocytes and lowered blood glucose levels in two mouse models of diabetes.[54] This initial discovery has led to the development of a newer generation of insulin mimetics which are orally active and more effective.[56]

One of the derivatives of L-783,281, known as compound 2, activates the insulin receptor tyrosine kinase with an EC_{50} of 300 nmol/l. Interestingly, this compound not only activates the signaling pathways associated with the insulin receptor but also sensitizes the insulin receptor kinase to insulin, an important property to avoid desensitization occurring during long-term exposure.[56,57] Another small molecule named DMAQ-B1 isolated from a mixture of metabolites produced by a tropical endophytic fungus, Pseudomassaria, was also found to act

as an orally active insulin mimic.[57] Similar non-peptide IGF-I mimetics have yet to be characterized. However, on the basis of the high degree of sequence homology between the insulin and IGF-I receptors, strategies used thus far to develop non-peptide insulin mimics should be applicable to IGF-I.

An alternative approach aimed at releasing bound IGF-I may also prove beneficial. For example, several isoquinoline analogs that bind to IGFBP-3 as well as to other IGFBPs have been characterized.[58] These small compounds are able to release biologically active IGF-I from the IGF-I–IGFBP-3 complex.[58] The human IGF-I analog [[Leu^{24,59,60}Ala^{31}]hIGF-I] is one of these molecules. This analog has high affinity for IGFBPs and no biological activity at the IGF-I receptor. It was shown to increase the levels of free, bioavailable IGF-I in the cerebrospinal fluid.[59] Moreover, the intracerebroventricular administration of this analog up to 1 h after an ischemic insult to the rat brain had a potent neuroprotective action, comparable to that of exogenously applied IGF-I.[59] Hence, the development of more potent and selective derivatives leading to the release of IGF-I bound to IGFBPs is warranted.

CONCLUSIONS

IGF-I is a trophic factor with multiple functions in the CNS. Apart from its effects on normal growth and development, IGF-I is a highly potent neuroprotective/neurorescuing agent. With age, alterations in its levels or that of its receptors, or in its signaling cascade, could result in significant losses in neuronal plasticity and resistance to insults such as those occurring in AD and stroke. The development of non-peptide, small-molecule IGF-I mimetics would constitute a major step forward toward the possible use of IGF-I-based therapies.

REFERENCES

1. Rinderknecht E, Humbel RE. The amino acid sequence of human insulin-like growth factor I and its structural homology with proinsulin. J Biol Chem 1978; 253: 2769–76

2. Rinderknecht E, Humbel RE. Primary structure of human insulin-like growth factor II. FEBS Lett 1978; 89: 283–6

3. Isaksson OG, Ohlsson C, Nilsson A, et al. Regulation of cartilage growth by growth hormone and insulin-like growth factor I. Pediatr Nephrol 1991; 5: 451–3

4. Daughaday WH, Rotwein P. Insulin-like growth factors I and II. Peptide, messenger ribonucleic acid and gene structures, serum, and tissue concentrations. Endocr Rev 1989; 10: 68–91

5. Humbel RE. Insulin-like growth factors I and II. Eur J Biochem 1990; 190: 445–62

6. de Pablo F, de la Rosa EJ. The developing CNS: a scenario for the action of proinsulin, insulin and insulin-like growth factors. Trends Neurosci 1995; 18: 143–50

7. Loddick SA, Rothwell NJ. Mechanisms of tumor necrosis factor alpha action on neurodegeneration: interaction with insulin-like growth factor-1. Proc Natl Acad Sci USA 1999; 96: 9449–51

8. Beilharz EJ, Russo VC, Butler G, et al. Co-ordinated and cellular specific induction of the components of the IGF/IGFBP axis in the rat brain following hypoxic–ischemic injury. Brain Res Mol Brain Res 1998; 59: 119–34

9. Gluckman PD, Guan J, Williams C, et al. Asphyxial brain injury – the role of the IGF system. Mol Cell Endocrinol 1998; 140: 95–9

10. Loddick SA, Liu XJ, Lu ZX, et al. Displacement of insulin-like growth factors from their binding proteins as a potential treatment for stroke. Proc Natl Acad Sci USA 1998; 95: 1894–8

11. Niblock MM, Brunso-Bechtold JK, Lynch CD, et al. Distribution and levels of insulin-like growth factor I mRNA across the life span in the Brown Norway x Fischer 344 rat brain. Brain Res 1998; 804: 79–86

12. Sonntag WE, Lynch C, Thornton P, et al. The effects of growth hormone and IGF-I deficiency on cerebrovascular and brain aging. J Anat 2000; 197: 575–85

13. Griffin RG, Kelliher M, Johnston JA, Williams CH, et al. Dysfunctional insulin-like growth factor-1 Akt signal transduction in Alzheimer's disease brain. Soc Neurosci Abstr 2000; 26: 20–47

14. Meng Y, Xu H, Wang R, et al. Impairment of signal transduction pathway on neuronal survival in brains of Alzheimer's disease. Zhonghua Bing Li Xue Za Zhi 2002; 31: 502–5

15. Cheng B, Mattson, MP. IGF-I and IGF-II protect cultured hippocampal and septal neurons against calcium-mediated hypoglycemic damage. J Neurosci 1992; 12: 1558–66

16. Dore S, Kar S, Quirion R. Insulin-like growth factor I protects and rescues hippocampal neurons against β-amyloid- and human amylin-induced toxicity. Proc Natl Acad Sci USA 1997; 94: 4772–7

17. Galli C, Meucci O, Scorziello A, et al. Apoptosis in cerebellar granule cells is blocked by high KCl, forskolin, and IGF-I through distinct mechanisms of action: the involvement of intracellular calcium and RNA synthesis. J Neurosci 1995; 15: 1172–9

18. Sortino MA, Canonico PL. Neuroprotective effect of insulin-like growth factor I in immortalized hypothalamic cells. Endocrinology 1996; 137: 1418–22

19. Zheng WH, Kar S, Dore S, Quirion R. Insulin-like growth factor-1 (IGF-I): a neuroprotective trophic factor acting via the Akt kinase pathway J Neural Transm Suppl 2000; 261–72

20. LeRoith D, Werner H, Beitner-Johnson D, Roberts CT Jr. Molecular and cellular aspects of the insulin-like growth factor I receptor. Endocr Rev 1995; 16: 143–63

21. Butler AA, Yakar S, Gewolb IH, et al. Insulin-like growth factor-I receptor signal transduction: at the interface between physiology and cell biology. Comp Biochem Physiol B Biochem Mol Biol 1998; 121: 19–26

22. Blakesley VA, Bulter AA, Koval AP, et al. IGF-I receptor function. In Rosen RG, Robert CT, eds. The IGF System: Molecular Biology, Physiology, and Clinical Applications. Totowa, NJ: Humana Press, 1999: 143–63

23. Adams TE, Epa VC, Garrett TP, Ward CW. Structure and function of the type 1 insulin-like growth factor receptor. Cell Mol Life Sci 2000; 57: 1050–93

24. Myers MG Jr, Grammer TC, Wang LM, et al. Insulin receptor substrate-1 mediates phosphatidylinositol 3′-kinase and p70S6k signaling during insulin, insulin-like growth factor-1, and interleukin-4 stimulation J Biol Chem 1994; 269: 28783–9

25. Chan TO, Rittenhouse SE, Tsichlis PN. AKT/PKB and other D3 phosphoinositide-regulated kinases: kinase activation by phosphoinositide-dependent phosphorylation. Annu Rev Biochem 1999; 68: 965–1014

26. Datta SR, Brunet A, Greenberg ME. Cellular survival: a play in three Akts. Genes Dev 1999; 13: 2905–27

27. Zheng WH, Kar S, Quirion R. Insulin-like growth factor-1-induced phosphorylation of the forkhead family transcription factor FKHRL1 is mediated by akt kinase in PC12 cells J Biol Chem 2000; 275: 39152–8

28. Zheng WH, Kar S, Quirion R. Stimulation of protein kinase C modulates insulin-like growth factor-1-induced akt activation in PC12 cells. J Biol Chem 2000; 275: 13377–85

29. Zheng WH, Kar S, Quirion R. Insulin-like growth factor-1-induced phosphorylation of transcription factor FKHRL1 is mediated by phosphatidylinositol 3-kinase/Akt kinase and role of this pathway in insulin-like growth factor-1-induced survival of cultured hippocampal neurons Mol Pharmacol 2002; 62: 225–33

30. Zheng WH, Kar S, Quirion R. FKHRL1 and its homologs are new targets of nerve growth factor Trk receptor signaling. J Neurochem 2002; 80: 1049–61

31. De Meyts P, Wallach B, Christoffersen CT, et al. The insulin-like growth factor-I receptor. Structure, ligand-binding mechanism and signal transduction. Horm Res 1994; 42: 152–9

32. Su B, Karin M. Mitogen-activated protein kinase cascades and regulation of gene expression. Curr Opin Immunol 1996; 8: 402–11

33. Leventhal PS, Russell JW, Feldman EL. IGFs and the nervous system. In Rosen RG, Robert CT, eds. The IGF System: Molecular Biology, Physiology, and Clinical Applications. Totowa, NJ: Humana Press, 1999: 425–55

34. Selkoe DJ. The cell biology of beta-amyloid precursor protein and presenilin in Alzheimer's disease. Trends Cell Biol 1998; 8: 447–53

35. Lackey BR, Gray SL, Henricks DM. Actions and interactions of the IGF system in Alzheimer's disease: review and hypotheses. Growth Horm IGF Res 2000; 10: 1–13

36. Roher AE, Lowenson JD, Clarke S, et al. beta-Amyloid-β(1–42) is a major component of cerebrovascular amyloid deposits: implications for the pathology of Alzheimer disease. Proc Natl Acad Sci USA 1993; 90: 10836–40

37. Harris ME, Hensley K, Butterfield DA, et al. Direct evidence of oxidative injury produced by the Alzheimer's beta-amyloid peptide (1–40) in cultured hippocampal neurons. Exp Neurol 1995; 131: 193–202

38. Gasparini L, Xu H. Potential roles of insulin and IGF-I in Alzheimer's disease. Trends Neurosci 2003; 26: 404–6

39. Gage SL, Keim SR. Low WC. Effects of insulin-like growth factor II (IGF-II) on transplanted cholinergic neurons from the fetal septal nucleus. Prog Brain Res 1990; 82: 73–80

40. Kar S, Seto D, Dore S, et al. Insulin-like growth factors-I and -II differentially regulate endogenous acetylcholine release from the rat

hippocampal formation. Proc Natl Acad Sci USA 1997; 94: 14054–9

41. Carro E, Trejo JL, Gomez-Isla T, et al. Serum insulin-like growth factor I regulates brain amyloid-beta levels. Nat Med 2002; 8: 1390–7

42. Hsiao K, Chapman P, Nilsen S, et al. Correlative memory deficits, Abeta elevation, and amyloid plaques in transgenic mice. Science 1996; 274: 99–102

43. Hong M, Lee VM. Insulin and insulin-like growth factor-1 regulate tau phosphorylation in cultured human neurons. J Biol Chem 1997; 272: 19547–53

44. Dik MG, Pluijm SM, Jonker C, et al. Insulin-like growth factor I (IGF-I) and cognitive decline in older persons. Neurobiol Aging 2003; 24: 573–81

45. Crews FT, McElhaney R, Freund G, et al. Insulin-like growth factor I receptor binding in brains of Alzheimer's and alcoholic patients. J Neurochem 1992; 58: 1205–10

46. Jafferali S, Dumont Y, Sotty F, et al. Insulin-like growth factor-I and its receptor in the frontal cortex, hippocampus, and cerebellum of normal human and Alzheimer Disease brains. Synapse 2000; 38: 450–9

47. Sonntag WE, Lynch C, Thornton P, et al. The effects of growth hormone and IGF-I deficiency on cerebrovascular and brain ageing. J Anat 2000; 197: 575–85

48. Thornton PL, Ingram RL, Sonntag WE. Chronic [D-Ala2]-growth hormone-releasing hormone administration attenuates age-related deficits in spatial memory. J Gerontol A Biol Sci Med Sci 2000; 55: B106–12

49. O'Kusky JR, Ye P, D'Ercole AJ. Insulin-like growth factor-I promotes neurogenesis and synaptogenesis in the hippocampal dentate gyrus during postnatal development. J Neurosci 2000; 20: 8435–42

50. Liu XF, Fawcett JR, Thorne RG, Frey WH. Non-invasive intranasal insulin-like growth factor-I reduces infarct volume and improves neurologic function in rats following middle cerebral artery occlusion. Neurosci Lett 2001; 308: 91–4

51. Liu XF, Fawcett JR, Thorne RG, et al. Intranasal administration of insulin-like growth factor-I bypasses the blood–brain barrier and protects against focal cerebral ischemic damage. J Neurol Sci 2001; 187: 91–7

52. Trejo JL, Carro E, Torres-Aleman I. Circulating insulin-like growth factor I mediates exercise-induced increases in the number of new neurons in the adult hippocampus. J Neurosci 2001; 21: 1628–34

53. Carro E, Trejo JL, Busiguina S, Torres-Aleman I. Circulating insulin-like growth factor I mediates the protective effects of physical exercise against brain insults of different etiology and anatomy. J Neurosci 2001; 21: 5678–84

54. Zhang B, Salituro G, Szalkowski D, et al. Discovery of a small molecule insulin mimetic with antidiabetic activity in mice. Science 1999; 284: 974–7

55. De Meyts P, Whittaker J. Structural biology of insulin and IGF1 receptors: implications for drug design. Nat Rev Drug Discov 2002; 1: 769–83

56. Salituro GM, Pelaez F, Zhang BB. Discovery of a small molecule insulin receptor activator. Recent Prog Horm Res 2001; 56: 107–26

57. Manchem VP, Goldfine ID, Kohanski RA, et al. A novel small molecule that directly sensitizes the insulin receptor in vitro and in vivo. Diabetes 2001; 50: 824–30

58. Chen C, Zhu YF, Liu XJ, et al. Discovery of a series of nonpeptide small molecules that inhibit the binding of IGF-I to IGF-binding proteins. J Med Chem 2001; 44: 4001–10

Chapter 8

The interrelationships between gait and cognitive function

N Giladi, PL Sheridan, JM Hausdorff

INTRODUCTION

Typically, gait and cognitive function are viewed, at least at first glance, as separate and more or less distinct processes. Here we briefly review some of the recent, less intuitive evidence that belies this perspective and that led us to change our thinking about these two key functions.

Walking is a motor task that is generally mastered during the second year of life. Unless a problem develops, gait is performed automatically even though the walking pattern is constantly adjusted in response to internal and external circumstances. A healthy child learns to adapt his gait to the environment around age 4. From this age until late in life, the gait and posture system is constantly confronted with environmental obstacles and sensory disturbances as well as with mental distractions and motor disturbances. Despite these challenges, a healthy person stays on his/her two feet and very rarely falls. This remarkable feat, the safe movement of an inherently unstable 'inverted pendulum', is the product of a highly sensitive, responsive and efficient mechanism that relies heavily on the sensory, motor and autonomic systems and, as discussed below, higher cognitive control.

COGNITIVE ASPECTS OF NORMAL WALKING

Although gait and mobility are generally considered over-learned and automatic functions, recent research highlights the importance of intact higher cognitive function and mental health in routine walking, particularly as we get older.[1–4] As the population ages, falls are taking their place as an important complication of aging, in part because of the cognitive disturbances that are seen in higher frequency in the elderly. Falls in older adults are a major health problem with significant social and economic ramifications, particularly among those with dementia.[5–7] Patients with Alzheimer's disease (AD), the most common cause of dementia, have a significantly increased risk of falls and fractures.[5,7,8] The prevalence of falls and serious morbidity in AD patients exceeds that of cognitively intact, age-matched peers, even though muscle strength and 'motor' control are generally intact in AD. A longitudinal study of AD and normal aging found that falls were more than three times more likely among AD subjects compared to age-matched controls.[7] The source of these walking difficulties and the increased risk of falls is not entirely clear.[9] We suggest that this points to and underscores the importance of cognitive function in routine walking.

Why is cognition so important for normal walking?

Although we may not realize it, walking in daily life is a continuous challenge that requires adjustment by higher cognitive processes. Executive functions encompass a variety of higher cognitive processes that modulate and use information from the posterior cortical sensory systems to produce behavior.[10–12] These include initiation or intention of action, planning, accessing working memory and attention. Attention is a dynamic executive function driven by sensory perception and the need to select a preferred stimulus for a particular action while ignoring the irrelevant.[11] The process of attention can be divided into separate functions such as response selection, divided attention and vigilance.[11] Actions are considered goal-directed behaviors involving movement.[10,13,14] Cognitive control of action involves integration of incoming sensory information with previously learned motor programs to formulate a new plan for movement, heavily relying on attentional processes.[10,13–16]

Under healthy conditions, gait is generally considered to be an automatic behavior, as are all previously learned, routine movements. However, the concept that routine or previously learned actions do not utilize executive functions such as attention is currently being challenged. Research using neuroimaging techniques (e.g. functional magnetic resonance imaging (fMRI), single photon emission computed tomography (SPECT)) has demonstrated activation of brain areas involved in the network of executive functions during performance of routine motor tasks.[14,17,18] Performance of simple motor tasks such as moving fingers on both hands simultaneously in sequence showed activation of brain areas involved in executive functions (dorsolateral prefrontal and cingulated cortices), suggesting that control of routine movement may require continuous input from posterior sensory systems and integration of this information with previously learned motor programs.[13]

A closer look at walking suggests that even routine ambulation is not automatic, but is a goal-directed action that requires executive function, particularly attention. Walking involves constant decision-making regarding the purpose, detailed planning of the route, speed, stride length, stride width and, more generally, the walking pattern (a form of dual tasking). This strategic planning is based on previous experience as well as new sensory or mental information acquired about the task and the environment as well as the physical condition of the person at the specific moment before gait is initiated. Once gait is initiated, the sensory systems provide continuous updates about the environment, the route, the destination and potential obstacles along with feedback on the actual motor performance and the motor state. All that information is processed centrally and adjustments in the gait pattern allow for safe and efficient performance. In order to perform all those tasks simultaneously, one has to rely heavily on attention capabilities, a subtype of executive function, especially the ability to divide attention. Walking under 'real life' conditions almost always involves dual (or triple) tasking and divided attention; walking typically occurs while we talk, look, stare, eat, drink, think, carry an object and/or take precautions not to trip over any obstacles.

Work by our group supports the idea that gait, especially under dual tasking conditions, relies upon executive function.[3,19] In a study of patients with AD, we found that executive function measures were not related to gait speed

Table 8.1 Association between executive function and stride-to-stride variability in patients with Parkinson's disease and controls under different 'dual task' conditions

Cognitive domain	Walking condition		
	Single task usual walking	'Easy' dual task	'Difficult' dual task
Executive functions	$r = -0.39$	$r = -0.53$	$r = -0.67$
	$p = 0.192$	$p = 0.016$	$p = 0.001$
Memory	$r = -0.17$	$r = -0.063$	$r = -0.003$
	$p = 0.589$	$p = 0.793$	$p = 0.989$

Pearson's correlation coefficients and the corresponding p values

during single or dual tasking (a simple task), but were related to stride variability during dual tasking.[19] Recently, we observed similar results in preliminary findings of a study of patients with Parkinson's disease and controls. In fact, as anticipated, the association between executive function and stride variability increased as the degree of difficulty of the dual task was increased (Table 8.1).

With various pathologies and with aging, the highly complex and efficient system that normally responds to sensory inputs and regulates walking under dual task conditions may be challenged. The accuracy of the sensory information (e.g. vision, vestibular or peripheral sensation) that finds its way to the brain decreases, as does the speed in which the feedback systems work. The motor system may not be able to execute tasks as quickly and accurately as it once did. These changes in function may produce feedback delays and uncoordinated movements not fully time locked to the internal or external situation. In addition to deteriorations in the efficiency of the afferent and efferent systems, the central processing may be slower and less efficient, creating an un-reliable system. Despite these challenges, many older adults walk normally; two-thirds of community-living older adults walk without falling in any given year. This is most likely to

reflect highly efficient compensatory mechanisms and protective redundancies. Unfortunately, however, any additional challenge, either physiological (dual tasking, unpredictable obstacle, etc.) or pathological (disease, drugs, etc.), may upset this balance and reveal a gait network that is working at its maximal capacity with no reserve and is unable to respond to prevent instability and falls.

GAIT DISTURBANCES AS A MARKER OF MENTAL DISTURBANCES

The brain networks responsible for normal walking include the spinal cord, brain stem, midbrain and basal ganglia, as well as the thalamus, limbic system and the entire cortex (visual, sensory–motor, associative and the frontal lobe (executive functions)). Much of the brain is involved in this basic daily task. Furthermore, walking can be viewed as an axial motor task that requires synchronization of activity between the two hemispheres. It is understandable then how a disturbance in brain activity, focal, generalized or unilateral, may impact the gait pattern. This may be particularly true in continuous walking when synchronization of bilateral muscle activation is needed over a long period of time.

Recent multi-year, prospective studies have shown precisely what could be anticipated from the above perspective. Gait changes either in pattern or in speed predicted the development of cognitive decline and dementia up to 6 years later.[20,21] In other words, simple changes in walking appeared 6 years before the development of dementia and they were significant, independent risk factors for future dementia. In fact, the neural networks associated with gait were found to be much more sensitive than the cognitive networks for identifying brain dysfunction of any kind.[20,21] These findings are significant for clinical practice because gait assessments are relatively simple to perform and the outcomes associated with an altered gait apparently go far beyond changes in the spatial–temporal parameters of walking.

These studies that demonstrated that gait changes predict cognitive decline used relatively basic methods for evaluating gait, e.g. visual observation or measurement of gait speed. One can speculate that more sensitive, quantitative systems of gait analysis would be able to detect more subtle gait disturbances and possibly predict cognitive dysfunction earlier and more precisely. However, the most sophisticated gait laboratories are not ideally suited for that purpose because they generally provide details of a single stride, but very little on locomotion and changes that occur from one stride to the next. Also they can be considered 'artificial' walking environments. In contrast, ambulatory gait assessment systems are much more suitable for the evaluation of continuous locomotion and gait dynamics. We have been using such a system for several years and quantitatively measuring the stride time and its fluctuations using force-sensitive insoles or shoes as subjects walk for several minutes, instead of just a few strides. Examination of the stride-to-stride variations in gait has already been shown to be a highly sensitive method for prospectively identifying those who are prone to fall, another symptom often caused by multi-level brain dysfunction.[22–24] We propose that gait dynamics in the form of stride-to-stride variations and, even more, its fractal index, may be an early and sensitive measure of brain dysfunction that can easily be used as a screening tool for the early detection of brain disturbances.[3,22,25,26]

MENTAL DISTURBANCES AS RISK FACTORS FOR GAIT DISTURBANCES AND FALLS

If one accepts the idea that walking relies upon executive and other mental functions, then it is not surprising that mental disturbances affect gait and can lead to an increased risk of falls. Patients with AD, even in the early, mild stages of the disease, have changes in gait speed,[27] but an abnormal stride-to-stride variation and an inability to maintain a stable walking pattern have been significantly associated with fall risk.[24] Among older adults with a 'higher-level' gait disorder,[28] stride-to-stride variability was associated with fear of falling and depressive symptoms.[29] Among older adults with mild functional impairment and those attending a geriatric outpatient clinic, stride variability was also associated with cognitive function and depressive symptoms.[22,30]

Depression has long been associated with changes in the frontal lobe and has been known to influence cognitive function and, more specifically, memory and executive functions[31,32]. Depression may also alter motor performance at the level of reaction time and sensory processing, indicating that it might contribute to motor disturbance via multiple systems[33,34]. In fact, the motor performance of patients with depression is similar to the bradykinetic features of patients with Parkinson's disease.[35] Patients with major depression walk more slowly and have slower initiation of movement compared to controls.[36] In a pilot study, patients with major depression and bipolar depression exhibited increased stride-to-stride variability in their walking pattern, compared to controls. This finding is consistent with the reasoning that gait stability relies upon intact cognitive and mental function.

Falls are one of the most serious complications of gait and postural disturbances. Based on the above analysis, it is only logical to predict that patients with mental disturbances and associated gait disturbances will also fall more frequently. Several studies have confirmed this hypothesis. As noted above, patients with AD fall much more frequently than age-matched controls.[5,7,8] Depressed adults fall more frequently and have a higher rate of hip fractures, compared to their non-depressed peers[37]. A 3-year follow-up study found that women who exhibited mental distress were at increased risk of hip fractures, even after adjusting for medication usage.[38]

This brief review highlights the networks that connect mental function and gait. The mutual dependence suggests why and how the evaluation of gait may be used to predict cognitive changes and, conversely, how changes in mental function influence gait.

REFERENCES

1. Brown RG, Marsden CD. Dual task performance and processing resources in normal subjects and patients with Parkinson's disease. Brain 1991; 114: 215–31

2. Camicioli R, Howieson D, Lehman S, Kaye J. Talking while walking: the effect of a dual task in aging and Alzheimer's disease. Neurology 1997; 48: 955–8

3. Hausdorff JM, Balash J, Giladi N. Effects of cognitive challenge on gait variability in patients with Parkinson's disease. J Geriatr Psychiatry Neurol 2003; 16: 53–8

4. Woollacott M, Shumway-Cook A. Attention and the control of posture and gait: a review of an emerging area of research. Gait Posture 2002; 16: 1–14

5. Ballard CG, Shaw F, Lowery K, et al. The prevalence, assessment and associations of falls in dementia with Lewy bodies and Alzheimer's disease. Dement Geriatr Cogn Disord 1999; 10: 97–103

6. Kannus P, Parkkari J, Koskinen S et al. Fall-induced injuries and deaths among older adults. J Am Med Assoc 1999; 281: 1895–9

7. Morris JC, Rubin EH, Morris EJ, Mandel SA. Senile dementia of the Alzheimer's type: an important risk factor for serious falls. J Gerontol 1987; 42: 412–17

8. Weller I. The relation between hip fracture and Alzheimer's disease in the Canadian national population health survey health institutions data, 1994–1995. A cross-sectional study. Ann Epidemiol 2004; 14: 319–24

9. Shaw FE, Bond J, Richardson DA, et al. Multifactorial intervention after a fall in older people with cognitive impairment and dementia presenting to the accident and emergency department: randomised controlled trial. Br Med J 2003; 326: 73

10. Fuster JM. Synopsis of function and dysfunction of the frontal lobe. Acta Psychiatr Scand 1999; 395 (Suppl): 51–7

11. Perry RJ, Hodges JR. Attention and executive deficits in Alzheimer's disease. A critical review. Brain 1999; 122: 383–404

12. Shallice T, Burgess P. The domain of supervisory processes and temporal organization of behaviour. Philos Trans R Soc Lond B Biol Sci 1996; 351: 1405–11

13. Jahanshahi M, Frith CD. Willed action and its impairments. Cog Neuropsychol 1998; 15: 483–533

14. Jueptner M, Stephan KM, Frith CD, et al. Anatomy of motor learning. I. Frontal cortex and attention to action. J Neurophysiol 1997; 77: 1313–24

15. Badgaiyan RD. Executive control, willed actions, and nonconscious processing. Hum Brain Mapp 2000; 9: 38–41

16. Passingham RE. Attention to action. Philos Trans R Soc Lond B Biol Sci 1996; 351: 1473–9

17. Jahanshahi M, Jenkins IH, Brown RG, et al. Self-initiated versus externally triggered movements. I. An investigation using measurement of regional cerebral blood flow with PET and movement-related potentials in normal and Parkinson's disease subjects. Brain 1995; 118: 913–33

18. Jueptner M, Frith CD, Brooks DJ, et al. Anatomy of motor learning. II. Subcortical structures and learning by trial and error. J Neurophysiol 1997; 77: 1325–37

19. Sheridan P, Solomont J, Kowall N, Hausdorff JM. Influence of executive function on locomotor function: divided attention increases gait variability in Alzheimer's disease. J Am Geriatr Soc 2003; 51: 1633–7

20. Marquis S, Moore MM, Howieson DB, et al. Independent predictors of cognitive decline in healthy elderly persons. Arch Neurol 2002; 59: 601–6

21. Verghese J, Lipton RB, Hall CB, et al. Abnormality of gait as a predictor of non-Alzheimer's dementia. N Engl J Med 2002; 347: 1761–8

22. Hausdorff JM, Rios D, Edelberg HK. Gait variability and fall risk in community-living older adults: a 1-year prospective study. Arch Phys Med Rehabil 2001; 82: 1050–6

23. Maki BE. Gait changes in older adults: predictors of falls or indicators of fear. J Am Geriatr Soc 1997; 45: 313–20

24. Nakamura T, Meguro K, Sasaki H. Relationship between falls and stride length variability in senile dementia of the Alzheimer type. Gerontology 1996; 42: 108–13

25. Goldberger AL, Amaral LA, Hausdorff JM, et al. Fractal dynamics in physiology: alterations with disease and aging. Proc Natl Acad Sci USA 2002; 99 (Suppl 1): 2466–72

26. Hausdorff JM, Mitchell SL, Firtion R, et al. Altered fractal dynamics of gait: reduced stride-interval correlations with aging and Huntington's disease. J Appl Physiol 1997; 82: 262–9

27. Alexander NB, Mollo JM, Giordani B, et al. Maintenance of balance, gait patterns, and obstacle clearance in Alzheimer's disease. Neurology 1995; 45: 908–14

28. Nutt JG, Marsden CD, Thompson PD. Human walking and higher-level gait disorders, particularly in the elderly. Neurology 1993; 43: 268–79

29. Giladi N, Herman T, Rieder-Grossover I, et al. The non-specific gait disorder of the elderly: is it a disorder or a syndrome? Mov Disord 2002; 17: S243

30. Hausdorff JM, Nelson ME, Kaliton D, et al. Etiology and modification of gait instability in older adults: a randomized controlled trial of exercise. J Appl Physiol 2001; 90: 2117–29

31. Feil D, Razani J, Boone K, Lesser I. Apathy and cognitive performance in older adults with depression. Int J Geriatr Psychiatry 2003; 18: 479–85

32. Hammar A, Lund A, Hugdahl K. Long-lasting cognitive impairment in unipolar major depression: a 6-month follow-up study. Psychiatry Res 2003; 118: 189–96

33. Nebes RD, Halligan EM, Rosen J, Reynolds CF III. Cognitive and motor slowing in Alzheimer's disease and geriatric depression. J Int Neuropsychol Soc 1998; 4: 426–34

34. Ortiz AT, Lopez-Ibor MI, Martinez CE, et al. Deficit in sensory motor processing in depression and Alzheimer's disease: a study with EMG and event related potentials. Electromyogr Clin Neurophysiol 2000; 40: 357–63

35. Rogers MA, Bradshaw JL, Phillips JG, et al., Parkinsonian motor characteristics in unipolar major depression. J Clin Exp Neuropsychol 2000; 22: 232–44

36. Lemke MR, Wendorff T, Mieth B, et al. Spatiotemporal gait patterns during over ground locomotion in major depression compared with healthy controls. J Psychiatr Res 2000; 34: 277–83

37. Stalenhoef PA, Diederiks JP, Knottnerus JA, et al. A risk model for the prediction of recurrent falls in community-dwelling elderly: a prospective cohort study. J Clin Epidemiol 2002; 55: 1088–94

38. Forsen L, Meyer HE, Sogaard AJ, et al. Mental distress and risk of hip fracture. Do broken hearts lead to broken bones? J Epidemiol. Commun Health 1999; 53: 343–7

Advances in gene transfer and pharmacological regulation of protein aggregation in the treatment of Alzheimer's and Parkinson's diseases

P Bar-On, E Rockenstein, M Hashimoto, E Masliah

INTRODUCTION

Alzheimer's disease (AD) and Parkinson's disease (PD) are the most common neurodegenerative disorders in the elderly affecting over 2 million people in the USA alone.[1] In recent years, it has become clear that AD and PD as well as other neurodegenerative diseases involve aggregation and deposition of misfolded proteins.[2] In AD the main component of the plaque core is the amyloid β peptide 1–42 (Aβ 1–42), a proteolytic product of the amyloid precursor protein (APP) metabolism,[3] whereas in PD, α-synuclein, originally identified in human brain as a precursor protein of the non-Aβ component (NAC) of the AD amyloid,[4-6] accumulates intracellularly in the neuronal perikaryon and synapses. The exact causes that trigger the abnormal folding and accumulation of proteins are not yet clear, and the mechanisms by which aggregated α-synuclein or Aβ promote synaptic dysfunction leading to neurodegeneration are under intense scrutiny. Nerve damage leading to synaptic loss and neuronal cell death probably result from the early conversion in intracellular compartments of normally non-toxic α-synuclein or Aβ monomers into toxic oligomers and protofibrils. In this view, new therapeutic strategies for the treatment of AD and PD are aimed at reducing Aβ 1–42 production (e.g. γ- and β-secretase inhibitors), rapid clearance of Aβ aggregates (e.g. vaccination), protecting neurons against toxic aggregate proteins (e.g. antioxidants, neurotrophic agents), blocking α-synuclein toxic oligomerization, and promoting α-synuclein protofibril degradation using antiamyloidogenic compounds and chaperones that will stimulate proteosomal degradation. In this regard, we characterized β-synuclein, the non-amyloidogenic homolog of α-synuclein, as an inhibitor of α-synuclein toxic conversion. Our results raise the intriguing possibility that β-synuclein might be a natural negative regulator of α-synuclein aggregation, and that a similar class of endogenous factors might modulate the toxic conversion of other molecules involved in neurodegeneration. Such an anti-amyloidogenic property of β-synuclein in combination with other treatments might also provide a novel strategy for the treatment of neurodegenerative disorders.

Notably, a majority of patients with AD also have α-synuclein-immunoreactive Lewy bodies (LBs) in the amygdala,[7,8] and a substantial proportion of them develop a form of parkinsonism: a condition denominated by dementia with LBs.[9] This suggests that factors involved in the pathogenesis of AD might promote the development of particularly aggressive forms of parkinsonism. We have recently shown that the Aβ 1–42 promotes the toxic conversion of α-synuclein and accelerates α-synuclein-dependent motor deficits.[10] Moreover, it is worth taking into account the fact that both these proteins are associated with the membrane and are affected by changes in cholesterol or lipid composition.[11,12] Therefore, further studies on membrane interactions and the impact of changes in the membrane during aging will help to elucidate the connection between both proteins in neurodegeneration, and efforts to gain better understanding of the relationship and the mechanisms that facilitate such pathological interactions between α-synuclein and Aβ will aid in the development of new treatment strategies for AD and PD.

Genetic transfer approaches have received recent consideration as a potential treatment for human central nervous system (CNS) and peripheral nervous system (PNS) neurodegenerative disorders, including AD and PD. There has been considerable progress in the development of safe and efficient viral vectors and lentiviral vectors, as well as in transplantation of genetically modified cells into the brain for expression and delivery of transgenes, neurotrophic factors, neurotransmitter-synthesized enzyme and cellular regulatory proteins for intervention of neurodegenerative diseases.

In this chapter the main objectives are to describe recent advances in gene transfer and pharmacological regulation of protein aggregation, based on the supposition that Aβ interacts with α-synuclein, with special emphasis on the role of abnormal interaction in intracellular membrane compartments.

ADVANCES IN GENE TRANSFER AND PHARMACOLOGICAL MANIPULATION OF PROTEIN AGGREGATION IN ALZHEIMER'S DISEASE AND DEMENTIA WITH LEWY BODIES

The memory loss in AD is associated with synaptic loss in the limbic system and is accompanied by formation of abundant neuritic plaques mostly consisting of Aβ peptide and neurofibrillary tangles. Early intracellular accumulation of Aβ oligomers is believed to be an initiating event for neuronal loss in AD. The role of the extracellular amyloid fibrils in the plaques is more controversial. In this case, three proteases: α-, β-, and γ-secretase which are involved in cleavage of the APP to Aβ, are one of the major targets for the development of drugs to treat AD. The most promising advances are the development of drugs that block the formation of the Aβ, such as β- and γ-secretase inhibitors and antiamyloidogenic compounds. A novel strategy is to regulate the clearance of Aβ by an immunological response, vaccination, or gene transfer of neprilysin.[13] Another approach is protecting neurons using antioxidants and nerve growth factor (NGF) transfer delivery.[14] Several recent studies have suggested brain cholesterol alterations as an important event in the progression of AD.[15,16] In this context, the interaction of Aβ with α-synuclein, their transport to the membrane, and their interaction following the changes in the lipid composition of membranes and altered membrane fluidity during aging provide a new strategy for drug development.

NGF is an important molecule that regulates neuronal survival and differentiation.[17,18] Nerve growth factor plays a role in the maintenance of the cholinergic neurotransmitter system in specific populations of neurons, including a group of cholinergic forebrain neurons.[17,18] This provides the rationale for the potential gene delivery of NGF to improve cognition in AD patients, who consistently demonstrate a loss of functional basal forebrain cholinergic neurons.[19] Studies have demonstrated that NGF can prevent lesion-induced basal forebrain cholinergic neuronal degeneration, and can reverse age-related degeneration in these neurons.[18] Long-term intraparenchymal delivery of NGF targeted to the primate cholinergic basal forebrain did not significantly increase β-amyloid deposition in aged monkeys, although it has been reported that NGF upregulates the expression of APP.[20] Administration of NGF by intracerebroventricular infusion or transplantation of NGF-secreting cells to the basal forebrain improved spatial memory in aged animals.[21] Using the adeno-associated-virus (AAV) vector system, basal forebrain neurons were transduced to produce NGF for long intervals (at least 9 months).[22]

Neprilysin, a zinc metalloendopeptidase that functions to degrade peptide signaling in the immune, circulatory and nervous systems,[23] has recently been identified as a major extracellular Aβ degradation enzyme in the brain.[24] Recent studies have shown that neprilysin knock-out mice exhibit a gene dose-dependent increase in Aβ levels in the brain.[25] Additionally, neprilysin is reduced in areas vulnerable to plaque formation.[26-29] Furthermore, down-regulation of neprilysin with chemical inhibitors results in increased Aβ concentrations in the brain.[24] Moreover, infection of primary neurons with a vector expressing neprilysin also reduced Aβ production in vitro.[30] To determine whether neprilysin can antagonize the deposition of Aβ in vivo, a lentiviral vector expressing the human neprilysin was tested in transgenic mouse models of amyloidosis. A unilateral intracerebral injection of lentiviral-neprilysin reduced Aβ deposits by half relative to the untreated side. Furthermore, lentiviral-neprilysin ameliorated neurodegenerative

alterations in the frontal cortex and hippocampus of these transgenic mice. Taken together, these studies suggest that neprilysin plays a key role in regulating the deposition and the clearance of Aβ.[13]

The interaction of α-synuclein with Aβ and the contribution of α-synuclein accumulation in AD plaques has been studied considerably in recent years, in an effort to elucidate the underlying mechanism.[31] The amyloid deposits are mainly composed of aggregates of the Aβ peptide with 40–42 residues,[3] whereas α-synuclein was originally identified in human brain as a precursor protein of the NAC of the AD amyloid.[4-6] Remarkably, the majority of patients with AD also have α-synuclein-immunoreactive LBs in the amygdala.[7,8] A substantial proportion of them develop parkinsonism leading to dementia with Lewy bodies.[9] It has been shown that α-synuclein and Aβ can interact in vitro,[32] and that Aβ stimulated α-synuclein aggregation.[10] Moreover, it was shown that Aβ promotes the intracellular accumulation of α-synuclein and accelerates α-synuclein-dependent motor deficits in double α-synuclein and mutant APP transgenic mice.[10] One possible mechanism for the interaction between Aβ with α-synuclein is that Aβ 1–42 accumulating in the intracellular pool might leak from the endomembranous compartment and interact directly with α-synuclein in the cytosol. Alternatively, secreted Aβ 1–42 might indirectly trigger α-synuclein accumulation by promoting oxidative stress. Thus, the combined actions of Aβ 1–42 and α-synuclein may result in leakiness and membrane damage that allows for a direct contact between Aβ 1–42 and α-synuclein in the cytosol. This effect of Aβ 1–42 on α-synuclein might be mediated by direct fibrillogenic interactions between these molecules,[33,34] by free radicals and/or by interactions with the mitochondrial membrane. Furthermore, Aβ 1–42 generates reactive oxygen species (ROS),[35] and growing evidence suggests that oxidative cross-linking of α-synuclein contributes to its toxic conversion.[36,37] Therefore, treatment with antioxidants in combination with β-synuclein and other antiaggregation compounds may be considered as a useful treatment strategy.

Another possible mechanism through which abnormal interactions between Aβ and α-synuclein may occur is when changes in cholesterol levels and lipid composition occur in the membrane. A number of epidemiological studies suggest that high levels of cholesterol may contribute to the pathogenesis of AD.[15,16] Individuals with elevated levels of cholesterol have an increased susceptibility to AD, and therefore cholesterol is considered a risk factor for AD.[15,16] Apolipoprotein E (apoE) is one of the major apolipoproteins in the plasma and the principal cholesterol carrier protein in the brain. Numerous independent studies have consistently confirmed that the apoE ε4 allele is the most prevalent risk factor for AD.[38] Studies in a transgenic mouse model expressing human APP suggest that apoE contributes to the deposition of Aβ.[39] Moreover, amyloid deposition was found to be strictly dependent on apoE expression levels in a dose-dependent manner.[16] Studies using animal models show a strong connection between cholesterol levels and Aβ generation. High cholesterol diet increased the level of Aβ accumulation in the brain.[40] In addition to *in vivo* results, strong biochemical evidence also supports a direct role of intracellular cholesterol on Aβ generation and deposition.[16,40] Several studies have indicated that changes in cholesterol levels, homeostasis, distribution and compartment impact both the processing of APP and the biogenesis of Aβ. Altered cholesterol distribution affects the activity of the secretase enzymes. It has been shown that cholesterol reduction promotes the non-amyloidogenic α-secretase pathway and the formation of neuroprotective α-secretase cleaved soluble APP, whereas increasing evidence suggests that β-secretase functions best in a high cholesterol environment.[42-48]

Drugs that lower cholesterol levels are currently being considered and tested as potential therapies for the treatment of AD. Recent evidence suggests that the cholesterol-lowering enzymes, termed statins, can inhibit Aβ production and reduce the prevalence of AD. In cells overexpressing APP, treatment with lovastatin resulted in higher expression of the α-secretase ADAM 10, a disintegrin and metalloprotease that was found to be the major target of the cholesterol effects on APP metabolism.[42,45]

The normal function of α-synuclein remains unclear so far, but recent reports suggest that it is involved in trafficking synaptic terminals and that its function includes interaction with lipids.[12] Moreover, it has been shown that α-synuclein binds to vesicles, and therefore it was proposed that α-synuclein has a role in vesicle function at synaptic terminals and that it may regulate the size of the synaptic vesicle pool.[49] In addition, it was found that α-synuclein has motifs homologous to fatty acid-binding proteins, suggesting that it might play a role in fatty acid transport between aqueous and phospholipid compartments in neuronal cells.[50] Protofibrils of α-synuclein, which seem to be the most toxic structure of α-synuclein, were shown to bind synthetic vesicles very tightly and transiently permeabilize and damage these vesicles.[51-53] Taken together, further studies on membrane interactions and the impact of changes in membrane composition during aging will help to elucidate the connection between Aβ and α-synuclein. An effective therapy treatment may ultimately consist of a combination of lipid regulation products in combination with statins or other cholesterol management products.

ADVANCES IN GENE TRANSFER AND PHARMACOLOGICAL MANIPULATION OF PROTEIN AGGREGATION IN PARKINSON'S DISEASE

Current gene therapy models for PD have focused mainly on two treatment strategies. The first strategy is the replacement of biosynthetic enzymes for dopamine synthesis, and the second strategy is the addition of neurotrophic factors for protection and restoration of dopaminergic neurons using neurotrophic factors and antioxidants.[54] New therapeutic strategies for the treatment of PD are aimed at blocking α-synuclein toxic oligomerization and protofibril formation using β-synuclein[55,56] and antioxidants, promoting α-synuclein protofibril degradation with proteosome targeting chaperones, and preventing α-synuclein translocation to the membrane, or extracting it from the pathological compartments.[55]

Many gene therapy experiments in PD were focused on replacement of dopamine biosynthetic enzymes. These studies involve transfecting the tyrosine hydroxylase (TH) gene.[57] Double transfection with TH and GTP-cyclohydrolase 1 (GCH1) appeared to improve L-dopa and dopamine production in rat models of PD.[58,59] Additional gene transfer studies have shown that double transfection of TH and aromatic-L-amino acid decarboxylase (AADC) have resulted in better biochemical and behavioral outcomes than transfection of TH alone.[60,61] Recent experiments of triple transfection of TH, GHC1 and AADC using the AAV delivery system have shown greater dopamine production *in vitro* and reduction of rotational behavior in a rat PD model *in vivo*.[62] Moreover, transfection of the vesicular monoamine transporter (VMAT) gene for dopamine storage within cells gave higher levels of dopamine production and storage.[63] Overall, the combination of oral administration of L-dopa with replacement therapy aimed at restoration of dopamine levels have not provided the protection against the progression of dopamine loss, and it is unlikely that this approach will be sufficient in the long term.

Delivery of neurotrophic factors to the CNS represents an important challenge for the treatment of neurodegenerative disorders for their neuroprotective and restorative properties. The members of the glial cell line-derived neurotrophic factor (GDNF) are the most potent and specific neurotrophic factors identified for dopaminergic neurons, because of their potent *in vivo* effects in animal models of PD.[64] In a rat model of PD, using recombinant viral vectors derived from adenovirus, AAV, or lentivirus have been shown to be effective for long-term delivery of GDNF in the nigrostriatal system.[22,65] Delivery of GDNF via these vectors into a 6-hydroxydopamine (6-OHDA) rat PD model, have shown both behavioral improvement as well as neuroprotection of dopaminergic neurons.[64,66] Moreover, delivery of GDNF to the striatum, prior to a 6-OHDA injection, provided both long-term protection of dopaminergic terminals and behavioral recovery.[67] Experiments using lentivirus-GDNF vector show that sustained GDNF delivery could improve behavioral performance in 1-methyl-4-phenyl-1,2,3,6-tetrahydropyridine (MPTP)-treated monkeys.[68] Injection of lentivirus-GDNF into the striatum and substantia nigra a week after treatment with MPTP showed reversal of motor deficits and prevention of dopaminergic neuronal loss in monkeys.[69]

Neuronal accumulation of misfolded α-synuclein has been proposed to be centrally involved in PD pathogenesis. This synaptic associated protein is natively unfolded and self-aggregates to form oligomers, protofibrils and fibrils with amyloid-like charateristics, that are the most abundant component of LBs. In view of evidence that α-synuclein toxic oligomers may initiate neurodegeneration, antiamyloido-genic compounds are under development. Among these, we have characterized β-synuclein, the non-amyloidogenic homolog of α-synuclein, as an inhibitor of aggregation of α-synuclein.[55] In a study utilizing doubly-transgenic mice expressing both α- and β-synuclein we found that β-synuclein ameliorated the motor deficits, neurodegenerative alterations and neuronal accumulation of α-synuclein observed in α-synuclein transgenic mice, a model system of Parkinson-like disease. Similarly, cell lines stably transfected with β-synuclein were resistant to α-synuclein accumulation when this latter molecule was expressed under the control of the inducible muristerone A system. Moreover, it has been shown that β-synuclein is natively unfolded in monomeric form, but structured in protofibrillar form. β-Synuclein protofibrils do not bind to, or permeabilize, synthetic vesicles, unlike protofibrils comprising α-synuclein. In addition, β-synuclein significantly inhibits the generation of A53T α-synuclein protofibrils and fibrils.[56] More recently, we have developed a β-synuclein-expressing lentiviral system that has shown a significant reduction of α-synuclein aggregation and toxic effects. Taken together, these findings suggest that β-synuclein might be a natural negative regulator of α-synuclein,[55] and homologs or derivatives of β-synuclein might have a therapeutic potential for the treatment of PD.

α-Synuclein is capable of self-aggregating to form both oligomers and fibrillar polymers with amyloid-like characteristics.[51] Most recent evidence suggests that there might be both low-molecular-weight non-toxic oligomers that associate with the cell membrane as well as higher molecular-weight toxic oligomers (protofibrils).[51-53] Association of non-toxic oligomers with components of the plasma membrane, such as polyunsaturated fatty acids, might play a role in synaptic plasticity.[70] In contrast, higher molecular-weight toxic oligomers form protofibrils that can potentially damage the cell membrane.[71,72] Recent evidence suggests that protofibrils differ considerably from fibrils with respect to their interactions with synthetic and biological membranes.[51-53] Protofibrillar α-synuclein, in contrast to the monomeric and the fibrillar forms, binds synthetic vesicles very tightly via a β-sheet-rich structure and transiently permeabilizes and damages these vesicles. The possibility that the toxicity of α-synuclein fibrillization may be derived from an oligomeric intermediate, rather than a fibril, has implications regarding the design of therapeutics for PD.[71] In this context, the relationship between mitochondrial dysfunction, α-synuclein aggregation and neurodegeneration is complex.[73] For example, it is widely proposed that in dementia with Lewy bodies, mitochondrial dysfunction promotes α-synuclein aggregation and neurodegeneration. Alternatively, the opposite situation might be at play, namely that α-synuclein aggregation might trigger mitochondrial damage. Recent findings showing that the release of cytochrome C from mitochondria promotes α-synuclein aggregation supports a role for mitochondrial pathology in α-synuclein accumulation.[74] Thus, effective therapies might be directed at reducing α-synuclein oligomerization and blocking protofibril generation by preventing α-synuclein translocation to the plasma membrane or by extracting α-synuclein from the membrane. In this context, we are currently testing a number of drug candidates and derivatives of the statin family as potential therapeutic agents for PD.

CONCLUDING REMARKS

Significant progress has been made in the field of gene therapy, and successful tools for gene transfer into the CNS have been developed.

However, further optimization in terms of timing, dosing and location of gene delivery in addition to regulation and prolongation of gene expression are needed. Today, most gene transfer experiments focus on transfer of neurotrophic factors in order to protect and restore neurons. New concepts for gene transfer such as genes to prevent toxic conversion/aggregation and apoptosis, and to detoxify free radicals, might be utilized as well, and eventually gene therapy might include a combination of antioxidants, neurotrophic factors, antiaggregation and apoptosis inhibitor genes.

Considerable progress has been made in understanding the mechanisms by which misfolded proteins lead to neurodegenerative diseases. However, further studies are necessary to elucidate the connection between Aβ and α-synuclein, as well as to understand cholesterol metabolism in the brain and the changes in cholesterol and lipid composition in neurodegenerative disorders.

REFERENCES

1. Katzman R, Saitoh T. Advances in Alzheimer's disease. FASEB J 1991; 5: 278–86

2. Shastry BS. Neurodegenerative disorders of protein aggregation. Neurochem Int 2003; 43: 1–7

3. Iwatsubo T, Odaka A, Suzuki N, et al. Visualization of A beta 42(43) and A beta 40 in senile plaques with end-specific A beta monoclonals: evidence for an initially deposited species in A beta 42(43). Neuron 1994; 13: 45–53

4. Ueda K, Masliah E, Xia Y, et al. Novel amyloid component (NAC) differentiates Alzheimer's disease from normal aging plaques. Soc Neurosci Abstr 1993; 19: 1254

5. Masliah E, Iwai A, Mallory M, et al. Altered presynaptic protein NACP is associated with plaque formation and neurodegeneration in Alzheimer's disease. Am J Pathol 1996; 148: 201–10

6. Iwai A. Properties of NACP/alpha-synuclein and its role in Alzheimer's disease. Biochim Biophys Acta 2000; 1502: 95–109

7. Lippa C, Fujiwara H, Mann D, et al. Lewy bodies contain altered alpha-synuclein in brains of many familial Alzheimer's disease patients with mutations in presenilin and amyloid precursor protein genes. Am J Pathol 1998; 153: 1365–70

8. Hamilton RL. Lewy bodies in Alzheimer's disease: a neuropathological review of 145 cases using alpha-synuclein immunohistochemistry. Brain Pathol 2000; 10: 378–84

9. Hansen L, Salmon D, Galasko D, et al. The Lewy body variant of Alzheimer's disease: a clinical and pathologic entity. Neurology 1990; 40: 1–7

10. Masliah E, Rockenstein E, Veinbergs I, et al. β amyloid peptides enhance α-synuclein accumulation and neuronal deficits in a transgenic mouse model linking Alzheimer's and Parkinson's disease. Proc Natl Acad Sci USA 2001; 98: 12245–50

11. Frears ER, Stephens DJ, Walters CE, et al. The role of cholesterol in the biosynthesis of beta-amyloid. Neuroreport 1999; 10: 1699–705

12. Jo E, McLaurin J, Yip C, et al. Alpha-synuclein membrane interactions and lipid specificity. J Biol Chem 2000; 275: 34328–34

13. Marr RA, Rockenstein E, Mukherjee A, et al. Neprilysin gene transfer reduces human amyloid pathology in transgenic mice. J Neurosci 2003; 23: 1992–6

14. Wyman T, Rohrer D, Kirigiti P, et al. Promoter-activated expression of nerve growth factor for treatment of neurodegenerative diseases. Gene Ther 1999; 6: 1648–60

15. Wolozin B. Cholesterol and Alzheimer's disease. Biochem Soc Trans 2002; 30: 525–9

16. Puglielli L, Tanzi RE, Kovacs DM. Alzheimer's disease: the cholesterol connection. Nat Neurosci 2003; 6: 345–51

17. Barde YA. Trophic factors and neuronal survival. Neuron 1989; 2: 1525–34

18. Tuszynski MH, Gabriel K, Gage FH, et al. Nerve growth factor delivery by gene transfer induces differential outgrowth of sensory, motor, and noradrenergic neurites after adult spinal cord injury. Exp Neurol 1996; 137: 157–73

19. Geschwind MD, Kessler JA, Geller AI, Federoff HJ. Transfer of the nerve growth factor gene into cell lines and cultured neurons using a defective herpes simplex virus vector. Transfer of the NGF gene into cells by a HSV-1 vector. Brain Res Mol Brain Res 1994; 24: 327–35

20. Tuszynski MH, Smith DE, Roberts J, et al. Targeted intraparenchymal delivery of human NGF by gene transfer to the primate basal forebrain for 3 months does not accelerate beta-amyloid plaque deposition. Exp Neurol 1998; 154: 573–82

21. Klein RL, Hirko AC, Meyers CA, et al. NGF gene transfer to intrinsic basal forebrain neurons increases cholinergic cell size and protects from age-related, spatial memory deficits in middle-aged rats. Brain Res 2000; 875: 144–51

22. Bjorklund A, Kirik D, Rosenblad C, et al. Towards a neuroprotective gene therapy for Parkinson's disease: use of adenovirus, AAV and lentivirus vectors for gene transfer of GDNF to the nigrostriatal system in the rat Parkinson model. Brain Res 2000; 886: 82–98

23. Turner AJ, Isaac RE, Coates D. The neprilysin (NEP) family of zinc metalloendopeptidases: genomics and function. Bioessays 2001; 23: 261–9

24. Iwata N, Tsubuki S, Takaki Y, et al. Identification of the major Abeta1–42-degrading catabolic pathway in brain parenchyma: suppression leads to biochemical and pathological deposition. Nat Med 2000; 6: 143–50

25. Iwata N, Tsubuki S, Takaki Y, et al. Metabolic regulation of brain Abeta by neprilysin. Science 2001; 292: 1550–2

26. Akiyama H, Kondo H, Ikeda K, et al. Immunohistochemical localization of neprilysin in the human cerebral cortex: inverse association with vulnerability to amyloid beta-protein (Abeta) deposition. Brain Res 2001; 902: 277–81

27. Reilly CE. Neprilysin content is reduced in Alzheimer brain areas. J Neurol 2001; 248: 159–60

28. Yasojima K, Akiyama H, McGeer EG, McGeer PL. Reduced neprilysin in high plaque areas of Alzheimer brain: a possible relationship to deficient degradation of beta-amyloid peptide. Neurosci Lett 2001; 297: 97–100

29. Yasojima K, McGeer EG, McGeer PL. Relationship between beta amyloid peptide generating molecules and neprilysin in Alzheimer disease and normal brain. Brain Res 2001; 919: 115–21

30. Hama E, Shirotani K, Masumoto H, et al. Clearance of extracellular and cell-associated amyloid beta peptide through viral expression of neprilysin in primary neurons. J Biochem (Tokyo) 2001; 130: 721–6

31. Wirths O, Bayer TA. Alpha-synuclein, Abeta and Alzheimer's disease. Prog Neuropsychopharmacol Biol Psychiatry 2003; 27: 103–8

32. Jensen P, Hojrup P, Hager H, et al. Binding of Aβ to α- and β-synucleins: identification of segments in α-synuclein/NAC precursor that bind Aβ and NAC. Biochem J 1997; 323: 539–46

33. El-Agnaf O, Irvine G. Review: Formation and properties of amyloid-like fibrils derived from alpha-synuclein and related proteins. J Struct Biol 2000; 130: 300–9

34. El-Agnaf O, Mahil D, Patel B, Austen B. Oligomerization and toxicity of beta-amyloid-42 implicated in Alzheimer's disease. Biochem Biophys Res Commun 2000; 273: 1003–7

35. Mattson M, Begley J, Mark R, Furukawa K. Abeta25–35 induces rapid lysis of red blood cells: contrast with Abeta 1–42 and examination of underlying mechanisms. Brain Res 1997; 771: 147–53

36. Hashimoto M, Hsu L, Xia Y, et al. Oxidative stress induces amyloid-like aggregate formation of NACP/α-synuclein in vitro. Neuroreport 1999; 10: 717–21

37. Giasson BI, Duda JE, Murray IV, et al. Oxidative damage linked to neurodegeneration by selective alpha-synuclein nitration in synucleinopathy lesions. Science 2000; 290: 985–9

38. Tanzi RE, Bertram L. New frontiers in Alzheimer's disease genetics. Neuron 2001; 32: 181–4

39. Bales KR, Verina T, Dodel RC, et al. Lack of apolipoprotein E dramatically reduces amyloid beta-peptide deposition. Nat Genet 1997; 17: 263–4

40. Refolo LM, Malester B, LaFrancois J, et al. Hypercholesterolemia accelerates the Alzheimer's amyloid pathology in a transgenic mouse model. Neurobiol Dis 2000; 7: 321–31

41. Lee SJ, Liyanage U, Bickel PE, et al. A detergent-insoluble membrane compartment contains A beta in vivo. Nat Med 1998; 4: 730–4

42. Bodovitz S, Klein WL. Cholesterol modulates alpha-secretase cleavage of amyloid precursor protein. J Biol Chem 1996; 271: 4436–40

43. Racchi M, Baetta R, Salvietti N, et al. Secretory processing of amyloid precursor protein is inhibited by increase in cellular cholesterol content. Biochem J 1997; 322: 893–8

44. Simons M, Keller P, De Strooper B, et al. Cholesterol depletion inhibits the generation of beta-amyloid in hippocampal neurons. Proc Natl Acad Sci USA 1998; 95: 6460–4

45. Kojro E, Gimpl G, Lammich S, et al. Low cholesterol stimulates the nonamyloidogenic pathway by its effect on the alpha-secretase ADAM 10. Proc Natl Acad Sci USA 2001; 98: 5815–20

46. Yip CM, Elton EA, Darabie AA, et al. Cholesterol, a modulator of membrane-associated Abeta-fibrillogenesis and neurotoxicity. J Mol Biol 2001; 311: 723–34

47. Yip CM, Darabie AA, McLaurin J. Abeta42-peptide assembly on lipid bilayers. J Mol Biol 2002; 318: 97–107

48. Arispe N, Doh M. Plasma membrane cholesterol controls the cytotoxicity of Alzheimer's disease AbetaP (1–40) and (1–42) peptides. FASEB J 2002; 16: 1526–36

49. Davidson W, Jonas A, Clayton D, George J. Stabilization of alpha-synuclein secondary structure upon binding to synthetic membranes. J Biol Chem 1998; 273: 9443–9

50. Sharon R, Goldberg MS, Bar-Josef I, et al. Alpha-synuclein occurs in lipid-rich high molecular weight complexes, binds fatty acids, and shows homology to the fatty acid-binding proteins. Proc Natl Acad Sci USA 2001; 98: 9110–15

51. Hashimoto M, Hernandez-Ruiz S, Hsu L, et al. Human recombinant NACP/α-synuclein is

aggregated and fibrillated in vitro: relevance for Lewy body disease. Brain Res 1998; 799: 301–6

52. Conway KA, Lee SJ, Rochet JC, et al. Acceleration of oligomerization, not fibrillization, is a shared property of both alpha-synuclein mutations linked to early-onset Parkinson's disease: implications for pathogenesis and therapy. Proc Natl Acad Sci USA 2000; 97: 571–6

53. Rochet J, Conway K, Lansbury PJ. Inhibition of fibrillization and accumulation of prefibrillar oligomers in mixtures of human and mouse alpha-synuclein. Biochemistry 2000; 39: 10619–26

54. Le HN, Frim DM. Gene therapy for Parkinson's disease. Expert Opin Biol Ther 2002; 2: 151–61

55. Hashimoto M, Rockenstein E, Mante M, et al. β-Synuclein inhibits alpha-synuclein aggregation: a possible role as an anti-parkinsonian factor. Neuron 2001; 32: 213–23

56. Park JY, Lansbury PT Jr. Beta-synuclein inhibits formation of alpha-synuclein protofibrils: a possible therapeutic strategy against Parkinson's disease. Biochemistry 2003; 42: 3696–700

57. During MJ, Naegele JR, O'Malley KL, Geller AI. Long-term behavioral recovery in parkinsonian rats by an HSV vector expressing tyrosine hydroxylase. Science 1994; 266: 1399–403

58. Bencsics C, Wachtel SR, Milstien S, et al. Double transduction with GTP cyclohydrolase I and tyrosine hydroxylase is necessary for spontaneous synthesis of L-DOPA by primary fibroblasts. J Neurosci 1996; 16: 4449–56

59. Mandel RJ, Rendahl KG, Spratt SK, et al. Characterization of intrastriatal recombinant adeno-associated virus-mediated gene transfer of human tyrosine hydroxylase and human GTP-cyclohydrolase I in a rat model of Parkinson's disease. J Neurosci 1998; 18: 4271–84

60. Imaoka T, Date I, Ohmoto T, Nagatsu T. Significant behavioral recovery in Parkinson's disease model by direct intracerebral gene transfer using continuous injection of a plasmid DNA-liposome complex. Hum Gene Ther 1998; 9: 1093–102

61. Fan DS, Ogawa M, Fujimoto KI, et al. Behavioral recovery in 6-hydroxydopamine-lesioned rats by co-transduction of striatum with tyrosine hydroxylase and aromatic L-amino acid decarboxylase genes using two separate adeno-associated virus vectors. Hum Gene Ther 1998; 9: 2527–35

62. Shen Y, Muramatsu SI, Ikeguchi K, et al. Triple transduction with adeno-associated virus vectors expressing tyrosine hydroxylase, aromatic-L-amino-acid decarboxylase, and GTP cyclohydrolase I for gene therapy of Parkinson's disease. Hum Gene Ther 2000; 11: 1509–19

63. Lee WY, Chang JW, Nemeth NL, Kang UJ. Vesicular monoamine transporter-2 and aromatic L-amino acid decarboxylase enhance dopamine delivery after L-3,4-dihydroxyphenylalanine administration in Parkinsonian rats. J Neurosci 1999; 19: 3266–74

64. Lin LF, Doherty DH, Lile JD, et al. GDNF: a glial cell line-derived neurotrophic factor for midbrain dopaminergic neurons. Science 1993; 260: 1130–2

65. Georgievska B, Kirik D, Rosenblad C, et al. Neuroprotection in the rat Parkinson model by intrastriatal GDNF gene transfer using a lentiviral vector. Neuroreport 2002; 13: 75–82

66. Bensadoun JC, Deglon N, Tseng JL, et al. Lentiviral vectors as a gene delivery system in the mouse midbrain: cellular and behavioral improvements in a 6-OHDA model of Parkinson's disease using GDNF. Exp Neurol 2000; 164: 15–24

67. Connor B, Kozlowski DA, Unnerstall JR, et al. Glial cell line-derived neurotrophic factor (GDNF) gene delivery protects dopaminergic

terminals from degeneration. Exp Neurol 2001; 169: 83–95

68. Gash DM, Zhang Z, Ovadia A, et al. Functional recovery in parkinsonian monkeys treated with GDNF. Nature 1996; 380: 252–5

69. Kordower JH, Emborg ME, Bloch J, et al. Neurodegeneration prevented by lentiviral vector delivery of GDNF in primate models of Parkinson's disease. Science 2000; 290: 767–73

70. Perrin R, Woods W, Clayton D, George J. Interaction of human alpha-synuclein and Parkinson's disease variants with phospholipids: structural analysis using site-directed mutagenesis. J Biol Chem 2000; 275: 34393–8

71. Volles MJ, Lee SJ, Rochet JC, et al. Vesicle permeabilization by protofibrillar alpha-synuclein: implications for the pathogenesis and treatment of Parkinson's disease. Biochemistry 2001; 40: 7812–19

72. Narayanan V, Scarlata S. Membrane binding and self-association of alpha-synucleins. Biochemistry 2001; 40: 9927–34

73. Hsu LJ, Sagara Y, Arroyo A, et al. α Synuclein promotes mitochondrial deficiencies and oxidative stress. Am J Pathol 2000; 157: 401–10

74. Hashimoto M, Takeda A, Hsu LJ, et al. Role of cytochrome C as a stimulator of α-synuclein aggregation in Lewy body disease. J Biol Chem 1999; 274: 28849–52

α- and β-Synucleins: two parent proteins that display similar anti-apoptotic phenotypes but distinct responses to 6-hydroxydopamine-induced toxicity

F Checler, C Alves da Costa

INTRODUCTION

α-Synuclein is a small cytoplasmic protein that is at the frontier of the study of Alzheimer's disease (AD) and Parkinson's disease (PD). α-Synuclein is the main component of Lewy bodies,[1–3] the main cerebral histopathological hallmark occurring in PD-affected brains.[4,5] The recent demonstration that a few mutations on α-synuclein trigger familial forms of PD[6,7] has clearly emphasized the likely central role of α-synuclein in this pathology. α-Synuclein is also the main non-amyloidogenic component of the senile plaques, the extracellular aggregates that invade cortical and subcortical areas in AD brains, particularly in AD cases associated with Lewy bodies.[8] The fact that α-synuclein could be envisioned as a common denominator of various neurodegenerative diseases led us to examine its putative contribution to cell death, a paradigm that appears to be exacerbated in both AD and PD.[9–11] Furthermore, we compared the α-synuclein-associated phenotype with that of β-synuclein, a parent protein thought to modulate α-synuclein function. While both proteins trigger anti-apoptotic phenotype, we have demonstrated that the dopaminergic toxin 6-hydroxydopamine (6OH-dopa) abolishes the protective function of α- but not β-synuclein.

Interestingly, we also established that the latter restores the 6OH-dopa-sensitive antiapoptotic function of α-synuclein.

MATERIALS AND METHODS

Wild-type (wt) and A53T-α-synuclein- and β-synuclein-expressing TSM1 cells have been described elsewhere.[12,13] The XTT assay, caspase activity measurements and p53 transcriptional activity have been described in detail.[14,15] Transient transfections were performed in TSM1 neurons with DAC30 containing 2 μg of cDNA encoding either α-synuclein or β-synuclein alone or in combination. Cells were used 48 h post-transfection. For the detection of α- and β-synucleins, equal amounts of protein (50 μg) were separated on Tris-tricine gels, Western blotted and probed with the anti-α- and anti-β-synuclein rabbit polyclonal antibodies (Affiniti Laboratories). Active caspase 3, p53 and β-tubulin immunoreactivities were analyzed by Western blot performed by means of anti-active caspase 3 (rabbit polyclonal, R&D System), anti-p53 (mouse monoclonal, Santa Cruz), and anti-β-tubulin (Sigma, Saint Quentin-Fallavier). Immunological complexes were revealed, as previously described.[14,15]

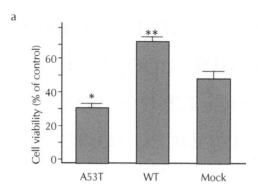

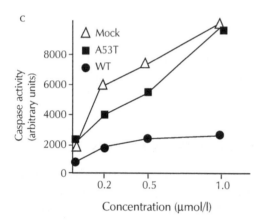

Figure 10.1 Wild-type α-synuclein but not 53T-synuclein is antiapoptotic in neuronal cells. (a) Mock-, α-synuclein- (wild type (WT)) or A53T-α-synuclein (A53T)-expressing TSM1 neurons were cultured in the absence (control) or in the presence of staurosporine (1 μmol/l, for 2 h). Cell viability was measured by the XTT assay as described in the Methods. Bars are means ± SEM of 14–18 experiments. * $p < 0.01$; ** $p < 0.001$; compared with Mock-treated cells. The same cell lines were treated with 1 μmol/l staurosporine for indicated times (b) or for 2 h with indicated staurosporine concentrations (c), then assayed for caspase activity. Points correspond to the Ac-DEVD-al-sensitive Ac-DEVD-7AMC-hydrolyzing activities and are the means of three independent determinations

RESULTS

α-Synuclein is antiapoptotic in neuronal cells: abolishment of protective function by the A53T-PD-linked mutation

Viability of TSM1 neuronal cells was examined by the XTT assay. Clearly, wt-α-synuclein protects TSM1 neurons from staurosporine-induced toxicity (Figure 10.1a) and etoposide-induced toxicity (not shown). Conversely, the A53T-α-synuclein-expressing TSM1 neurons appear more susceptible to toxic stimuli (Figure 10.1a). Staurosporine induces caspase 3 activation in a time dependent (Figure 10.1b) and dose-dependent (Figure 10.1c) manner.

Interestingly, wt-α-synuclein drastically lowered staurosporine-induced caspase activation (Figure 10.1b and c). Here again, the A53T mutation abolished the antiapoptotic function exhibited by wt-α-synuclein (Figure 10.1b and c) (for details see reference 12).

α-Synuclein lowers p53 expression and transcriptional activity

Caspase 3 has been previously identified as a downstream effector of p53-mediated cell death. This led us to examine whether the anti-apoptotic phenotype associated with α-synuclein could be linked to a down-regulation of p53 expression and activity. Indeed, α-synuclein overexpression lowered p53-like immunoreactivity (Figure 10.2a) and transcriptional activity (Figure 10.2b). Furthermore, α-synuclein-associated down-regulation of p53 was further confirmed by the drastic decrease of p21^{waf} promoter activation (Figure 10.2c), a well known p53 targeted gene.[15]

6-Hydroxydopamine abolishes α-synuclein antiapoptotic function

6OH-dopa is a dopaminergic toxin often used to trigger PD-like pathology in mouse models of the disease. TSM1 neurons respond to 6OH-dopa by a drastic stimulation (about 6-fold increase) of their endogenous caspase 3 activity (Figure 10.3a, shaded bars). Interestingly, 6OH-dopa abolished α-synuclein-mediated inhibition of caspase 3 activity (Figure 10.3a). This was accompanied by the restoration of 'normal' p53 expression (Figure 10.3b). Strikingly, 6OH-dopa but not staurosporine, increased α-synuclein-like immunoreactivity in a time- and concentration-dependent manner (Figure 10.3c) (for details see reference 15). Work is in progress to identify the mechanisms by which 6OH-dopa could modulate α-synuclein levels in TSM1 neuronal cells.

β-Synuclein is antiapoptotic, lowers p53 levels but remains insensitive to 6OH-dopa-induced toxicity in neurons

β-Synuclein also behaves as a modulator of neuronal cell death and mimics the α-synuclein phenotype. Thus, β-synuclein drastically inhibited staurosporine-induced caspase 3 activation (Figure 10.4a) and diminished p53 expression (Figure 10.4b). Unlike for α-synuclein, 6OH-dopa did not abolish β-synuclein anti-apoptotic function (Figure 10.5a).

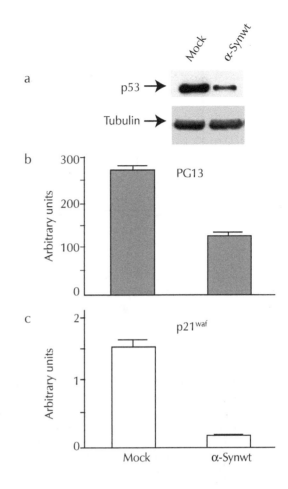

Figure 10.2 Wild-type α-synuclein decreases p53 expression and transcriptional activity in neuronal cells. (a) p53-like immunoreactivity monitored (see Methods) in Mock- or α-synuclein (α-Synwt)-expressing TSM1 neurons. (b and c) Mock- and α-synuclein-expressing neurons were transiently transfected with β-galactosidase and PG13 (b)- or p21^{waf-1} (c)-luciferase cDNAs. Forty eight hours after transfection, luciferase and galactosidase activities were monitored as described[15]

Of most interest is our observation that β-synuclein not only remained insensitive to 6OH-dopa but also restored the anti-apoptotic phenotype of α-synuclein in the presence of the

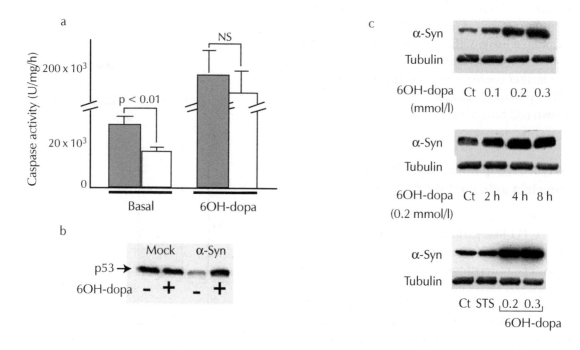

Figure 10.3 6OH-dopa abolishes α-synuclein anti-apoptotic phenotype. Mock (shaded bars)- or α-synuclein wild type (α-Syn) (empty bars)-cells were treated for 8 h with 0.2 mmol/l of 6OH-dopa then caspase 3 activity (a) and p53-like immunoreactivity (b) were monitored as described in the Methods. Bars are the means ± SEM of 6–10 independent experiments. Note that caspase activity is about six times higher in 6OH-dopa-treated Mock-transfected cells than in untreated controls. NS, not statistically significant. (c) α-Synuclein-like immunoreactivity monitored in α-synuclein wild type cells treated for 8 h with the indicated concentrations of 6OH-DOPA (top panel), for the indicated times with 0.2 mmol 6OH-dopa (middle panel) or with 1 μmol/l of staurosporine (lower panel)

dopaminergic toxin (Figure 10.5b) (for details see reference 13).

DISCUSSION

Several lines of enquiry have suggested that α-synuclein contributes to PD pathology. First, it appears that PD is associated with cell death stigmata. That α-synuclein could contribute to this phenomenon is underlined by the observations that mutations on this protein accelerate PD onset and progression,[6,7] exacerbate propensity to aggregation[16–18] and increase apoptosis in cells.[19,20] Our data suggest

to some extent that PD pathology could be due to loss of function of α-synuclein. Thus, this protein appears antiapoptotic in neurons but this phenotype is abolished by PD-associated mutations. This anti-apoptotic function is also prevented by 6OH-dopa, a dopaminergic toxic derivative. Several authors have reported on the presence of 6OH-dopa *in vivo*.[21,22] Although natural 6OH-dopa production is still controversial, it is clear that the machinery able to 'convert' dopamine into its toxic species exists in dopaminergic neurons.[23] The fact that 6OH-dopa contributes to PD by abolishing the α-synuclein antiapoptotic function would explain

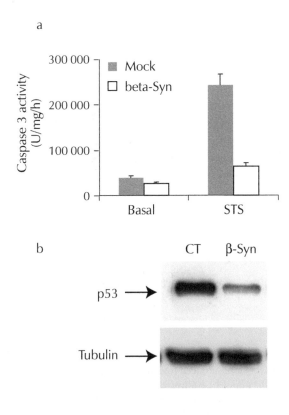

a

b

p53 →

Tubulin →

Figure 10.4 β-Synuclein (β-Syn) inhibits stauro-sporine-stimulated caspase activation and decreases p53 expression in neuronal cells. (a) Caspase 3 activity in Mock (shaded bars) and β-synuclein-expressing cells (white bars), in the absence (basal) or in the presence of staurosporine (STS, 1 μmol/l, for 2 h). Bars represent the Ac-DEVD-al sensitive caspase 3-like activity and are the means ± SEM of eight determinations carried out in duplicate. (b) p53-like immunoreactivity monitored in Mock- (CT) or β-synuclein (β-Syn)-expressing TSM1 neurons. Protein charge was controlled by β-tubulin analysis

A physiological means to protect α-synuclein function from dopaminergic dysfunction and thereby to contribute to the delay of PD onset could be β-synuclein. Our data indicate that this protein is also antiapoptotic but, unlike α-synuclein, it maintains this potential in the presence of 6OH-dopa. This molecular protection of α-synuclein function is in agreement with more macroscopic observations indicating that β-synuclein fragments can inhibit α-synuclein aggregation.[24] Furthermore, β-synuclein when expressed with α-synuclein in double transgenic mice drastically reduced the phenotypic alterations triggered by overexpression of α-synuclein alone.[25] The above observations are all in agreement with the fact that the β-synuclein/α-synuclein mRNA ratio is altered in Lewy bodies.[26]

Two pathways for putative strategies aimed at delaying or preventing PD are suggested by our study. First, is the inhibition of p53 activity (since expression of this oncogene is drastically lowered by α-synuclein and is augmented when α-synuclein function is altered). This is in good agreement with a recent paper showing that pifithrin-α, a selective inhibitor of p53 transcriptional activity, improves motor deficits in a murine model of parkinsonism.[27] Second, is gene therapy consisting of the delivery of the β-synuclein gene into targeted brain areas. At first sight, although many putative problems could occur, particularly because of the yet unknown function of β-synuclein, the second approach could be more specific and would avoid possible side-effects associated with the blockade of the tumor suppressor p53.

ACKNOWLEDGEMENTS

We wish to thank Dr B. Vogelstein (Johns Hopkins University, Baltimore, USA) for providing us with the PG13-luciferase construct.

the selectivity of the lesions occurring in PD. Thus, while most of the neurons display α-synuclein, only the dopaminergic cells of the mesocorticolimbic and nigrostriatal pathways bear the potential of producing 6OH-dopa.

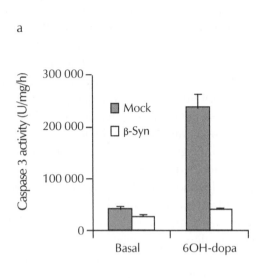

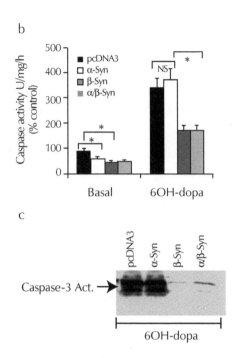

Figure 10.5 Cross-talk between α- and β-synuclein (Syn) for 6OH-dopa-induced toxicity. (a) Mock (shaded bars)- or β-Syn (empty bars)-expressing cells were treated for 8 h with 0.2 mmol/l of 6-hydroxydopamine (6OH-dopa), then caspase 3 activity was measured as described in the Methods. Bars are the means ± SEM of ten independent determinations carried out in duplicate. (b) TSM1 neurons were transiently transfected with empty pcDNA3 vector or containing the cDNAs of α-syn, β-syn or α-synuclein and β-synuclein (α/β-syn). After 48 h of transfection, cells were treated for 8 h in the absence (Basal) or in the presence of 0.2 mmol/l of 6OH-dopa and recovered for caspase-3 activity (Act.) measurements. Note that the means concerning cells transfected either with pcDNA3 or α-Syn when treated with 6OH-dopa are not significantly different (NS). (c) Active caspase 3 immunoreactivity in the above indicated transiently transfected cells of a representative experiment after treatment with 0.2 mmol/l 6OH-dopa

We wish to thank Dr Eliezer Masliah (University of California, San Diego, USA) for providing β-synuclein cDNA. E.M. is supported by grant AG18440. C.A.C. was supported by Aventis Pharma. This work was supported by the INSERM and CNRS.

REFERENCES

1. Wakabayashi K, Matsumoto K, Takayama K, et al. NACP, a presynaptic protein, immunoreactivity in Lewy bodies in Parkinson's disease. Neurosci Lett 1997; 239: 45–8

2. Takeda A, Mallory M, Sundsmo M, et al. Abnormal accumulation of NACP/α-synuclein in neurodegenerative disorders. Am J Pathol 1998; 152: 367–72

3. Hashimoto M, Masliah E. Alpha-synuclein in Lewy body disease and Alzheimer's disease. Brain Pathol 1999; 9: 707–20

4. Goedert M, Spillantini MG, Davies SW. Filamentous nerve cell inclusions in neurodegenerative diseases. Curr Opin Neurobiol 1998; 8: 619–32

5. Trojanowski JQ, Goedert M, Iwatsubo T, Lee VM-Y. Fatal attractions: abnormal protein aggregation and neuron death in Parkinson's disease and Lewy body dementia. Cell Death Diff 1998; 5: 832–7

6. Polymeropoulos MH, Lavedan C, Leroy E, et al. Mutation in the α-synuclein gene identified in families with Parkinson disease. Science 1997; 276: 2045–7

7. Krüger R, Kuhn W, Müller T, et al. Ala30Pro mutation in the gene encoding α-synuclein in Parkinson's disease. Nat Genet 1998; 18: 106–8

8. Yokota O, Terada S, Ishizu H, et al. NACP/α-synuclein, NAC, and β-amyloid pathology of familial Alzheimer's disease with the E184D presenilin-1 mutation: a clinicopathological study of two autopsy cases. Acta Neuropathol 2002; 104: 637–48

9. Cotman CW. Apoptosis decision cascades and neuronal degeneration in Alzheimer's disease. Neurobiol Aging 1998; 19: S29–S32

10. Anglade P, Vyas S, Javoy-Agid F, et al. Apoptosis and autophagy in nigral neurons of patients with Parkinson's disease. Histol Histopathol 1997; 12: 25–31

11. Hirsch E, Hunot S, Faucheux B, et al. Dopaminergic neurons degenerate by apoptosis in Parkinson's disease. Mov Disord 1999; 14: 383–5

12. Alves da Costa C, Ancolio K, Checler F. Wild-type but not Parkinson's disease-related Ala53Thr-α-synuclein protect neuronal cells from apoptotic stimuli. J Biol Chem 2000; 275: 24065–9

13. Alves da Costa C, Masliah E, Checler F. β-synuclein displays an antiapoptotic p53-dependent phenotype and protects neurons from 6-hydroxydopamine-induced caspase 3 activation: cross-talk with α-synuclein and implication for Parkinson's disease. J Biol Chem 2003; 278: 37330–5

14. Alves da Costa C, Paitel E, Mattson MP, et al. Wild-type and mutated presenilin-2 trigger p53-dependent apoptosis and down-regulate presenilin-1 expression in HEK293 human cells and in murine neurons. Proc Natl Acad Sci USA 2002; 99: 4043–8

15. Alves da Costa C, Paitel E, Vincent B, Checler F. α-Synuclein lowers p53-dependent apoptotic response of neuronal cells: abolishment by 6-hydroxydopamine and implication for Parkinson's disease. J Biol Chem 2002; 277: 50980–4

16. Baba M, Nakajo S, Tu P-H, et al. Aggregation of α-synuclein in Lewy bodies of sporadic Parkinson's disease and dementia with Lewy bodies. Am J Pathol 1998; 152: 879–84

17. Ostrerova-Golts N, Petrucelli L, Hardy J, et al. The A53T α-synuclein mutation increases iron-dependent aggregation and toxicity. J Neurosci 2000; 20: 6048–54

18. Narhi L, Wood SJ, Steavenson S, et al. Both familial Parkinson's disease mutations accelerate α-synuclein aggregation. J Biol Chem 1999; 274: 9843–6

19. Lee M, Hyun D-H, Halliwell B, Jenner P. Effect of the overexpression of wild-type or mutant α-synuclein on cell susceptibility to insult. J Neurochem 2001; 76: 998–1009

20. Giasson BI, Duda JE, Quinn SM, et al. Neuronal α-synucleinopathy with severe movement disorder in mice expressing A53T human α-synuclein. Neuron 2002; 34: 521–33

21. Curtius HC, Wolhensberger M, Steinmann B, Redweik S. Mass fragmentography of dopamine and 6OH-dopamine. Application to the determination of dopamine in human brain biopsies from the caudate nucleus. J Chromatogr 1974; 99: 529–40

22. Jellinger K, Linert L, Kienzl E, et al. Chemical evidence for 6-hydroxydopamine to be an endogenous toxic factor in the pathogenesis of Parkinson's disease. J Neural Transm 1995; 46: 297–314

23. Blum D, Torch S, Lambeng N, et al. Molecular pathways involved in the neurotoxicity of 6OH-DOPA and MPTP: contribution to the apoptotic theory in Parkinson's disease. Prog Neurobiol 2001; 65: 135–72

24. Windisch M, Hutter-Paier B, Rockenstein E, et al. Development of a new treatment for Alzheimer's disease and Parkinson's disease using anti-aggregatory β-synuclein-derived peptides. J Mol Neurosci 2002; 19: 63–9

25. Hashimoto M, Rockenstein E, Mante M, et al. β-Synuclein inhibits α-synuclein aggregation: a possible role as an anti-Parkinsonian factor. Neuron 2001; 32: 213–23

26. Rockenstein E, Hansen LA, Mallory M, et al. Altered expression of the synuclein family mRNA in Lewy body and Alzheimer's disease. Brain Res 2001; 914: 48–56

27. Duan W, Zhu X, Ladenheim B, et al. p53 inhibitors preserve dopamine neurons and motor function in experimental parkinsonism. Ann Neurol 2002; 52: 597–606

Chapter 11

Functional genomics and pharmacogenetics in Alzheimer's disease

R Cacabelos, Y Kubota, C Isaza, J Henao, L Fernández-Novoa,
VRM Lombardi, L Corzo, V Pichel

INTRODUCTION

Alzheimer's disease (AD) is a heterogeneous disorder in which more than 50 different genes distributed across the human genome may be involved.[1,2] It's phenotypic features and current biological markers[3] are inconsistent and do not always correlate with a defined genotypic profile. This suggests that environmental factors and epigenetic phenomena may also contribute to the premature phenotypic expression of dementia, represented by its neuropathological hallmarks (amyloid deposition in senile plaques and brain vessels, neurofibrillary tangle (NFT) formation, synaptic loss, neuronal death) and clinical symptoms (memory deficit, behavioral changes, functional decline). Furthermore, 60–80% of the therapeutic failures in AD can be potentially attributed to problems associated with both pharmacogenetic and pharmacogenomic factors. In order to advance towards a mature genomic medicine of dementia, we have to incorporate functional genomics, proteomics, pharmacogenomics, high-throughput screening methods, combinatorial chemistry and bioinformatics to the AD field with the prospective view of improving diagnostics and therapeutics by using the modern tools provided by these disciplines.[4] This is particularly important in complex/polygenic multifactorial disorders in which genetic factors are modulated by both environmental and epigenetic phenomena, as might be the case in more than 90% of the central nervous system (CNS) disorders with clinical onset in adulthood and the elderly.[2] Recent studies have clearly shown that the therapeutic response in AD is genotype-specific and that many clinical features of AD are genotype-related.[5,6]

STRUCTURAL AND FUNCTIONAL GENOMICS

AD-related genes can be classified into those with demonstrated mutations following a Mendelian inheritance pattern (mutational genetics) (e.g. *APP, PS1, PS2*), susceptibility genes or polymorphic loci potentially contributing to AD predisposition (susceptibility genetics) (*APOE, A2M, LRP1, IL1A, ACE, NOS3*) and defective genes linked to mitochondrial DNA (mtDNA) with heteroplasmic transmission.[1,4,5]

Primary loci associated with AD include the following: the *APP* gene (21q21.2-q21) encoding the amyloid precursor protein (APP); the presenilin-1 (*PS1*) and presenilin-2 (*PS2*) genes located on chromosomes 14 (14q24.3) and 1 (1q31-q42), respectively, encoding very similar integral membrane proteins with multiple transmembrane domains, whose mutations can cause familial AD3 and fAD4; and polymorphic variants in the *APOE* gene (19q13.2) associated with risk (APOE-4 allele) or protection (APOE-2 allele) for AD.[1,5-10] Since mutations in *APP*, *PS1* and *PS2* genes account for less than 10% of AD cases and the APOE locus is apparently neither necessary nor sufficient to cause AD, it seems plausible that other genetic loci may be involved in AD, possibly in combination with environmental factors and/or epigenetic phenomena.[1,5,7] Some candidate genes with polymorphic loci and/or mutations potentially associated with AD and with other forms of dementia include the following: the macro-tubule-associated protein tau gene (*MAPT*) (17q21.1) whose missense mutations and splicing defects can lead to frontotemporal dementia and familial progressive subcortical gliosis; a common polymorphism (-15Ala/Thr) in the signal peptide of the α-1-antichymotrypsin (*AACT*) gene (14q24.3-q32.1) encoding the plasma protease inhibitor AACT; a polymorphism in the butyrylcholinesterase (BCHE) gene (3q26.1-q26.2) (*BCHE-K*); the α-2-macro-globulin (*A2M*) gene (12p13.3-p12.3); the low-density lipoprotein (LDL)-related protein (*LRP1*) gene (12q13.1-q13.3); the type 5 AD-linked chromosome 12 gene; the bleomycin hydrolase (*BMH*) gene (17q11.1-q11.2); the *FOS* gene (14q24.3); the interleukin-1 (IL-1) gene cluster (2q14); the tumor necrosis factor (TNF-α) gene (6p21.3); the nitric oxide synthase 3 (*NOS3*) gene (7q36); the angiotensin I converting enzyme gene (*ACE*) (17q23); the β-site amyloid β-A4 precursor protein-cleaving enzyme gene (*BACE*) (11q23.3) (BACE1, BACE2, β-secretase, memapsin-2, ASP2, p501); the cystatin C gene (*CST3*) (20p11.2); the methyl-enetetrahydrofolate reductase gene (*MTHFR*)

(1p36.3); mitochondrial DNA-associated genes; and other AD-related candidate genes including the insulin-degrading enzyme gene (*IDE*) (10q24) associated with type 6 AD (*AD6*); the AD2 gene (19cen-q13.2) associated with type 2 AD (*AD2*); the glycogen synthase kinase 3β gene (*GSK3B*); the *CYP46* (14q) encoding cholesterol 24-hydrolase; and the α-synuclein gene (*SNCA*) (4q21.3-q22), encoding a 35-amino acid protein also called NAC (non-Aβ component of AD amyloid).[1,5,7]

It is highly plausible that many of these genes interact with each other to regulate specific metabolic pathways either confluent with, or different from, the amyloid cascade.[1,5,7,11,12]

Alzheimer's disease-related genomic clusters and genetic variation

According to the information collected during the past 30 years regarding genetic factors in dementia,[1] AD might be the result of a multistep process of mutations in regulatory genes associated with genomic susceptibility factors and epigenetic alterations that induce a loss of balanced polygenic expression in the CNS. New findings also indicate that AD might result from an overwhelming increase in genetic variation surpassing an optimality threshold supposedly established by natural selection. This specula-tion implies that excessive genomic variation might lead to the activation of a genomically regulated mechanism of accelerated neuronal destruction, prematurely to eliminate the most evolved cells in nature.[5,7,13]

The design of matrix models integrating allele and genotype combinations with two (bigenic), three (trigenic), four (tetragenic) and five (pentagenic) or more AD-related genes has yielded genomic clusters of 18, 36, 108 and 972 different genotypes, respectively, which have been used for studies of functional genomics and pharmacogenomics in dementia.[5,7,13,14] With these models we have studied the genetic variation rate in AD, comparing the number of genomic clusters present in the AD population and that of the normal population with no family history of dementia.[13]

Single nucleotide repeats (SNPs) are the most common forms of genetic variation. Any two unrelated individuals differ by approximately one base pair change in every 1000 bp. Given that there are 3×10^9 bp in the human genome, the frequency of genetic variation equates to 3×10^6 differences between any two unrelated individuals.[15] The allelic architecture of complex disorders shows a highly differentiated genomic variation (GV).[16] GV is relevant for the understanding of etiopathogenesis and treatment, since approximately 40–60% of therapeutic failures might be attributed to GV-related factors. Variation in genomic structures related to disease susceptibility, drug metabolism and/or environmental responses is often specific to socially defined populations.[17] Genetic variations in AD may have a protective or pathogenic role in the expression of the disease.

According to our calculations, the AD population shows about a 3–5 times higher GV rate than the control population and more than 80% of AD patients exhibit a genomic profile significantly different from the control population.[5,7,13] Furthermore, the expressed/repressed genotype ratio is 1.2 in AD and 0.4 in controls, indicating that AD patients express more genetic variants than the control population.[5,7,13]

GENOTYPE–PHENOTYPE CORRELATIONS

A practical approach to understand the potential influence of a particular gene or a genomic cluster on a specific phenotype is to study genotype–phenotype correlations[1,2] (Table 11.1). Combining congenic mapping with microarray expression profiling provides an opportunity to establish functional links between genotype and phenotype for complex traits.[18] It is accepted that APOE-related polymorphic variants, especially the APOE-4 allele, are major risk factors for AD,[1,19] and some authors have attempted to correlate the presence of the

Table 11.1 Issues of potential interest in the functional genomics and pharmacogenomics of Alzheimer's disease (AD). From reference 37

Issue	Evidence	Potential
Genetics	more than 50 different genes are associated with AD in the human genome	80–90%
	mutational/Mendelian genetics	
	susceptibility genetics	5–20%
	polymorphic variants	60–80%
Genetic variation	the AD population shows a higher genetic variation than the normal population without family history of dementia	60–80%
Environmental factors	education, nutrition, life style, accidents and many other environmental factors influence the phenotypic expression of dementia	10–40%

continued

Table 11.1 *continued*

Issue	*Evidence*	*Potential*
Cerebrovascular factors	stroke and cerebrovascular dysfunction are major risk factors for dementia	60–80%
Medical conditions	many different medical conditions influence AD, exerting deleterious effects on brain function and neuronal survival (e.g. diabetes, hypertension, dyslipidemia, atherosclerosis, hypotension, folic acid deficiency, vitamin B_{12} deficiency, ferropenic anemia, hypothyroidism)	10–20%
Epigenetic phenomena	lack of evidence at present, but high probability of influence based on recent data related to other complex disorders	?
Genotype–phenotype correlations	APOE-4 vs. brain atrophy	confirmed
	APOE-4 vs. brain bioelectrical activity	confirmed
	APOE-4 vs. cerebrovascular dysfunction	confirmed
	APOE-4 vs. cognitive decline	confirmed
	APOE-4 vs. age of onset	confirmed
	APOE-4 vs. behavioral changes	confirmed
	APOE-4 vs. immunological function	confirmed
	APOE-4 vs. lymphocyte apoptosis	confirmed
	APOE-4 vs. blood pressure	confirmed
	APOE-4 vs. lipid metabolism	confirmed
	APOE-4 vs. β-amyloid deposition	confirmed
	APOE-4 vs. microglial nitric oxide production	confirmed
	APOE-4 vs. serum ApoE levels	confirmed
	PS-1 vs. β-amyloid deposition	confirmed
	PS-2 vs. β-amyloid deposition	confirmed
	TAU vs. tau protein hyperphosphorylation	confirmed
	CYP46 vs. β-amyloid deposition	confirmed
	CYP46 vs. tau protein hyperphosphorylation	confirmed
Pharmacogenetics	CYP2D6 vs. drug safety and efficacy	15–30%
	poor metabolizers	8–10%
	extensive metabolizers	70–85%
	ultrarapid metabolizers	7–10%
Pharmacogenomics	APOE-4 vs. Tacrine	confirmed
	APOE-4 vs. donepezil	confirmed
	APOE-4 vs. Anapsos	confirmed
	APOE-4 vs. CDP-choline	confirmed
	APOE-4 vs. Memantine	no effect
	PS-1 vs. Memantine	confirmed
	APOE-4 vs. multifactorial therapy	confirmed
	PS-1 vs. multifactorial therapy	no effect
	PS-2 vs. multifactorial therapy	confirmed
	Trigenic cluster (APOE + PS1 + PS2) vs. multifactorial therapy	confirmed

APOE-4 allele with phenotypic traits represented by the pathogenic hallmarks and clinical features of dementia, obtaining very variable results.[1,2,19] We have previously demonstrated that the APOE genotype influences the phenotypic expression of different clinical symptoms (cognitive decline, behavioral changes, functional disability), biological parameters (brain atrophy, lymphocyte apoptosis, serum ApoE and β-amyloid protein levels), and therapeutic responses in AD.[1,2,5,7,13,14]

APOE-related brain atrophy

The association between brain volume and intelligence seems to be of genetic origin[20] and the influence of genetics on brain structure has been recently demonstrated.[21] Most CNS regions tend to show age-dependent changes associated with brain atrophy which is currently region-specific. In AD, brain atrophy is circumscribed to frontoparietotemporal regions and hippocampal formation. In a recent study,[22] clear APOE-related changes were found in different brain regions measured by computed tomography (CT) analysis in the Spanish population with dementia. Significant differences appear between subjects with: APOE-3/3 (6.80 ± 2.82 CT units) and APOE-3/4 genotypes (7.12 ± 2.60 U) in interventricular distance (IVD) ($p < 0.002$); APOE-2/3 and APOE-3/4 in left temporal atrophy (LTA) ($p < 0.04$); APOE-3/4 and APOE-4/4 in LTA ($p < 0.05$); and APOE-2/3 and APOE-3/4 in right temporal atrophy (RTA) ($p < 0.02$)[22] (Figure 11.1). In general, APOE-4 carriers show an anticipated age-dependent brain atrophy reflected by an increase in both the interventricular distance and the interhippocampal distance which is more significant in AD than in the general aged population (Figure 11.1).

APOE-related brain function

Several studies have demonstrated that APOE-4 carriers tend to develop an early-onset AD with an accelerated clinical course characterized by a rapid cognitive decline and poorer response to conventional treatments.[1,23] Brain bioelectrical activity deteriorates progressively in parallel with GDS staging,[6] showing an increase in delta and theta activity and a decrease in alpha and beta activity;[6] however, brain activity slowing can be reversed by drugs with cognition-enhancing capacity.[23]

We have investigated the phenotypic profile of brain mapping in healthy subjects of different ages ($x = 55.24 \pm 17.71$ years; range 9–96 years) associated with the APOE genotype. A total of 2828 qEGG recordings were distributed in the following groups according to the frequency of the APOE genotypes: APOE-2/2 ($n = 63$, $F = 2.23\%$); APOE-2/3 ($n = 278$, $F = 13.36\%$); APOE-2/4 ($n = 84$, $F = 2.97\%$); APOE-3/3 ($n = 1337$, $F = 47.28\%$); APOE-3/4 ($n = 903$, $F = 31.93\%$); and APOE-4/4 ($n = 63$, $F = 2.23\%$). In all subjects both delta and theta activity increased with age, whereas alpha and beta activity decreased with age. However, a clear phenotypic variation in brain mapping activity has been identified in association with APOE-related polymorphisms. Brain function significantly deteriorates in APOE-4/4 subjects as depicted by a dramatic increase in delta ($21.26 \pm 11.78\%$, $p < 0.0001$), and theta relative power ($33.89 \pm 33.89\%$, $p < 0.0001$) accompanied by a significant decrease in alpha ($22.74 \pm 12.54\%$, $p < 0.0001$) and beta power ($7.29 \pm 4.20\%$, $p < 0.001$) as compared with the other APOE genotypes and the average value of the whole population. These data clearly indicate that brain function exhibits an APOE-associated phenotypic variation pattern in the general population in which APOE-4/4 carriers show a premature decline (Figure 11.2).

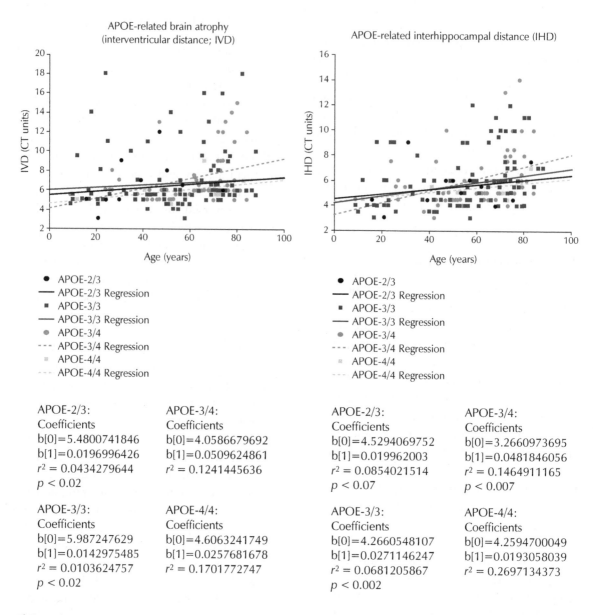

Figure 11.1 Age-dependent APOE-related brain atrophy in the general population and in Alzheimer's disease. CT, computed tomography

APOE-related brain hemodynamics

It is clear that cerebrovascular dysfunction and stroke tend to accumulate with age. However, age-dependent hemodynamic changes in the CNS have not been well documented as yet in association with genomic factors. We have investigated several hemodynamic parameters in the major arteries of the circle of Willis by using transcranial Doppler ultrasonography in a

APOE-related delta power
APOE-related qEEG delta activity in healthy subjects

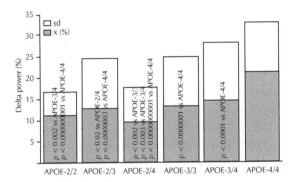

APOE-related theta power
APOE-related qEEG theta activity in healthy subjects

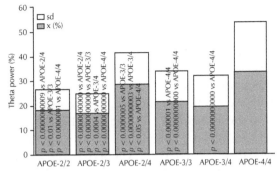

APOE-related alpha power
APOE-related qEEG alpha activity in healthy subjects

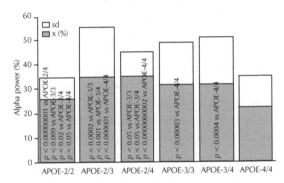

APOE-related beta power
APOE-related qEEG beta activity in healthy subjects

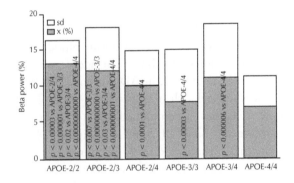

Figure 11.2 APOE-related brain activity mapping in the general population

population of 382 patients of both sexes (age 52.04 ± 22.17 years; range 1–88 years). As a prototype analysis we have evaluated hemodynamic parameters in the middle cerebral arteries (MCA) including mean velocity (Mv), systolic velocity (Sv), diastolic velocity (Dv), the pulsatility index of Gossling (PI = (Sv – Dv)/Mv) and the resistance index of Pourcelot (RI = (Sv – Dv)/Sv). Mv in the left (L-MCA-Mv) and right (R-MCA-Mv) cerebral arteries were 55.08 ± 17.68 and 54.81 ± 16.89 cm/s, respectively. PI and RI values were the following: L-MCA-PI = 0.87 ± 0.20; L-MCA-RI = 0.56 ± 0.07; R-MCA-PI = 0.86 ± 0.19; R-MCA-RI = 0.56 ± 0.07.

Mv significantly decreased with age in both L-MCA ($r^2 = 0.36$, $p < 0.0001$) and R-MCA ($r^2 = 0.37$, $p < 0.0001$). In contrast, both the PI and RI significantly increased with age according to the following correlation values: L-MCA-PI $r^2 = 0.36$, $p < 0.0001$; L-MCA-RI $r^2 = 0.26$, $p < 0.0001$; R-MCA-PI $r^2 = 0.25$, $p < 0.007$; and R-MCA $r^2 = 0.30$, $p < 0.0001$. These data clearly indicate that brain hemodynamics progressively deteriorate with age, showing an age-dependent decrease in brain blood flow velocity together with an increase in both PI and RI, reflecting a gradual resistance to flow, probably due to the hardening of arteries, physicochemical changes in the cerebrovascular tree and mechanical changes in brain tissue.

In the same population we have studied APOE-related brain hemodynamics. No significant changes in brain blood flow were found among the different APOE genotypes in terms of absolute values. However, when brain blood flow was assessed as a function of age of subjects with the APOE-4/4 genotype, the results showed the most marked decline in L-MCA-Mv ($r^2 = 0.74$) as compared with APOE-2/3 ($r^2 = 0.30$, $p < 0.05$), APOE-3/3 ($r^2 = 0.26$, $p < 0.0001$), and APOE-3/4 genotypes ($r^2 = 0.38$, $p < 0.0001$). Subjects with the APOE-3/4 genotype showed the highest age-dependent PI values ($r^2 = 0.41$, $p < 0.0001$). These data clearly indicate that the APOE-3/4 and APOE-4/4 genotypes seem to influence brain blood flow, reducing brain perfusion in an age-dependent manner.[24] In contrast, in AD patients, APOE-4 carriers showed a clear reduction in brain blood flow velocities accompanied by a significant increase in both PI and RI (Figure 11.3), indicating that APOE-4 influences brain cerebrovascular function, probably through a dysregulation in lipid metabolism and induction of atheromatosis and vascular endothelial dysfunction.[25]

APOE-related changes in lipid metabolism and vascular risk factors

Vascular risk factors, including diabetes, hypertension and high levels of lipids (cholesterol, triglycerides) in blood are major risk factors for stroke, AD and vascular dementia.[25] Serum glucose levels did not show any significant difference among the APOE genotypes, although APOE-4/4 carriers tended to show higher levels of glucose. Serum total cholesterol levels were significantly higher in APOE-4/4 than in the other groups. High-density lipo-

protein (HDL)-cholesterol levels were significantly higher in APOE-2/4 and APOE-4/4; and LDL- cholesterol levels were significantly elevated in the APOE-4/4 group. Blood pressure is currently elevated in APOE-3/4 and APOE-4/4 carriers, and the heart rate is slightly faster in APOE-4/4.[25] A polymorphism of the CYP46 gene encoding cholesterol 24-hydroxylase is associated with increased β-amyloid load in brain tissues as well as with increased cerebrospinal fluid levels of β-amyloid peptides and phosphorylated tau protein.[26] Furthermore, both the total amount and the distribution of cholesterol within neurons impact amyloid biogenesis, probably through APOE-related mechanisms.[26]

All these data together, and additional information from other sources, suggest that the APOE-4 carriers show to some extent: increased brain atrophy; faster decline in brain function; dysregulation of lipid metabolism; excessive cardiovascular and hypertensive loads; nitric oxide dysfunction; and severe brain hemodynamic alterations reflected by decrease in brain blood flow velocity and increase in both PI and RI (brain hypoperfusion plus microvascular dysfunction).[25,28]

PHARMACOGENETICS

Although drugs effect a complex phenotype that depends on many factors, it is estimated that genetics account for 20–95% of variability in drug disposition and pharmacodynamics.[29] Drug metabolism includes phase I reactions (i.e. oxidation, reduction, hydrolysis) and phase II conjugation reactions (i.e. acetylation, glucuronidation, sulfation, methylation).[30] The typical paradigm for the pharmacogenetics of phase I drug metabolism is represented by the cytochrome P450 enzymes, a superfamily of microsomal drug-metabolizing enzymes.

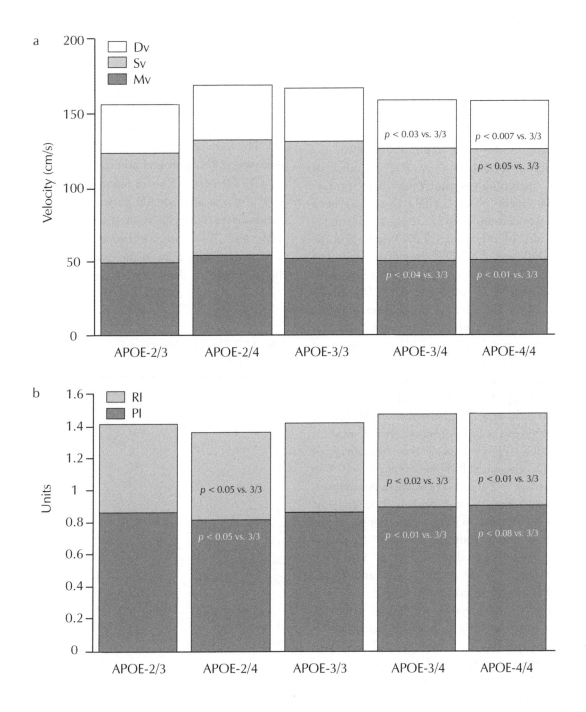

Figure 11.3 APOE-related cerebrovascular hemodynamics in Alzheimer's disease. (a) APOE-related brain blood flow velocity; (b) APOE-related blood flow pulsatility index (PI) and resistance index (RI). From R. Cacabelos and V. Pichel, EuroEspes Biomedical Research Center

The *CYP2D6* gene in Alzheimer's disease

The cytochrome P450 (CYP) enzymes are responsible for the metabolism of xenobiotic substances and many drugs of very diverse chemical structure.[31] There are more than 30 gene families involved in the metabolism of foreign compounds in humans. The *CYP2D6* isoenzyme is the most important pathway for the biotransformation of a large number of drugs, including psychotropics and cardiovascular agents. The *CYP2D* locus has been mapped to chromosome 22 (22q13.1-13.2) and is conformed by the active *CYP2D6* gene and the *CYP2D8P* and *CYP2D7P* pseudogenes.[32] The *CYP2D6* locus is highly polymorphic, with approximately 70 different *CYP2D6* alleles identified in the general population showing deficient (poor metabolizers, PM), normal (extensive metabolizers, EM) or increased enzymatic activity (ultrarapid metabolizers, UM). Remarkable interethnic differences exist in the frequency of the PM and UM phenotypes, as well as in the types of alleles responsible for the expression of the PM phenotype. For example, it has been reported that the frequency of CYP2D6-associated PM phenotypes is 5–10% in Caucasians, 1–2% in Black African populations and fewer than 1% in Orientals. Likewise, the frequency of UMs with multiple copies of the *CYP2D6* gene (mainly the *CYP2D6*2* allele) is about 1–4% in the Northern European population, 7–10% in Spaniards and up to 20–29% in African groups.[32]

In CNS disorders the CYP2D6 polymorphism is particularly important, because it is involved in the vast majority of the biotransformation processes of antidepressants and antipsychotics, including novel classes of antidepressants and the new generation of unconventional antipsychotics and cholinesterase inhibitors. In the first study performed in the Spanish population we have found that the most frequent *CYP2D6* allele is the functional allele *1 (75%) whereas other nonfunctional alleles showed the following frequencies: *CYP2D6*4 = 15.6%, CYP2D6*5 = 3%, CYP2D6*3 = 0.7%* and *CYP2D6*6 = 0.7%* (Table 11.2). No *CYP2D6*7* and *CYP2D6*8* alleles have been found in the Spanish population with AD. The frequency of the duplicate *1 or *2xN allele was 4.8%. This preliminary genotyping of the *CYP2D6* gene in Spain reflects the fact that 83.8% of the Spanish AD patients are normal metabolizers (NM), 8.6% are poor metabolizers (PM) and 7.4% are ultrarapid metabolizers (UM), suggesting that, in the case of drugs for the treatment of dementia, at least 10–20% of

Table 11.2 The *CYP2D6* gene in the Spanish population with Alzheimer's disease

	n	Frequency
Alleles (n = 268)		
*1	194	0.723
*3	2	0.007
*4	42	0.157
*5	8	0.03
*6	2	0.007
*7	0	0.00
*8	0	0.00
*10	8	0.03
Duplicate	12	0.045
Genotypes (n = 134)		
*1/*1	68	0.507
*1/*3	2	0.015
*1/*4	31	0.231
*1/*5	8	0.06
*1/*6	2	0.015
*1/*10	3	0.022
*4/*4	5	0.037
*4/*10	1	0.007
*10/*10	2	0.015
*1xN/*2 or *1/*1xN	12	0.09

the failures observed in clinical trials and approximately 20–35% of the problems related to drug efficacy and safety might be attributed to genetic variants in the *CYP2D6* gene and/or related genes currently neglected in this particular population (Figure 11.4).

PHARMACOGENOMICS

A few reports have shown that the therapeutic response in AD is genotype-specific.[5,7,13,14] Some studies have indicated that the presence of the *APOE-4* allele differentially affects the quality and size of drug responsiveness in AD patients treated with cholinergic enhancers (tacrine, donepezil).[5,7,13,14,33,34] For example, *APOE-4* carriers show a less significant therapeutic response to tacrine (60%) than patients with no *APOE-4*.[33,34] In contrast, other studies do not support the hypothesis that APOE and gender are predictors of the therapeutic response of AD patients to tacrine.[35] An APOE-related differential response has also been observed in patients treated with other compounds devoid of acetylcholinesterase inhibiting activity (CDP-choline, anapsos),[23] suggesting that APOE-associated factors may influence drug activity in the brain either directly acting on neural mechanisms (choline acetyltransferase activity, nicotinic-receptor binding, neurotransmission modulation, amyloid deposition, tau degradation or phosphorylation) or indirectly influencing diverse metabolic pathways (cholesterol internalization, apoE/LDL receptor regulation, or neuronal membrane phospholipid homeostasis).[1,5,6,13,25]

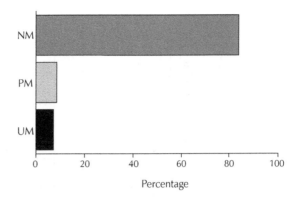

Figure 11.4 The CYP2D6 gene in Alzheimer's disease, related to normal metabolizers (NM), poor metabolizers (PM) and ultrarapid metabolizers (UM)

The application of pharmacogenomics at the preclinical level in drug development (transgenic models, biochips, DNA microarrays) would help to find drugs with etiopathogenic activity operating on specific biochemical pathways (drug target) involved in amyloid deposition (secretases), neurofibrillary tangle formation (tau hyperphosphorylation), neuronal apoptosis (caspases), free radical formation (antioxidants), nitric oxide (NO)-related endothelial dysfunction (NO inhibitors, NO-releasing nonsteroidal anti-inflammatory drugs), neuro-immunological dysregulation (cytokine inhibitors) and the like.[25,36] Pharmacogenetic studies would help to develop drugs devoid of adverse events by understanding their metabolic pathways and the CYP family of gene-related products involved in drug metabolism. Finally, clinical pharmacogenomics would be essential to define efficacy, optimizing the therapeutic outcome[5,7,13,14,25,36,37] (Table 11.1; Figure 11.5).

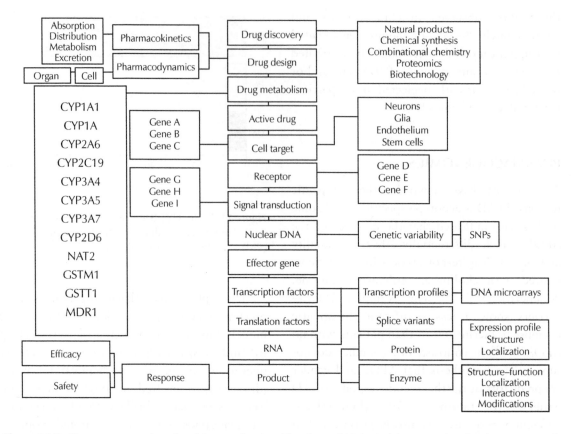

Figure 11.5 Pharmacogenomics-related drug evaluation. Flowchart of biological factors and molecular events to take into account in the design of protocols for pharmacogenomic studies in drug development

REFERENCES

1. Cacabelos R. Handbook of Neurogeriatrics. Alzheimer Disease and Other Dementias. Epidemiology and Genetics. Barcelona, Spain: Masson, 1999

2. Cacabelos R. Psychogeriatric research. A conceptual introduction to geriatric neuroscience. Psychogeriatrics 2001; 1: 158–88

3. Frank RA, Galsko D, Hampel H, et al. Biological markers for therapeutic trials in Alzheimer's disease. Proceedings of the biological markers working group; NIA initiative on neuroimaging in Alzheimer's disease. Neurobiol Aging 2003; 24: 521–36

4. Guttmacher AE, Collins FS. Genome medicine – a primer. N Engl J Med 2002; 347: 1512–20

5. Cacabelos R. Pharmacogenomics in Alzheimer's disease. Min Rev Med Chem 2002; 2: 59–84

6. Cacabelos R. Diagnosis of Alzheimer's disease: defining genetic profiles (genotype vs phenotype). Acta Neurol Scand 1996; 165: 72–84

7. Cacabelos R. Pharmacogenomics for the treatment of dementia. Ann Med 2002; 34: 357–79

8. Hardy J, Gwinn-Hardy K. Genetic classification of primary degenerative disease. Science 1998; 282: 1075–9

9. Tanzi RE, Kovacs DM, Kim TW, et al. The gene defects responsible for familial Alzheimer's disease. Neurobiol Dis 1996; 3: 159–68

10. Schellenberg GD, D'Souza I, Poorkaj P. The genetics of Alzheimer's disease. Curr Psychiatry Rep 2000; 2: 158–64

11. Price DL, Sisodia SS. Mutant genes in familial Alzheimer's disease and transgenic models. Ann Rev Neurosci 1998; 21: 479–505

12. Van Gassen G, Annaert W. Amyloid, presenilins, and Alzheimer's disease. Neuroscientist 2003; 9: 117–26

13. Cacabelos R, Fernández-Novoa L, Lombardi V, Takeda M. Genetic variation and pharmacogenomics in Alzheimer disease. Psychiatr Neurol Jap 2003; 105: 47–67

14. Cacabelos R, Alvarez A, Fernández-Novoa L, Lombardi VRM. A pharmacogenomic approach to Alzheimer's disease. Acta Neurol Scand 2000; 176: 12–19

15. Jazwinska EC. Exploiting human genetic variation in drug discovery and development. Drug Dis Today 2001; 6: 198–205

16. Johnson GCL, Todd JA. Strategies in complex disease mapping. Cur Opin Genet Dev 2000; 10: 330–4

17. Foster MW, Sharp RR. Race, ethnicity, and genomics: social classifications as proxies of biological heterogeneity. Genome Res 2002; 12: 844–50

18. Eaves IA, Wicker LS, Ghandour G, et al. Combining mouse congenic strains and microarray gene expression analyses to study a complex trait: the NOD mouse model of type 1 diabetes. Genome Res 2002; 12: 232–44

19. Saunders AM, Trowers MK, Shimkets RA, et al. The role of apolipoprotein E in Alzheimer's disease: pharmacogenomic target selection. Biochem Biophys Acta 2000; 1502: 85–94

20. Posthuma D, De Geus EJC, Baaré WFC, et al. The association between brain volume and intelligence is of genetic origin. Nature Neurosci 2002; 5: 83–4

21. Thompson PM, Cannon TD, Narr KL, et al. Genetic influences on brain structure. Nature Neurosci 2001; 4: 1253–8

22. Etcheverría I, Amado L, Pichel V, Cacabelos R. Differential brain atrophy profile associated with the APOE genotype in the Spanish population. 6th International Conference on Stroke and 3rd Conference of the Mediterranean Stroke Society, Monaco, Monte Carlo, 2003: 47

23. Cacabelos R, Alvarez XA, Lombardi V, et al. Pharmacological treatment of Alzheimer disease: from phychotropic drugs and cholinesterase inhibitors to pharmacogenomics. Drugs Today 2000; 36: 415–99

24. Etcheverría I, Amado L, Pichel V, Cacabelos R. Age- and APOE-dependent cerebrovascular changes in the Spanish population. 6th International Conference on Stroke and 3rd Conference of the Mediterranean Stroke Society, Monaco, Monte Carlo, 2003: 32

25. Cacabelos R, Fernández-Novoa L, Lombardi V, et al. Cerebrovascular risk factors in Alzheimer disease: brain hemodynamics and pharmacogenomic implications. Neurol Res 2003; 25: 567–80

26. Papassotiropoulos A, Streffer JR, Tsolaki M, et al. Increased brain β-amyloid load, phosphorylated tau, and risk of Alzheimer disease associated with an intronic CYP46 polymorphism. Arch Neurol 2003; 60: 29–35

27. Puglielli L, Tanzi RE, Kovacs DM. Alzheimer's disease: the cholesterol connection. Nature Neurosci 2003; 6: 345–51

28. De la Torre JC. Alzheimer disease as a vascular disorder. Stroke 2002; 33: 1152–62

29. Evans WE, McLeod HL. Pharma-cogenomics–drug disposition, drug targets, and side effects. N Engl J Med 2003; 348: 538–49

30. Weinshilboum R. Inheritance and drug response. N Engl J Med 2003; 348: 529–37

31. Nebert DW, Russell DW. Clinical importance of the cytochrome P450. Lancet 2002; 360: 1155–62

32. Isaza CA, Henao J, López AM, Cacabelos R. Isolation, sequence and genotyping of the drug metabolizer CYP2D6 gene in the Colombian population. Meth Find Exp Clin Pharmacol 2000; 22: 695–705

33. Poirier J. Apolipoprotein E4, cholinergic integrity and the pharmacogenetics of Alzheimer's disease. J Psychiatr Neurosci 1999; 24: 147–53

34. Farlow MR, Lahiri DK, Poirier J, et al. Treatment outcome of tacrine therapy depends on apolipoprotein genotype and gender of the subjects with Alzheimer's disease. Neurology 1998; 50: 669–77

35. Rigaud AS, Traykov L, Caputo L, et al. The apolipoprotein E epsilon 4 allele and the response to tacrine therapy in Alzheimer's disease. Eur J Neurol 2000; 7: 255–8

36. Cacabelos R, Fernández-Novoa L, Pichel V, et al. Pharmacogenomic studies with a combination therapy in Alzheimer disease. In Takeda M, ed. Molecular Neurobiology of Alzheimer Disease and Related Disorders. Tokyo, Japan: Karger, 2004: 94–107

37. Cacabelos R. The application of functional genomics to Alzheimer's disease. Pharmaco-genomics 2003; 4: 597–621

Chapter 12

The genetics of tau and neurodegenerative disease

B Kraemer, I D'Souza, GD Schellenberg

INTRODUCTION

Tau is a microtubule-associated protein enriched in neuronal axons. Tau's ability to bind, polymerize and stabilize microtubules is important for neuronal morphogenesis as well as axonal function such as axonal transport. Hyperphosphorylated tau forms paired helical filaments that aggregate as intraneuronal structures called neurofibrillary tangles (NFTs).[1,2] NFTs or insoluble tau aggregates a group of sporadic and familial neurodegenerative and movement disorders called 'tauopathies', which include Alzheimer's disease (AD), progressive supranuclear palsy, corticobasal degeneration, Pick's disease and frontotemporal dementia with parkinsonism – chromosome 17 type (FTDP-17). Autosomal dominant mutations cause FTDP-17, which comprises a group of clinically heterogeneous syndromes with broad overlapping behavioral, cognitive and motor abnormalities.[3–6]

TAU PROTEIN AND DISEASE

Although tau is expressed from a single gene, its expression in the central nervous system (CNS) is complex and developmentally regulated. Alternative splicing of exons 2, 3 and 10 generates six isoforms in the adult human brain. These exons are excluded in the fetal brain, which expresses only the shortest isoform. Exons 9–12 each contain an 18-amino acid imperfect, microtubule-binding repeat sequence (R1–R4, Table 12.1), separated by inter-repeat (IR) regions of 13–14-amino acids. Exon 10 inclusion adds an extra microtubule-binding repeat to generate four-repeat tau, whereas three-repeat tau isoforms lack exon 10 seqeunces. The four/three repeat ratio in the adult human brain is roughly 1. Since four-repeat tau assembles microtubules more efficiently and binds microtubules three-fold more strongly than three-repeat tau, the development-specific expression of different tau isoforms represents different functional prerequisites for tau–microtubule interactions in fetal and adult neurons. At least 30 missense, silent, deletion and intronic mutations in the human tau gene (*MAPT*) have been reported[2,7] (Table 12.1). These mutations fall into two functional classes: one class alters the biochemical function of tau, and the second class alters the 4R/3R isoform ratio by affecting E10 splicing. Biochemical mutations that increase or decrease mutant tau's affinity for and stabilization of microtubues

Table 12.1 Location of FTDP-17 mutations in tau exons (E1–E13) and intron 10 (I10). Protein domains 'N-ter' and 'C-ter' represent N- and C-terminal, respectively. Microtubule (MT)-repeat and interrepeat sequences are represented by 'R' and 'IR', respectively. RNA elements represent splicing regulatory sequences as explained in the text. Mutations that increase or decrease E10 splicing (E10+) are shown by 'arrows' or by '?', where results from *in vitro* assays are ambiguous

	Mutation	RNA elements	E10+	Protein domain	
E1	R5L			N-ter	
	R5H			N-ter	
E9	K257V			R1	
	I260V			R1	
	L266V			R1	
	G272V			R1	
E10	N279K	PPE	↑	IR1-2	
	Δ280K	PPE	↓	IR1-2	
	L284L	ACE	↑	—	
	N296N	ESS	↑		MT-
	N296H	ESS	↑	—	binding
	Δ296N-homozygous	ESS	?	IR1-2	region
	P301L			R2	
	P301S			R2	
	S305S	5'ss	↑	IR2-3	
	S305N	5'ss	↑	IR2-3	
E11	L315L			—	
	L315R			IR2-3	
E12	R320F			R3	
	V337M			IR3-4	
	E342V	unknown	↑	IR3-4	
	K369I			IR4	
E13	G389R			C-ter	
	R406W			C-ter	
I10	E10+3	5'ss	↑		
	E10+11	ISS	↑		
	E10+12	ISS	↑		
	E10+13	ISS	↑		
	E10+14	ISS	↑		
	E10+16	ISS	↑		
	E10+19	ISM	↓		

occur in constitutive exons E1 (R5L, R5H), E9 (G257V, G266V, G272V), E11 (S230F), E12 (V337M) and E13 (R406W); these mutations are present in all six tau isoforms.[4,7–15] Mutations Δ280K, N296H, Δ296N, P301S and P301L in alternatively spliced exon 10, affect the biochemical properties of only 4R isoforms. Splicing mutations deregulate E10 inclusion and alter 4R/3R ratios (N279K, Δ280K, L284L, N296N, N296H, Δ296N, S305N, S305S and seven intronic mutations).[4,9,10,12,13,16–19] Some mutations (N279K, Δ280K, Δ296N) appear to affect both E10 splicing and microtubule-binding properties. Interestingly, although mutation E342V is located in E12, it appears to increase E10 inclusion and decrease inclusion of E2/E3 in RNA analyzed from patient brain.[20] One theory is that the mutation disrupts an existing splicing enhancer sequence in E12. Constitutive recognition and splicing-in of mutant E12 may be kinetically slower, allowing more time for E10 to be recognized and committed to splicing. A third category of mutations (Δ280K and P301L) appear to increase the ability of tau to self-aggregate as paired helical filaments.[21] Mutagenesis and *in vitro* splicing analyses show that E10 splicing is complex. Balanced E10 inclusion requires at least ten *cis*-acting splicing regulatory sequences that include splicing enhancer and inhibitor sequences including weak 5′ and 3′ splice sites.[9] The 5′ end of E10 contains three non-redundant exon splicing enhancer (ESE) sequences: a SC35-like, a polypurine enhancer (PPE) and an A/C-rich enhancer (ACE) sequence. Downstream of the ESE region is an exon splicing silencer (ESS). A bipartite regulatory sequence is present immediately downstream of the 5′ splice site in I10 and is composed of the intron splicing silencer (ISS) and the intron splicing modulator (ISM) elements. Fifteen different FTDP-17 mutations[14,15] disrupt six of these splicing regulatory sequences and include the PPE (N279K, Δ280K), ACE (L284L), ESS (Δ296N, N296N, N296H), 5′ splice site (S305N, S305S, E10+3), ISS (E10+11, E10+12, E10+13, E10+14, E10+16) and ISM (E10+19). The fact that these mutations cause severe neurodegenerative disease demonstrates the functional and mechanistic significance of these regulatory elements *in vivo*. Furthermore, *trans*-acting factors that associate with these splicing regulatory sequences may act as genetic modifiers of disease, which may explain the variable clinical and neuropathological phenotypes associated with FTDP-17.

ANIMAL MODELS OF TAUOPATHY

To understand how tau mutations cause disease, we have used transgenic animals to model tauopathy. Animal modeling is one of the basic methods for research into the cause and molecular mechanisms of human disease and we have used this approach to model the neuropathological phenotypes associated with FTDP-17 and other tauopathies. To identify critical steps in tau-induced neurodegeneration and test different hypotheses of pathogenesis, we generated a transgenic animal disease model for tauopathy in *Caenorhabditis elegans*. As an intensively studied organism, the worm *C. elegans* offers a number of distinct advantages for modeling human neurodegenerative diseases including small size, short generation time, rapid generation of transgenic lines, robust classical genetics, a simple thoroughly characterized nervous system and well-studied behavior. This neurodegenerative disease model should allow both classical genetic and transgenic approaches to be applied to understanding the molecular mechanisms of tau aggregation and resulting neurodegeneration. Similarities between the neuronal defects seen in tau transgenic *C. elegans* and tauopathy patients suggest that worms will be a viable organism for modeling the consequences of tau aggregation and neurotoxicity. Indeed, *C. elegans* has been used to model the pathological aggregation of Aβ seen in AD[22–24] and huntingtin aggregation seen in Huntington's disease.[25,26] Thus, use of these *C. elegans* models may provide general insights into the mechanisms of how neurotoxic aggregation of protein causes diseases in humans.

In transgenic *C. elegans*, pan-neuronal expression of normal or FTDP-17 mutant tau cDNA sequences recapitulated several features of tauopathy.[27] Tau transgenic worms exhibited altered behavior (uncoordinated movement), accumulation of insoluble phosphorylated tau, age-dependent loss of axons and neurons, and structural damage of axonal tracks characteristic of degenerating neurons. This degenerative phenotype was more severe in transgenic lines expressing FTDP-17 mutant tau when compared to lines expressing normal tau. Thus, this transgenic model exhibits features that mimic the tau-induced neurodegeneration seen in FTDP-17. In this worm model, transgene expression caused defective cholinergic transmission by disrupting pre-synaptic cholinergic signaling. Also, abnormal behavior occurred prior to accumulation of insoluble tau and neuronal loss, suggesting that aggregated tau is not required for tau-induced neuronal dysfunction[27] (Figure 12.1).

Transgenic animal models for tauopathy have been described in mice (reviewed in references 28–30), flies[31,32] and worms.[27] Collectively, these animal models recapitulate many features of authentic human tauopathies including behavioral deficits, tau hyperphosphorylation, tau aggregation, NFT pathology, axonopathy, neuronal loss and shortened lifespan. Furthermore, these models have shed light on the role of tau in neurodegeneration and promise to illuminate the mechanisms of tau-induced neurodegeneration.

In one model utilizing *Drosophila melanogaster*, neuronal expression of tau resulted in tau phosphorylation, premature death, late-onset neurodegeneration and loss of cholinergic neurons in the absence of NFT; these phenotypes are exacerbated by FTDP-17 mutations $^{R}406^{W}$ and $^{V}337M$.[31] Likewise in worms, FTDP-17 mutations $^{P}301^{L}$ and $^{V}337M$ exacerbate the phenotypes caused by normal

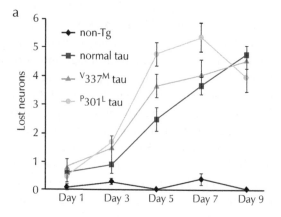

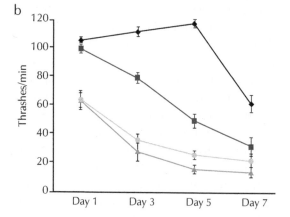

Time	Thrashes/min (mean ± SEM)	Insoluble tau (arbitrary units)
Day 1	27.6 ± 3.3	0.3
Day 3	11.9 ± 2.3	22.5
Day 5	4.6 ± 1.4	60.0

Figure 12.1 Tau induced phenotypes in *Caenorhabditis elegans* (adapted from reference 27). (a) Neuronal expression of human tau causes loss of g-aminobutyric acid (GABA)ergic neurons in the ventral nerve cord. (b) Tau induces behavioral defects in locomotion. FTDP-17 mutations cause impaired locomotion prior to the onset of significant neurodegeneration. (c) Association between behavioral deficits and insoluble tau. Expression of $^{V}337M$ tau induces behavioral defects prior to the accumulation of any detectable insoluble tau. The progressive decline of locomotion parallels the accumulation of insoluble tau. Tg, transgenic

human tau, and cause post-adulthood neuro-degeneration in the absence of fibrillar tau. In another fly model, overexpression of tau in the eye primordium in combination with tau phosphorylation by glycogen synthase kinase-3β caused developmental defects of the eye neurodegeneration in the eye and neurofibrillary pathology.[32] Similarly, neuronal expression of normal tau is sufficient to cause neuro-degeneration in *C. elegans*, although in the absence of tangles. Furthermore, prominent motor and behavioral defects distinguish our *C. elegans* model, from both *Drosophila* models, which lack a distinct behavioral phenotype.

In contrast, many of the transgenic mouse models share obvious behavioral defects comparable to those seen in the worm model. For instance, mice overexpressing [V]337[M] mutated human tau exhibited locomotory/-spatial behavior abnormalities in an elevated plus maze, consistent with hippocampal neurodegeneration;[33] similarly, mice over-expressing either the normal isoforms of human tau[33,35] or [P]301[L] mutated tau[35] exhibited hind-limb clasping defects consistent with motor neuron degeneration. Expression of human tau in mouse neurons resulted in biochemical changes in tau, including phos-phorylation and accumulation of insoluble tau as demonstrated.[33,35–38] As with both worm and fly models, tau transgenic mice displayed clear evidence of neuodegeneration.[37–40] Strikingly, some tau transgenic mouse lines show clear evidence of fibrillar tau,[35,36,38] while others do not exhibit fibrillar tau.[37,40] However, some of the transgenic mouse models described above exhibited signs of neuropathological changes in the absence of fibrillar tau, suggesting that NFTs may not be necessary for tau to induce neurodegeneration. Thus, a variety of transgenic animal models show that abnormal tau function and/or low-level tau aggregation in the absence of NFTs is sufficient to cause tau-induced neuronal dysfunction and neurodegeneration. This suggests that the neurotoxic tau species in tauopathy is not the NFT, but rather monomeric abnormal tau or low-level tau aggregates.

ANIMAL MODELS AS A TOOL FOR UNDERSTANDING HUMAN DISEASE

This *C. elegans* model for tau pathology provides a number of interesting avenues for future investigation. Classical genetic screens to identify modifiers of the tau-induced phenotype should reveal genes involved in formation of pathological tau. Such modifier genes may have homologs in humans that also act in the formation of pathological tau and may be potential points for therapeutic intervention. More significantly, the tauopathy phenotype in these transgenic worms is robust enough and has sufficient verisimilitude to human disease to enable development of rapid *in vivo* screens for drugs that may have therapeutic benefit for treating AD, FTDP-17 and other human neurodegenerative diseases with prominent tau pathologies. Given the reported feasibility of high throughput screening of *C. elegans*, this approach should be viable.

REFERENCES

1. Lee VMY, Goedert M, Trojanowski JQ. Neurodegenerative tauopathies. Ann Rev Neurosci 2001; 24:1121–59

2. Ingram EM, Spillantini MG. Tau gene mutations: dissecting the pathogenesis of FTDP-17. Trends Mol Med 2002; 8: 555–62

3. Foster NL, Wilhelmsen K, Sima AAF, et al. Frontotemporal dementia and parkinsonsim linked to chromosome 17: a consensus conference. Ann Neurol 1997; 41:706–15

4. Hutton M, Lendon CL, Rizzu P, et al. Association of missense and 5'-splice-site mutations in tau with the inherited dementia FTDP-17. Nature 1998; 393: 702–5

5. Poorkaj P, Bird TD, Wijsman E, et al. Tau is a candidate gene for chromosome 17 frontotemporal dementia. Ann Neurol 1998; 43: 815–25

6. Spillantini MG, Murrell JR, Goedert M, et al. Mutation in the tau gene in familial multiple system tauopathy with presenile dementia. Proc Natl Acad Sci USA 1998; 95: 7737–41

7. Barghorn S, Zhengfischhofer Q, Ackmann M, et al. Structure, microtubule interactions, and paired helical filament aggregation by tau mutants of frontotemporal dementias. Biochemistry 2000; 39: 11714–21

8. Barghorn S, Mandelkow E. Toward a unified scheme for the aggregation of tau into Alzheimer paired helical filaments. Biochemistry 2002; 41: 14885–96

9. D'Souza I, Poorkaj P, Hong M, et al. Missense and silent tau gene mutations cause front temporal dementia with parkinsonism–chromosome 17 type by affecting multiple alternative RNA splicing regulatory elements. Proc Natl Acad Sci USA 1999; 96:5598–603

10. Grover A, Houlden H, Baker M, et al. 5' splice mutations in tau associated with the inherited dementia FTDP-17 affect a stem–loop structure that regulates alternative splicing of exon 10. J Biol Chem 1999; 274: 15134–43

11. Hong M, Zhukareva V, Vogelsberg-Ragaglia V, et al. Mutation-specific functional impairments in distinct tau isoforms of hereditary FTDP-17. Science 1998; 282: 1914–17

12. Jiang ZH, Cote J, Kwon JM, et al. Aberrant splicing of tau pre-mRNA caused by intronic mutations associated with the inherited dementia frontotemporal dementia with parkinsonism linked to chromosome 17. Mol Cell Biol 2000; 20: 4036–48

13. Clark LN, Poorkaj P, Wszolek Z, et al. Pathogenic implications of mutations in the tau gene in pallido-ponto-nigral degeneration and related neurodegenerative disorders linked to chromosome 17. Proc Natl Acad Sci USA 1998; 95: 13103–7

14. Murrell JR, Koller D, Foroud T, et al. Familial multiple-system tauopathy with presenile dementia is localized to chromosome 17. Am J Hum Genet 1997; 61: 1131–8

15. Spillantini MG, Yoshida H, Rizzini C, et al. A novel tau mutation (N296N) in Familial Dementia with swollen achromatic neurons and corticobasal inclusion bodies. Ann Neurol 2000; 48: 939–43

16. Gao QS, Memmott J, Lafyatis R, et al. Complex regulation of tau exon 10, whose missplicing causes frontotemporal dementia. J Neurochem 2000; 74: 490–500

17. Spillantini MG, Murrell JR, Goedert M, et al. Mutation in the tau gene in familial multiple system tauopathy with presenile dementia. Proc Natl Acad Sci USA 1998; 95: 7737–41

18. Pastor P, Pastor E, Carnero C, et al. Familial atypical progressive supranuclear palsy associated with homozygosity for the delN296 mutation in the tau gene. Ann Neurol 2001; 49: 263–7

19. Stanford PM, Shepherd CE, Halliday GM, et al. Mutations in the tau gene that cause an increase in three repeat tau and frontotemporal dementia. Brain 2003; 126: 814–26

20. Lippa CF, Zhukareva V, Kawarai T, et al. Frontotemporal dementia with novel tau pathology and a Glu342Val tau mutation. Ann Neurol 2000; 48: 850–8

21. von Bergen M, Barghorn S, Li L, et al. Mutations of tau protein in frontotemporal dementia promote aggregation of paired helical filaments by enhancing local beta-structure. J Biol Chem 2001; 276: 48165–74

22. Davis JA, Naruse S, Chen H, et al. An Alzheimer's disease-linked PS1 variant rescues the developmental abnormalities of PS1-deficient embryos. Neuron 1998; 20: 603–9

23. Levitan D. Effects of SEL-12 presenilin on LIN-12 localization and function in Caenorhabditis elegans. Development 1998; 125: 3599–606

24. Link CD. Expression of human beta-amyloid peptide in transgenic Caenorhabditis elegans. Proc Natl Acad Sci USA 1995; 92: 9368–72

25. Faber PW, Alter JR, MacDonald ME, Hart AC. Polyglutamine-mediated dysfunction and apoptotic death of a Caenorhabditis elegans sensory neuron. Proc Natl Acad Sci USA 1999; 96: 179–84

26. Parker JA, Connolly JB, Wellington C, Hayden M, Dausset J, Neri C. Expanded polyglutamines in Caenorhabditis elegans cause axonal abnormalities and severe dysfunction of PLM mechanosensory neurons without cell death. Proc Natl Acad Sci USA 2001; 98:13318–13323

27. Kraemer BC, Zhang B, Leverenz JB, Thomas JH, Trojanowski JQ, Schellenberg GD. Neurodegeneration and defective neurotransmission in a Caenorhabditis elegans model of tauopathy. Proc Natl Acad Sci U S A 2003; 100:9980–5

28. Goedert M, Hasegawa M. The tauopathies – Toward an experimental animal model. Am J Pathol 1999; 154:1–6

29. Hutton M, Lewis J, Dickson D, Yen SH, McGowan E. Analysis of tauopathies with transgenic mice. Trends Mol Med 2001; 7:467–70

30. Hutton M, Lewis J, Dickson D, et al. Analysis of tauopathies with transgenic mice. Trends Mol Med 2001; 7: 467–70

31. Wittmann CW, Wszolek MF, Shulman JM, et al. Tauopathy in Drosophilia: neurogeneration without neurofibrillary tangles. Science 2001; 293: 711–14

32. Copeland MP, Daly E, Hines V, et al. Psychiatric symptomatology and prodromal Alzheimer's disease. Alzheimer Dis Assoc Dis 2003; 17: 1–8

33. Tanemura K, Murayama M, Akagi T, et al. Neurodegeneration with tau accumulation in a transgenic mouse expressing V337M human tau. J Neurosci 2002; 22: 133–41

34. Ishihara T, Higuchi M, Zhang B, et al. Attenuated neurodegenerative disease phenotype in tau transgenic mouse lacking neurofilaments. J Neurosci 2001; 21: 6026–35

35. Lewis J, McGowan E, Rockwood J, et al. Neurofibrillary tangles, amyotrophy and progressive motor disturbance in mice expressing mutant (P301L) tau protein. Nat Genet 2000; 25: 402–5

36. Gotz J, Chen F, Barmettler R, Nitsch RM. Tau filament formation in transgenic mice expressing P301L tau. J Biol Chem 2001; 276: 529–34

37. Probst A, Gotz J, Wiederhold KH, et al. Axonopathy and amyotrophy in mice transgenic for human four-repeat tau protein. Acta Neuropathologica 2000; 99: 469–81

38. Allen B, Ingram E, Takao M, et al. Abundant tau filaments and nonapoptotic neurodegeneration in transgenic mice expressing human P301S tau protein. J Neurosci 2002; 22: 9340–51

39. Ishihara T, Hong M, Zhang B, et al. Age-dependent emergence and progression of a tauopathy in transgenic mice overexpressing the shortest human tau isoform. Neuron 1999; 24: 751–62

40. Spittaels K, Van den Haute C, Van Dorpe J, et al. Prominent axonopathy in the brain and spinal cord of transgenic mice over expressing four-repeat human tau protein. Am J Pathol 1999; 155: 2153–65

Amyloid plaques and neurofibrillary tangles in a triple transgenic model: qualitative similarities with human Alzheimer's neuropathology

S Oddo, FM LaFerla

INTRODUCTION

Alzheimer's disease (AD), the most common neurodegenerative disorder, is characterized by the presence of two pathological hallmarks: extracellular plaques, mainly formed by the amyloid-β (Aβ) peptide and neurofibrillary tangles.[1] The Aβ peptide is derived via endoproteolysis from the β-amyloid precursor protein (APP). Rare mutations in the APP gene lead to autosomal dominant early-onset familial Alzheimer's disease (FAD).[2] The vast majority of autosomal dominant FAD cases are due to mutations in the presenilin (PS1 and PS2) gene.[3,4] Clinical mutations in these three genes affect Aβ metabolism, either leading to an increase in total Aβ levels or altering the Aβ42/40 ratio (reviewed by Hardy[5]). As for the other hallmark lesion, neurofibrillary tangles, this is composed of aggregates of the tau protein, which can be hyperphosphorylated at specific residues. Tau is encoded by a single gene on chromosome 17, which can be alternatively spliced to produce six different tau protein isoforms. The tau gene is not genetically linked to AD, but rather to another form of dementia called frontotemporal dementia with parkinsonism linked to chromosome 17 (FTDP-17).[6–10] Notably, the aggregates caused by mutations in the tau gene are qualitatively similar to those found in the AD brain (reviewed by Higuchi and collaborators[11]).

Several transgenic models have been generated that recapitulate key elements of AD neuropathology, but to date, no model fully mimics the complete neuropathological spectrum.[12] Although a single missense mutation in either the APP, PS1, or PS2 gene is sufficient to induce an aggressive form of AD in humans, this has not been the case following the introduction of these mutant alleles into genetically modified mice. Likewise, Down's syndrome patients, who harbor an increased concentration of the APP gene, almost invariably develop the complete gamut of AD neuropathology by their fifth decade.[13,14] Whereas mutant APP overexpression in transgenic mice allows for the successful modeling of amyloid deposition, surprisingly, the introduction of missense mutations in the APP, PS1, or PS2 genes (or their increased expression) has generally proved insufficient for inducing the complete spectrum of AD neuropathology in genetically altered mice – most notably characterized by the paucity of neurofibrillary pathology. Consequently, the development of both plaques and tangles has required aggressive biotechnological approaches, such as the development of genetically modified mice harboring multiple transgenes.

To mimic AD hallmark lesions in a mouse model and to study their neuropathological consequences, we generated a triple transgenic mouse model (3xTg-AD) that contains clinically relevant mutations in the PS1, APP and tau transgenes. The 3xTg-AD mice develop both plaques and tangles in an age-dependent manner in AD-relevant brain regions.[15] Here we show that the Aβ plaques and neurofibrillary tangles that develop in the 3xTg-AD mice are qualitatively similar to lesions found in human AD brain specimens. The development of both plaques and tangles in AD-relevant brain regions and the fact that these aggregates are qualitatively similar to those found in AD brain indicates that this model is suitable for investigating the molecular mechanisms linking plaques and tangles, and for studying the efficacy of therapeutic compounds.

RESULTS AND DISCUSSION

We previously described the generation and characterization of the 3xTg-AD mice, using an approach that allowed us simultaneously to introduce plaque- and tangle-encoding transgenes into mice, without altering their genetic background.[15] Specifically, we microinjected two independent transgenes encoding human APP with the Swedish mutation and human tau with the P301L mutation, both under the control of the Thy1.2 regulatory element, into single-cell embryos harvested from homozygous PS1$_{M146V}$ knockin (PS1-KI) mice. The APP and tau transgenes are overexpressed, with steady-state levels approaching three- and six-fold their endogenous counterparts in both hemizygous and homozygous mice, respectively. The inclusion of

the PS1 mutation acts to increase the Aβ42/40 ratio.[16]

We reported that the accumulation of intracellular Aβ immunoreactivity was the first pathological manifestation evident in the brains of the 3xTg-AD mice, occurring around 3–4 months of age in cortical regions, followed shortly thereafter in the CA1 region of the hippocampus. Extracellular amyloid plaques first became evident in the cortex by 6 months and emerged in the hippocampus by 9–12 months. Likewise, there was a temporal and regional hierarchy to the development of the neurofibrillary pathology, with conformational and phosphorylation-specific modifications to tau first detectable in the hippocampus at about 10–12 months of age, and then later emerging in the cortex.[15,17]

To determine whether the plaques and tangles present in the 3xTg-AD mice were qualitatively similar to those found in AD brain specimens, we immunostained brains from 22-month-old 3xTg-AD mice, the most advanced age that we have investigated thus far. By this timepoint, we found that the mice exhibited profound Aβ pathology, including extensive fibrillar deposits, as indicated by thioflavin staining in both the hippocampus and the cortex (Figure 13.1h). Likewise, at this age, the 3xTg-AD mice contained tangles in both the hippocampus and the cortex (Figure 13.1a and d). Thus, this model reproduces two of the most important neuropathological features of AD – plaques and tangles.

Figure 13.1 shows the extensive Aβ pathology that occurs in the hippocampus and cortex of the 3xTg-AD mice. By contrast, age- and gender-matched non-transgenic mice failed to show these deposits (Figure 13.1g). In the AD brain, the main component of amyloid plaques is Aβ42, which can be found in both diffuse and neuritic plaques. Immunostaining with Aβ42-specific antibodies revealed that many of these

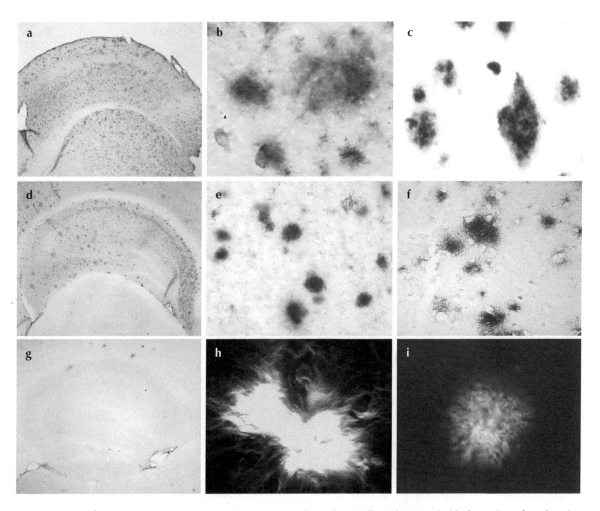

Figure 13.1 Aβ plaques in the 3xTg-AD mice are immunohistochemically indistinguishable from those found in the Alzheimer's disease (AD) brain. Free-floating sections (50 μm) were obtained from brains fixed in 4% paraformaldehyde and stained with monoclonal antibody anti-Aβ 1560 (1:3000), obtained from Chemicon, and polyclonal Aβ 42 (1:200) antibody, obtained from Biosource. (a) and (d) Cortex and the hippocampus of 22-month-old 3xTg-AD mice stained with 1560, respectively. (b) A high magnification of (a). (c) 1560 positive plaques in sections from AD brain. (e) and (f) Aβ42-positive plaques in the brain of a 3xTg-AD mouse and AD human, respectively. (g) The brain of an age-matched non-transgenic mouse. (h) and (i) Fibrillary plaques stained with thioflavin in the brain of a 3xTg-AD mouse, and in a specimen from AD brain, respectively. Original magnifications: 2.5×(a, d), 5×(g), 40×(b, c, e, f), 150× (i), 250×(h)

amyloid structures in the 3xTg-AD brains were Aβ42 immunoreactive (Figure 13.1e). Notably, many of the amyloid deposits contained an extensive β-pleated sheet structure, as evidenced by their reactivity with thioflavin (Figure 13.1h). Again, these thioflavin-positive structures appeared to be similar in the transgenic and human brain samples (see Figure 13.1h and i).

Tau phosphorylation is controlled in the brain by a balance between the activity of different kinases and phosphatases. In different tauopathies, including AD, tau is

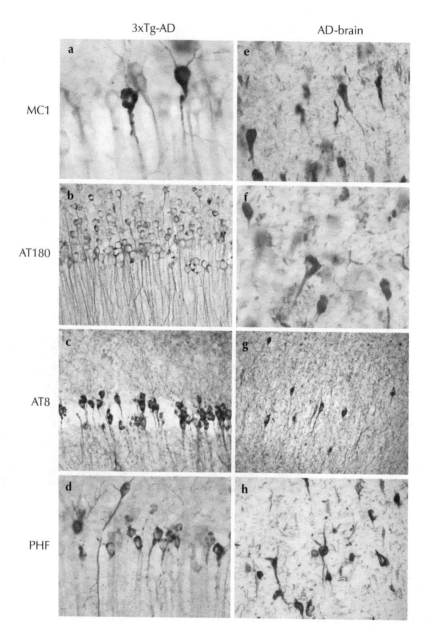

3xTg-AD AD-brain

MC1

AT180

AT8

PHF

Figure 13.2 In the 3xTg-AD mouse, tau is hyperphosphorylated at specific residues analogous to those found in postmortem human Alzheimer's disease (AD) brain specimens. Tau immunoreactive lesions in the 3xTg-AD mouse are qualitatively similar to those found in human AD brains, following immunostaining with the conformational-specific marker MC1 (a, e), and phosphospecific antibodies: AT180 (b, f), which detects phosphorylated tau proteins at threonine 231 residues; AT8 (c, g), which detects phosphorylated tau proteins at serine 202 and threonine 205 residues; and PHF1 (d, h), which detects phosphorylated tau proteins at serine 396 and 404 residues. As in AD brain, in the 3xTg-AD mice tau is mislocated and is accumulated mainly in dendrites and cell bodies of affected neurons. Primary antibodies were applied at dilutions of 1:500 for MC1, AT180 and AT8; 1:1000 for PHF1. Original magnifications: 20× (n, g, c); 40× (e, f, d, h); 60× (a)

hyperphosphorylated at specific threonine and serine residues. Besides reducing its ability to bind to microtubules, hyperphosphorylation leads to tau dislocation, and accumulation of this form of the protein becomes immunoreactive in dendrites and cell bodies.[18]

Previously, we reported that tau was hyperphosphorylated in the 3xTg-AD brains and that this hyperphosphorylation exhibited a hierarchical pattern. In other words, different threonine and serine residues become phosphorylated at different time points during aging. Initially, many neurons in the 3xTg-AD mice are immunoreactive for the conformational-specific antibody MC1; this antibody typically reacts with 'early' pathological stages assumed by the tau protein.[15]

We compared the phosphorylation status of tau in the brains of 3xTg-AD mice with that occurring in human AD brains (Figure 13.2). Different monoclonal antibodies raised against specific phosphorylated tau epitopes were used, including AT180, AT8 and PHF1. Comparison of the immunoreactive characteristics of these antibodies revealed that neurons immunopositive for AT180, AT8 and PHF1 were qualitatively similar between the mouse and human specimens, with flame-shaped neurons and dystrophic neurites present in both samples. Likewise, as in AD, the localization of tau is altered and accumulates mainly in the somato-dendritic compartment of cells, as opposed to its typical axonal localization.

In conclusion, we have demonstrated that the 3xTg-AD mice develop both plaques and tangles in AD-relevant brain regions. Moreover, both hallmark lesions of AD are qualitatively similar to those present in the AD brain, which should allow for a detailed investigation into the molecular mechanisms linking plaques and tangles.

ACKNOWLEDGEMENTS

We thank the Institute for Brain Aging and Dementia at the University of California, Irvine for the postmortem AD brain specimens and Antonella Caccamo for excellent technical assistance. This work was supported by grants from the Alzheimer's Association, and from the National Institutes of Health (AG17968 and AG0212982).

REFERENCES

1. Selkoe DJ. Alzheimer's disease: genes, proteins, and therapy. Physiol Rev 2001; 81: 741–66

2. Goate A, Chartier-Harlin MC, Mullan M, et al. Segregation of a missense mutation in the amyloid precursor protein gene with familial Alzheimer's disease. Nature 1991; 349: 704–6

3. Sherrington R, Rogaev EI, Liang Y, et al. Cloning of a gene bearing missense mutations in early-onset familial Alzheimer's disease. Nature 1995; 375: 754–60

4. Levy-Lahad E, Wasco W, Poorkaj P, et al. Candidate gene for the chromosome 1 familial Alzheimer's disease locus. Science 1995; 269: 973–7

5. Hardy J. Amyloid, the presenilins and Alzheimer's disease. Trends Neurosci 1997; 20: 154–9

6. Clark LN, Poorkaj P, Wszolek Z, et al. Pathogenic implications of mutations in the tau gene in pallido-ponto-nigral degeneration and

related neurodegenerative disorders linked to chromosome 17. Proc Natl Acad Sci USA 1998; 95: 13103–7

7. Foster NL, Wilhelmsen K, Sima AA, et al. Frontotemporal dementia and parkinsonism linked to chromosome 17: a consensus conference. Conference Participants. Ann Neurol 1997; 41: 706–15

8. Hutton M, Lendon CL, Rizzu P, et al. Association of missense and 5′-splice-site mutations in tau with the inherited dementia FTDP-17. Nature 1998; 393: 702–5

9. Poorkaj P, Bird TD, Wijsman E, et al. Tau is a candidate gene for chromosome 17 fronto-temporal dementia. Ann Neurol 1998; 43: 815–25

10. Spillantini MG, Murrell JR, Goedert M, et al. Mutation in the tau gene in familial multiple system tauopathy with presenile dementia. Proc Natl Acad Sci USA 1998; 95: 7737–41

11. Higuchi M, Lee VM, Trojanowski JQ. Tau and axonopathy in neurodegenerative disorders. Neuromolecular Med 2002; 2: 131–50

12. Wong PC, Cai H, Borchelt DR, Price DL. Genetically engineered mouse models of neurodegenerative diseases. Nat Neurosci 2002; 5: 633–9

13. Coyle JT, Oster-Granite ML, Gearhart JD. The neurobiologic consequences of Down syndrome. Brain Res Bull 1986; 16: 773–87

14. Mann DM. The pathological association between Down syndrome and Alzheimer disease. Mech Ageing Dev 1988; 43: 99–136

15. Oddo S, Caccamo A, Shepherd JD, et al. Triple-transgenic model of Alzheimer's disease with plaques and tangles: intracellular Abeta and synaptic dysfunction. Neuron 2003; 39: 409–21

16. Scheuner D, Eckman C, Jensen M, et al. Secreted amyloid beta-protein similar to that in the senile plaques of Alzheimer's disease is increased in vivo by the presenilin 1 and 2 and APP mutations linked to familial Alzheimer's disease. Nat Med 1996; 2: 864–70

17. Oddo S, Caccamo A, Kitazawa M, et al. Amyloid deposition precedes tangle formation in a triple transgenic model of Alzheimer's disease. Neurobiol Aging 2004; 24: 1063–70

18. Kowall NW, Kosik KS. Axonal disruption and aberrant localization of tau protein characterize the neuropil pathology of Alzheimer's disease. Ann Neurol 1987; 22: 639–43

Chapter 14

Apolipoprotein E and Alzheimer's disease: what has a decade told us?

KA Crutcher

INTRODUCTION

The apolipoprotein E (apoE) genotype is the single most important genetic risk factor identified so far for sporadic Alzheimer's disease (AD). The presence of the ε4 allele, confers a much greater risk of AD compared with the more common ε3 allele and may also be implicated in other degenerative diseases. If the ε2 allele is the basis of comparison, apoE may account for the vast majority of AD risk. The initial discovery of this risk factor a decade ago has since been replicated in numerous laboratories. However, remarkably little progress has been made in understanding how apoE confers increased risk of AD or other diseases. Although the role of apoE in AD is widely assumed to be indirect, through modification of amyloid deposition or clearance, there is also evidence that it may make a direct contribution to neuropathology. Elucidation of the physiological role of apoE in the central nervous system (CNS) and its contribution to neurodegenerative disease should clarify the suitability of apoE as a novel therapeutic target in AD.

There is no disagreement that AD represents a daunting and looming menace, but there is little agreement on what course of action should be taken to fight this mind-robbing malady. It has been a century since the disease was first identified as a distinct entity and almost four decades since candidate molecular mechanisms were proposed to account for the distinctive pathology. However, the first indication of a genetic risk factor that might apply to most cases of the disease emerged only a decade ago and the candidate gene (apoE) was a surprise, even though the protein had been studied for some time. In spite of the fact that apoE has been confirmed as a highly significant risk factor in the disease, relatively little effort has been focused on understanding its role. The fact that such unexpected discoveries occur and the slow rate at which such discoveries are incorporated into research programs should give us pause in projecting future successes in this arena. What follows is a consideration of several questions that would seem to be relevant to developing a therapeutic strategy for AD if apoE is really the most important genetic risk factor.

IS APOLIPOPROTEIN E THE SINGLE MOST IMPORTANT GENETIC RISK FACTOR FOR ALZHEIMER'S DISEASE?

The reports in 1993 of a genetic linkage between apoE and risk of AD represented a landmark in the search for genetic risk factors.[1–4] This finding was soon replicated in many studies.[5–13] Although the strength of the association varies according to ethnicity and other variables, there is increasing acceptance of the view that this locus may account for the majority of the genetic risk of 'non-familial' forms of AD.[14] The absolute risk is difficult to assess, partly because of the variability across populations but also because of a very simple yet profound question regarding the appropriate baseline for calculating risk.

The baseline is usually taken to be the most common genotype in the population under study, in this case the ε3 allele. On this basis, possession of ε4 increases AD risk several-fold. By the same argument, possession of the least common allele, ε2, is commonly viewed as conferring protection against the disease when compared with possession of the ε3 or ε4 allele. However, the assumption that disease risk should be based on comparison with the most common genotype is arbitrary. One could argue that risk should be assessed in comparison with the genotype that exhibits the lowest incidence of disease. If so, possession of either ε3 or ε4 confers greater risk of disease relative to ε2. On this basis, apoE could potentially account for 90% of the genetic risk associated with this disease.[14] In addition, studies that have failed to demonstrate an increased risk when comparing possession of ε4 with ε3 might well reveal significant effects if ε2 is taken as the basis for comparison.

This is not a trivial issue because much rests on the conclusion that the single most important genetic risk factor has already been identified. If true, there is little justification for continued search for genes that confer comparable or significant risk of the disease. This is not to say that additional genetic risk factors do not exist or that important loci will not be identified that interact with, and potentially modify, the risk

attributed to the apoE genotype. Nevertheless, if the primary genetic risk factor is now known, attention should be focused on defining the mechanism through which this risk is mediated.

WHAT KILLS NEURONS IN ALZHEIMER'S DISEASE?

Most investigators agree that the cognitive deficits in AD are due to the disruption of neuronal connections and/or the degeneration of nerve cells in specific brain regions.[15] Assuming that the loss of neurons and their connections is central to the disease process, it is reasonable to look for some contribution of apoE either to the pathway leading to nerve cell death or to the ability of the brain to respond to or repair such damage.

However, the cause of synaptic and neuronal loss in AD remains controversial. One of the most popular hypotheses over the past decade is that some form of the amyloid peptide is a direct cause of neuronal degeneration.[16] The assumption that some form of amyloid is neurotoxic underlies many of the current therapeutic approaches to the disease. However, in spite of the tremendous effort invested in this area, the amyloid hypothesis does not appear to be sufficient to account for all of the available aspects of AD pathogenesis, especially pertaining to the question of neuronal degeneration.[17] Alternative hypotheses regarding the role of amyloid in the brain have been proposed, some of which posit a beneficial role for this peptide.[18] Certainly, as far as genetic risk factors are concerned, mutations in the amyloid precursor protein (APP) account for a small minority of AD cases.

If the amyloid peptide, or some variation of it, accounts for neuronal degeneration in AD, then it is reasonable to search for a role for apoE in modifying the effects of the amyloid peptide.

In fact, numerous studies have demonstrated an interaction between amyloid and apoE, and there is clear evidence for isoform-specific effects of apoE on amyloid deposition in transgenic mice.[19–24] If amyloid deposition drives the other pathological changes in AD, ultimately leading to neuronal degeneration, then studies of the role of apoE in this process are warranted. If, however, amyloid deposition is a consequence, not a cause, of underlying neuronal or synaptic dysfunction, attention should be focused on other mechanisms of apoE-related neuro-degeneration and/or repair.

WHAT IS THE ROLE OF APOLIPOPROTEIN E IN ALZHEIMER'S DISEASE?

ApoE is well known as a carrier of lipid, and has been studied in that capacity for many years. It mediates uptake of lipoproteins through several cell-surface receptors including the low-density lipoprotein (LDL) receptor, the LDL-receptor-related protein (LRP) and the gp330 receptor.[25–33] The three major isoforms of apoE in humans (E2, E3 and E4) differ from each other by, at most, two amino acids[34–37] and the corresponding alleles are designated ε2, ε3 and ε4.

One of the first hints that apoE may be involved in AD pathology came from its immunohistochemical localization to senile plaques and tangles.[38] There have been several studies since then, in which apoE immuno-staining in AD brain has been reported,[39–44] but it was the genetic linkage analysis that led to the identification of the ε4 allele as a significant risk factor for AD.[4] Perhaps not surprisingly, the original reports were met with some skepticism because there was no obvious biological explanation for the association. However, the consistency of the results cannot be ignored and

there are now several groups pursuing hypotheses regarding apoE's contribution to the disease process.

Given the precedence and prominence of the amyloid hypothesis, it is not surprising that much of this work has focused on the impact of apoE on amyloid. In fact, an early suggestion was that apoE is involved through the 'binding, transport, and targeting of βA4 (or other peptides)'[39] or through 'a decreased ability to clear βA4 from the neuropil, due to altered apoE–βA4 interactions'.[5] The biochemical details of the interaction between apoE and amyloid continue to be investigated,[45,46] but the physiological relevance of these interactions remains to be established and, as noted above, the primacy of amyloid in causing neuronal degeneration is still contested.

Another early suggestion was that apoE is involved in tangle formation,[47] supported, in part, by the finding that the E3 isoform binds tau, thus preventing its abnormal phosphorylation.[48] Again, a number of investigators have been pursuing the possibility that apoE modifies tau or other cytoskeletal components, thereby contributing to tangle formation.[49–58] However, a consistent biochemical mechanism by which apoE could influence cytoskeletal structures has not yet emerged.

A third general hypothesis regarding apoE in AD is that isoform-specific differences in promotion of neurite outgrowth may contribute to a relative failure of regenerative repair with E4,[59] so that the association of the E4 isoform with AD is actually due to the absence of the E3 isoform. In fact, several *in vitro* studies have demonstrated that apoE exhibits isoform-specific effects on neurite outgrowth,[60–63] which are consistent with the general hypothesis that apoE plays a role in neuronal growth and that apoE4 may serve this role less efficiently.

Yet another hypothesis that is conceptually consistent with the latter mechanism is that apoE exhibits an isoform-specific ability to protect the brain through antioxidant activity.[64–70] The general conclusion from these studies is that apoE4 is less capable of protecting against oxidative damage. Of course, if this hypothesis is correct, the question of what generates the oxidative injury in AD remains unanswered.

IS APOLIPOPROTEIN E3 BENEFICIAL OR IS APOLIPOPROTEIN E4 DETRIMENTAL?

One conceptual distinction between the several hypotheses regarding the role of apoE is the extent to which disease risk can be ascribed to the absence of a beneficial function of one form of the protein versus the presence of a negative function. This is a very difficult question to answer and relates back to the conundrum raised above in the argument regarding the appropriate baseline for evaluating disease risk. If one assumes that the risk of disease, and any corresponding mechanism, should be evaluated against the ε2-carrying population, then it seems reasonable that there will be an isoform-associated mechanism that shows either a decreasing positive effect E2 > E3 > E4 or an increasing negative effect E4 > E3 > E2. The answer to this question also has direct bearing on the search for therapies. The goal of enhancing a beneficial effect, either through conversion of the detrimental to the beneficial form of the protein or through increased expression of the beneficial form, is likely to require a different strategy than the goal of inhibiting a detrimental effect. An interesting theoretical question is whether or not the absence of apoE, whatever the isoform, would increase or decrease the risk of AD. Of course, the loss of apoE-mediated lipid transport would presumably result in greater cardiovascular disease, as demonstrated in apoE-null mice. Assuming one did not die from heart disease, would the absence of apoE make it more or less likely for one to get AD?

The argument hinges on the 'normal' role of apoE, which is often taken to be its well-studied effects on lipid metabolism. However, if apoE is conferring risk through some other cellular pathway, it is possible that some beneficial function shows up in another (presumably post-reproductive) context as a pleiotropic negative effect.[71] The ε4 allele has been implicated in increased severity of AD pathology for both plaques and tangles,[40,72–74] but whether this is a loss or gain of function is difficult to establish. There is also some indication that expression of E4 may give rise to increased neuropathology following CNS injury.[75–77]

An example of a potential negative role for apoE is the isoform-specific neurotoxicity that has been described by several groups.[78–83] ApoE has also been found to exhibit various effects on cells that belie a simple role in lipid transport. For example, apoE has now been shown to activate intracellular signaling pathways.[84–87] Signaling effects appear to be mediated by LRP, pointing to the possibility of isoform-specific differences in intracellular signaling.[88–91]

Also relevant to the question of negative or positive effects of apoE: promoter polymorphisms associated with increased apoE expression may increase disease risk, regardless of isoform (reviewed by Bullido and Valdivieso[92]). Collectively, these results suggest that both E3 and E4 can contribute to disease risk, with a greater contribution from the E4 isoform. The possibility that E4 has a dominant negative effect is also consistent with emerging evidence for worse outcomes associated with other neurological insults.[93–100]

WHERE DO WE GO FROM HERE?

AD is an emerging healthcare issue. Although current therapies are having some immediate benefit in a subset of patients, it is not yet clear whether this will have a significant impact on the incidence of the disease or ultimate financial burden. Until there is a clearer understanding of the underlying cause(s) of the disease, it will be difficult to devise a strategy for developing effective treatments. The lack of consensus on specific disease mechanisms, even if there is currently majority support for the amyloid hypothesis, suggests that less is understood about the etiology of this disease than might be assumed from the available literature. The absence of bona fide animal models makes the task even more difficult. There is considerable debate as to whether any of the preclinical models are sufficiently developed to justify clinical trials based on such models. If AD is a uniquely human malady, for which an argument can be made, a complete animal model may never be found. If so, we may need to face the prospect that effective therapies will not emerge from preclinical studies but, rather, from clinical studies based on hypotheses that can only be truly studied in humans. Perhaps the next decade will provide new surprises that, when combined with current efforts, will open new therapeutic avenues. Unraveling the contribution of apoE to the disease is likely to be important to this process.

REFERENCES

1. Saunders AM, Roses AD. Apolipoprotein E4 allele frequency, ischemic cerebrovascular disease, and Alzheimer's disease. Stroke 1993; 24: 1416–17

2. Saunders AM, Strittmatter WJ, Schmechel D, et al. Association of apolipoprotein E allele epsilon 4 with late-onset familial and sporadic Alzheimer's disease. Neurology 1993; 43: 1467–72

3. Saunders AM, Schmader K, Breitner JC, et al. Apolipoprotein E epsilon 4 allele distributions in late-onset Alzheimer's disease and in other amyloid-forming diseases. Lancet 1993; 342: 710–11

4. Corder EH, Saunders AM, Strittmatter WJ, et al. Gene dose of apolipoprotein E type 4 allele and the risk of Alzheimer's disease in late onset families. Science 1993; 261: 921–3

5. Rebeck GW, Reiter JS, Strickland DK, Hyman BT. Apolipoprotein E in sporadic Alzheimer's disease: allelic variation and receptor interactions. Neuron 1993; 11: 575–80

6. Strittmatter WJ, Roses AD. Apolipoprotein E and Alzheimer disease. Proc Natl Acad Sci USA 1995; 9295: 4725–7

7. Hardy J. Apolipoprotein E in the genetics and epidemiology of Alzheimer's disease. Am J Med Genet 1995; 60: 456–60

8. Farrer LA, Abraham CR, Volicer L, et al. Allele epsilon 4 of apolipoprotein E shows a dose effect on age at onset of Pick disease. Exp Neurol 1995; 136: 162–70

9. Bennett C, Crawford F, Osborne A, et al. Evidence that the APOE locus influences rate of disease progression in late onset familial Alzheimer's disease but is not causative. Am J Med Genet 1995; 60: 1–6

10. Martinoli MG, Trojanowski JQ, Schmidt ML, et al. Association of apolipoprotein epsilon 4 allele and neuropathologic findings in patients

with dementia. Acta Neuropathol (Berl) 1995; 90: 239–43

11. St Clair D, Rennie M, Slorach E, et al. Apolipoprotein E epsilon 4 allele is a risk factor for familial and sporadic presenile Alzheimer's disease in both homozygote and heterozygote carriers. J Med Genet 1995; 32: 642–4

12. Schellenberg GD. Progress in Alzheimer's disease genetics. Curr Opin Neurol 1995; 8: 262–7

13. Martins RN, Clarnette R, Fisher C, et al. ApoE genotypes in Australia: roles in early and late onset Alzheimer's disease and Down's syndrome. Neuroreport 1995; 6: 1513–16

14. Ashford JW, Mortimer JA. Non-familial Alzheimer's disease is mainly due to genetic factors. J Alzheimers Dis 2002; 4: 169–77

15. Terry RD. Neuropathological changes in Alzheimer disease. Prog Brain Res 1994; 101: 383–90

16. Selkoe DJ. Alzheimer's disease is a synaptic failure. Science 2002; 298: 789–91

17. Neve RL, Robakis NK. Alzheimer's disease: a re-examination of the amyloid hypothesis. Trends Neurosci 1998; 21: 15–19

18. Robinson SR, Bishop GM. Abeta as a bio-flocculant: implications for the amyloid hypothesis of Alzheimer's disease. Neurobiol Aging 2002; 23: 1051–72

19. Holtzman DM, Bales KR, Wu S, et al. Expression of human apolipoprotein E reduces amyloid-beta deposition in a mouse model of Alzheimer's disease. J Clin Invest 1999; 103: R15–21

20. Bales KR, Verina T, Dodel RC, et al. Lack of apolipoprotein E dramatically reduces amyloid beta-peptide deposition. Nat Genet 1997; 17: 263–4

21. Bales KR, Verina T, Saura J, et al. Apolipoprotein E and amyloid deposition in transgenic mice. Soc Neurosci Abstr 1998; 24: 1502

22. Bales KR, Verina T, Cummins DJ, et al. Apolipoprotein E is essential for amyloid deposition in the APP(V717F) transgenic mouse model of Alzheimer's disease. Proc Natl Acad Sci USA 1999; 96: 15233–8

23. Holtzman DM, Bales KR, Tenkova T, et al. Apolipoprotein E isoform-dependent amyloid deposition and neuritic degeneration in a mouse model of Alzheimer's disease. Proc Natl Acad Sci USA 2000; 97: 2892–7

24. Irizarry MC, Cheung BS, Rebeck GW, et al. Apolipoprotein E affects the amount, form, and anatomical distribution of amyloid beta-peptide deposition in homozygous APP(V717F) transgenic mice. Acta Neuropathol (Berl) 2000; 100: 451–8

25. Cummings BJ, Cotman CW. Image analysis of beta-amyloid load in Alzheimer's disease and relation to dementia severity. Lancet 1995; 346: 1524–8

26. Mahley RW, Hui DY, Innerarity TL, Weisgraber KH. Two independent lipoprotein receptors on hepatic membranes of dog, swine, and man. Apo-B, E and apo-E receptors. J Clin Invest 1981; 68: 1197–206

27. Mahley RW, Innerarity TL, Weisgraber KH, et al. Cellular and molecular biology of lipoprotein metabolism: characterization of lipoprotein receptor–ligand interactions. Cold Spring Harb Symp Quant Biol 1986; 51: 821–8

28. Mahley RW, Innerarity TL, Rall SJ, Weisgraber KH. Lipoproteins of special significance in atherosclerosis. Insights provided by studies of type III hyperlipoproteinemia. Ann NY Acad Sci 1985; 454: 209–21

29. Innerarity TL, Friedlander EJ, Rall SJ, Weisgraber KH, Mahley RW. The receptor-binding domain of human apolipoprotein E. Binding of apolipoprotein E fragments. J Biol Chem 1983; 258: 12341–7

30. Innerarity TL, Weisgraber KH, Rall SJ, Mahley RW. Functional domains of apolipoprotein E and apolipoprotein B. Acta Med Scand Suppl 1987; 715: 51–9

31. Weisgraber KH, Innerarity TL, Rall SJ, Mahley RW. Receptor interactions controlling lipoprotein metabolism. Can J Biochem Cell Biol 1985; 63: 898–905

32. Weisgraber KH, Innerarity TL, Rall SJ, Mahley RW. Apolipoprotein E: receptor binding properties. Adv Exp Med Biol 1985; 63: 159–71

33. Weisgraber KH, Mahley RW. Characterization of apolipoprotein E-containing lipoproteins. Methods Enzymol 1986; 129: 145–66

34. Weisgraber KH, Rall SJ, Mahley RW. Human E apoprotein heterogeneity. Cysteine–arginine interchanges in the amino acid sequence of the apo-E isoforms. J Biol Chem 1981; 256: 9077–83

35. Weisgraber KH, Innerarity TL, Rall SJ, Mahley RW. Atherogenic lipoproteins resulting from genetic defects of apolipoproteins B and E. Ann NY Acad Sci 1990; 598: 37–48

36. Weisgraber KH. Apolipoprotein E: structure–function relationships. Adv Protein Chem 1994; 45: 249–302

37. Westerlund JA, Weisgraber KH. Discrete carboxyl-terminal segments of apolipoprotein E mediate lipoprotein association and protein oligomerization. J Biol Chem 1993; 268: 15745–50

38. Namba Y, Tomonaga M, Kawasaki H, et al. Apolipoprotein E immunoreactivity in cerebral amyloid deposits and neurofibrillary tangles in Alzheimer's disease and kuru plaque amyloid in Creutzfeld-Jacob disease. Brain Res 1991; 541: 163–6

39. Strittmatter WJ, Saunders AM, Schmechel D, et al. Apolipoprotein E: high-avidity binding to beta-amyloid and increased frequency of type 4 allele in late-onset familial Alzheimer disease. Proc Natl Acad Sci USA 1993; 90: 1977–81

40. Schmechel DE, Saunders AM, Strittmatter WJ, et al. Increased amyloid beta-peptide deposition in cerebral cortex as a consequence of apolipoprotein E genotype in late-onset Alzheimer disease. Proc Natl Acad Sci USA 1993; 90: 9649–53

41. Yamaguchi H, Ishiguro K, Sugihara S, et al. Presence of apolipoprotein E on extracellular neurofibrillary tangles and on meningeal blood vessels precedes the Alzheimer beta-amyloid deposition. Acta Neuropathol (Berl) 1994; 88: 413–19

42. Gearing M, Schneider JA, Robbins RS, et al. Regional variation in the distribution of apolipoprotein E and A beta in Alzheimer's disease. J Neuropathol Exp Neurol 1995; 54: 833–41

43. Dickson TC, Saunders HL, Vickers JC. Relationship between apolipoprotein E and the amyloid deposits and dystrophic neurites of Alzheimer's disease. Neuropathol Appl Neurobiol 1997; 23: 483–91

44. Styren SD, Kamboh MI, DeKosky ST. Expression of differential immune factors in temporal cortex and cerebellum: the role of alpha-1-antichymotrypsin, apolipoprotein E, and reactive glia in the progression of Alzheimer's disease. J Comp Neurol 1998; 396: 511–20

45. Sanan DA, Weisgraber KH, Russell SJ, et al. Apolipoprotein E associates with beta amyloid peptide of Alzheimer's disease to form novel monofibrils. Isoform apoE4 associates more efficiently than apoE3. J Clin Invest 1994; 94: 860–9

46. Strittmatter WJ, Weisgraber KH, Huang DY, et al. Binding of human apolipoprotein E to synthetic amyloid beta peptide: isoform-specific effects and implications for late-onset Alzheimer disease. Proc Natl Acad Sci USA 1993; 90: 8098–102

47. Strittmatter WJ, Saunders AM, Goedert M, et al. Isoform-specific interactions of apolipoprotein E with microtubule-associated protein tau: implications for Alzheimer disease. Proc Natl Acad Sci USA 1994; 91: 11183–6

48. Strittmatter WJ, Weisgraber KH, Goedert M, et al. Hypothesis: microtubule instability and paired helical filament formation in the Alzheimer disease brain are related to apolipoprotein E genotype. Exp Neurol 1994; 125: 163–71; discussion 172–4

49. Huang DY, Weisgraber KH, Goedert M, et al. ApoE3 binding to tau tandem repeat I is abolished by tau serine262 phosphorylation. Neurosci Lett 1995; 192: 209–12

50. Fleming LM, Weisgraber KH, Strittmatter WJ, et al. Differential binding of apolipoprotein E

isoforms to tau and other cytoskeletal proteins. Exp Neurol 1996; 138: 252–60

51. Tesseur I, Van Dorpe J, Spittaels K, et al. Expression of human apolipoprotein E4 in neurons causes hyperphosphorylation of protein tau in the brains of transgenic mice. Am J Pathol 2000; 156: 951–64

52. Huang Y, Liu XQ, Wyss-Coray T, et al. Apolipoprotein E fragments present in Alzheimer's disease brains induce neuro-fibrillary tangle-like intracellular inclusions in neurons. Proc Natl Acad Sci USA 2001; 98: 8838–43

53. Ljungberg MC, Dayanandan R, Asuni A, et al. Truncated apoE forms tangle-like structures in a neuronal cell line. Neuroreport 2002; 13: 867–70

54. Brecht WJ, Harris FM, Tesseur I, et al. ApoE proteolysis and hyperphosphorylation of tau in transgenic mice expressing apoE4 in neurons. Soc Neurosc Abstr 2002; 592: 13

55. Tesseur I, Van Dorpe J, Bruynseels K, et al. Prominent axonopathy and disruption of axonal transport in transgenic mice expressing human apolipoprotein E4 in neurons of brain and spinal cord. Am J Pathol 2000; 157: 1495–510

56. Fleming LM, Weisgraber KH, Strittmatter WJ, et al. Differential binding of apolipoprotein E isoforms to tau and other cytoskeletal proteins. Exp Neurol 1996; 138: 252–60

57. Zhang D, McQuade J-A, Shockley K, et al. Proteolysis of apolipoprotein E and Alzheimer's disease pathology. Alzheimer's Rep 2001; 4: 67–80

58. Kobayashi M, Ishiguro K, Katoh-Fukui Y, et al. Phosphorylation state of tau in the hippo-campus of apolipoprotein E4 and E3 knock-in mice. Neuroreport 2003; 14: 699–702

59. Poirier J. Apolipoprotein E in animal models of CNS injury and in Alzheimer's disease. Trends Neurosci 1994; 17: 525–30

60. Nathan BP, Bellosta S, Sanan DA, et al. Differential effects of apolipoproteins E3 and E4 on neuronal growth in vitro. Science 1994; 264: 850–2

61. Bellosta S, Nathan BP, Orth M, et al. Stable expression and secretion of apolipoproteins E3 and E4 in mouse neuroblastoma cells produces differential effects on neurite outgrowth. J Biol Chem 1995; 270: 27063–71

62. Holtzman DM, Pitas RE, Kilbridge J, et al. Low density lipoprotein receptor-related protein mediates apolipoprotein E-dependent neurite outgrowth in a central nervous system-derived neuronal cell line. Proc Natl Acad Sci USA 1995; 92: 9480–4

63. Nathan BP, Chang KC, Bellosta S, et al. The inhibitory effect of apolipoprotein E4 on neurite outgrowth is associated with micro-tubule depolymerization. J Biol Chem 1995; 270: 19791–9

64. Keller JN, Lauderback CM, Butterfield DA, et al. Amyloid beta-peptide effects on syn-aptosomes from apolipoprotein E-deficient mice. J Neurochem 2000; 74: 1579–86

65. Miyata M, Smith JD. Apolipoprotein E allele-specific antioxidant activity and effects on cytotoxicity by oxidative insults and beta-amyloid peptides. Nat Genet 1996; 14: 55–61

66. Mazur-Kolecka B, Frackowiak J, Kowal D, et al. Oxidative protein damage in cells engaged in beta-amyloidosis is related to apoE genotype. Neuroreport 2002; 13: 465–8

67. Pedersen WA, Chan SL, Mattson MP. A mechanism for the neuroprotective effect of apolipoprotein E: isoform-specific modification by the lipid peroxidation product 4-hydroxy-nonenal. J Neurochem 2000; 74: 1426–33

68. Ramassamy C, Averill D, Beffert U, et al. Oxidative damage and protection by anti-oxidants in the frontal cortex of Alzheimer's disease is related to the apolipoprotein E genotype. Free Radic Biol Med 1999; 27: 544–53

69. Ramassamy C, Averill D, Beffert U, et al. Oxidative insults are associated with apolipoprotein E genotype in Alzheimer's disease brain. Neurobiol Dis 2000; 7: 23–37

70. Hoy A, Leininger-Muller B, Jolivalt C, Siest G. Effect of apolipoprotein E on cell viability in a human neuroblastoma cell line: influence of oxidation and lipid-association. Neurosci Lett 2000; 285: 173–6

71. Wozniak MA, Itzhaki RF, Faragher EB, et al. Apolipoprotein E-epsilon 4 protects against severe liver disease caused by hepatitis C virus. Hepatology 2002; 36: 456–63

72. Polvikoski T, Sulkava R, Haltia M, et al. Apolipoprotein E, dementia, and cortical deposition of beta-amyloid protein. N Engl J Med 1995; 333: 1242–7

73. Ghebremedhin E, Schultz C, Braak E, Braak H. High frequency of apolipoprotein E epsilon4 allele in young individuals with very mild Alzheimer's disease-related neurofibrillary changes. Exp Neurol 1998; 153: 152–5

74. Ghebremedhin E, Schultz C, Thal DR, et al. Gender and age modify the association between APOE and AD-related neuropathology. Neurology 2001; 56: 1696–701

75. Laskowitz DT, Horsburgh K, Roses AD. Apolipoprotein E and the CNS response to injury. J Cereb Blood Flow Metab 1998; 18: 465–71

76. Sheng H, Laskowitz DT, Bennett E, et al. Apolipoprotein E isoform-specific differences in outcome from focal ischemia in transgenic mice. J Cereb Blood Flow Metab 1998; 18: 361–6

77. Sabo T, Lomnitski L, Nyska A, et al. Susceptibility of transgenic mice expressing human apolipoprotein E to closed head injury: the allele E3 is neuroprotective whereas E4 increases fatalities. Neuroscience 2000; 101: 879–84

78. Jordan J, Galindo MF, Miller RJ, et al. Isoform-specific effect of apolipoprotein E on cell survival and beta-amyloid-induced toxicity in rat hippocampal pyramidal neuronal cultures. J Neurosci 1998; 18: 195–204

79. DeMattos RB, Levine JM, Williams DL. Localization of apolipoprotein E in the cytoplasm of Neuro-2a cells is cytotoxic. Soc Neurosci Abstr 1997; 23: 826

80. Michikawa M, Yanagisawa K. Apolipoprotein E4 induces neuronal cell death under conditions of suppressed de novo cholesterol synthesis. J Neurosci Res 1998; 54: 58–67

81. Marques MA, Tolar A, Crutcher KA. Apolipoprotein E exhibits isoform-specific neurotoxicity. Alzheimer's Res 1997; 3: 1–6

82. Soulie C, Ferreira S, Delacourte A, Caillet-Boudin ML. ApoE and amyloid/apoE effects on human neuroblastoma SKNSH-SY 5Y cells. Soc Neurosci Abstr 1999; 25: 1348

83. Veinbergs I, Everson A, Sagara Y, Masliah E. Neurotoxic effects of apolipoprotein E4 are mediated via dysregulation of calcium home-ostasis. J Neurosci Res 2002; 67: 379–87

84. Ohkubo N, Mitsuda N, Tamatani M, et al. Apolipoprotein E4 stimulates cAMP response element-binding protein transcriptional activity through the extracellular signal-regulated kinase pathway. J Biol Chem 2001; 276: 3046–53

85. Muller W, Meske V, Berlin K, et al. Apolipoprotein E isoforms increase intra-cellular Ca^{2+} differentially through an omega-agatoxin IVa-sensitive Ca^{2+}-channel. Brain Pathol 1998; 8: 641–53

86. Tolar M, Keller JN, Chan S, et al. Truncated apolipoprotein E (apoE) causes increased intra-cellular calcium and may mediate apoE neuro-toxicity. J Neurosci 1999; 19: 7100–10

87. Qui Z, Crutcher KA, Hyman BT, Rebeck GW. ApoE isoforms affect neuronal NMDA calcium responses and toxicity via receptor-mediated processes. Neuroscience 2003; 122: 291–303

88. Nimpf J, Schneider WJ. From cholesterol transport to signal transduction: low density lipoprotein receptor, very low density lipo-protein receptor, and apolipoprotein E receptor-2. Biochim Biophys Acta 2000; 1529: 287–98

89. Herz J. Lipoprotein receptors: beacons to neurons? Trends Neurosci 2001; 24: 193–5

90. Herz J. The LDL receptor gene family: (un)expected signal transducers in the brain. Neuron 2001; 29: 571–81

91. Cooper JA, Howell BW. Lipoprotein receptors: signaling functions in the brain? Cell 1999; 97: 671–4

92. Bullido MJ, Valdivieso F. Apolipoprotein E gene promoter polymorphisms in Alzheimer's disease. Microsc Res Tech 2000; 50: 261–7

93. Teasdale GM, Nicoll JA, Murray G, Fiddes M. Association of apolipoprotein E polymorphism with outcome after head injury. Lancet 1997; 350: 1069–71

94. Tardiff BE, Newman MF, Saunders AM, et al. Preliminary report of a genetic basis for cognitive decline after cardiac operations. The Neurologic Outcome Research Group of the Duke Heart Center. Ann Thorac Surg 1997; 64: 715–20

95. Sorbi S, Nacmias N, Piacentini S, et al. ApoE as a prognostic factor for post-traumatic coma. Nat Med 1995; 1: 852

96. Slooter AJ, Tang MX, van Duijn CM, et al. Apolipoprotein E epsilon4 and the risk of dementia with stroke. A population-based investigation. J Am Med Assoc 1997; 277: 818–21

97. Mcarron MO, Muir KW, Weir CJ, et al. The apolipoprotein E epsilon4 allele and outcome in cerebrovascular disease. Stroke 1998; 29: 1882–7

98. Jordan BD, Relkin NR, Ravdin LD, et al. Apolipoprotein E epsilon4 associated with chronic traumatic brain injury in boxing. J Am Med Assoc 1997; 278: 136–40

99. Friedman G, Froom P, Sazbon L, et al. Apolipoprotein E-epsilon4 genotype predicts a poor outcome in survivors of traumatic brain injury. Neurology 1999; 52: 244–8

100. Alberts MJ, Graffagnino C, McClenny C, et al. ApoE genotype and survival from intracerebral haemorrhage. Lancet 1995; 346: 575

Comparison of the effects of apolipoprotein E4 on presynaptic and cytoskeletal plasticity following environmental stimulation

O Levi, DM Michaelson

INTRODUCTION

Alzheimer's disease (AD) is associated with genetic risk factors, of which the allele E4 of apolipoprotein E (apoE4) is the most prevalent,[1-3] and is affected by environmental factors such as education in early life and socioeconomic background.[4-6] The extent to which the phenotypic expression of the apoE genotype is affected by environmental factors and the mechanisms underlying such interactions are not known.

Environmental effects on neuronal and cognitive performance of rodents can be assessed by exposure to an enriched environment, which consists of social interactions, a running wheel and toys, and which increases synaptogenesis and improves learning and memory (for review, see Van Praag *et al.*[7]). Exposure of mice transgenic for human apoE on a mouse null-apoE background to an enriched environment revealed that young mice transgenic for apoE3, which is the benign AD apoE allele, improved their learning and memory. In contrast, mice transgenic for apoE4 were not so affected by the environmental stimulation, and their cognitive performance was similar to that of the non-enriched apoE3 transgenic mice.[8]

Furthermore, these cognitive effects were associated with increased hippocampal levels of the presynaptic protein synaptophysin, of the apoE3 but not of the apoE4 transgenic mice. In contrast, the cortical synaptophysin levels of the apoE3 and apoE4 transgenic mice were similarly elevated following environmental stimulation.[8]

The neuronal cytoskeleton plays a key role in numerous neuronal plasticity-related functions, which include neurite extension and retraction.[9-11] *In vitro* cell culture studies have revealed that neurite outgrowth is enhanced by apoE3 and inhibited by apoE4, and that these effects are associated with isoform-specific effects of apoE on neuronal microtubules and on the extent of polymerization of tubulin.[12] In the present study we investigated the extent to which impaired hippocampal synaptogenesis in apoE4 transgenic mice following environmental stimulation was associated with changes in the levels of cytoskeletal proteins. This was pursued by immunoblot measurements of the levels of tubulin and actin in the cortex and hippocampus of apoE3 and apoE4 transgenic mice, which were exposed to regular and enriched environments, and by comparing them to the corresponding synaptophysin levels.

EXPERIMENTAL PROCEDURES

Transgenic mice

Human apoE3 and apoE4 transgenic mice were generated on an apoE-deficient C57BL/6J background utilizing human apoE3 and apoE4 transgenic constructs as previously described.[13] The experiments were performed with the apoE3-453 and apoE4-81 lineages which express similar levels of brain apoE and which were back-bred with genetically homogeneous apoE-deficient mice (Jackson Laboratories, Bar Harbor, ME, USA; catalog no. N10JAX) for more than ten generations. The mice, which were heterozygous for the human apoE transgene and homozygous for mouse apoE deficiency, were genotyped by polymerase chain reaction (PCR) as previously described.[8]

Immunoblot analysis

The presently studied hippocampal and cortical brain samples were from the same animals that were previously used for showing that apoE4 impairs hippocampal plasticity in an isoform-specific manner, and blocks the environmental stimulation of synaptogenesis and memory.[8] Equal amounts of hippocampal and cortical homogenates of mice of each of the different groups (10 μg protein/lane for actin and tubulin and 1 μg/lane for synaptophysin) were loaded onto 12% polyacrylamide sodium dodecyl sulfate (SDS) gels that contained 26 lanes (Criterion system from BioRad, Hercules, CA, USA). The gels were then electrophoresed, blotted and stained with antitubulin (1 : 1000 from MabGenics, Gissen, Germany); antiactin (dilution 1 : 2500 from Santa-Cruz Biotechnology, Santa-Cruz, CA, USA); and antisynaptophysin (1 : 10000 from Sigma, St Louis, MO, USA) monoclonal antibodies. The resulting intensities of the corresponding immunoblot bands were determined utilizing the BIS-202 BioImaging System as previously described.[8] The use of wide 26-lane gels enabled the quantitative comparison, on the same gel, of up to 24 individual samples and two standards.

RESULTS AND DISCUSSION

The synaptophysin, tubulin and actin levels in the hippocampi and cortices of apoE3 and apoE4 transgenic mice are presented in Figure 15.1. As can be seen, environmental stimulation induced a three-fold increase in hippocampal synaptophysin of the apoE3 transgenic mice, whereas that of the apoE4 mice was unaffected by this treatment ($p < 0.002$ for group × treatment and for the difference between environmentally stimulated and regular apoE3 transgenic mice). In contrast, cortical synaptophysin levels were elevated in both mouse groups following environmental stimulation ($p < 0.001$ for the effect of treatment and for comparison of the environmentally stimulated and regular apoE3 transgenic mice and of the corresponding apoE4 transgenic mice). These findings suggest that the apoE4-mediated impairments in hippocampal plasticity are brain area-specific.

Environmental stimulation also affected the levels of tubulin in the hippocampus of the apoE transgenic mice. This effect, however, was much smaller than the observed changes in synaptophysin levels (i.e. less than 50% vs. up to 300%). Furthermore, statistical analysis of the results revealed a marginal effect of the environmental treatment ($p = 0.05$), and no effect of either group or group × treatment. Examination of the cortical tubulin levels revealed that they were unaffected by environmental stimulation in both the apoE3 and apoE4 transgenic mice.

Hippocampal actin levels were not affected either by the apoE genotype or by environmental

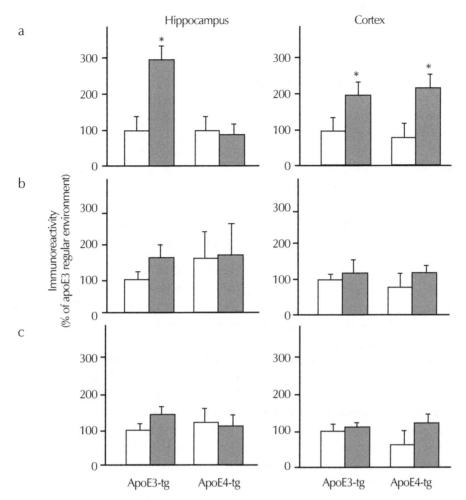

Figure 15.1 The effect of environmental stimulation on the levels of synaptophysin (a), tubulin (b) and actin (c) in the hippocampi and cortices of apolipoprotein (apo)E3 (ApoE3-tg) and apoE4 (ApoE4-tg) transgenic mice. Hippocampal and cortical homogenates were immunoblotted with antisynaptophysin (1 : 10 000), antitubulin (1 : 1000) and antiactin (1 : 2500) monoclonal antibodies, after which the resulting immunoblot bands were quantified by computerized densitometry as previously described.[8] Results shown are the means ± SD of four mice in each group and are presented relative to the sham-treated apoE3 transgenic mice. 100% = the mean of the sham-treated apoE3 transgenic mice. *$p < 0.001$

stimulation (Figure 15.1). There was, however, a small but significant reduction in the basal cortical levels of the apoE4 transgenic mice ($p < 0.01$), which was alleviated by environmental stimulation (Figure 15.1). In contrast, the cortical actin levels of the apoE3 transgenic mice were unaffected by environmental stimulation and were similar to those of the apoE4 mice following such treatment.

These findings suggest that the marked effects of environmental stimulation on brain synaptophysin levels are not associated with similar changes in the levels of actin and tubulin. The results further suggest that the isoform and brain area-specific inhibitory effects of apoE4 on hippocampal synaptophysin are not associated with parallel effects on the levels of actin and tubulin.

Previous neuronal cell culture studies revealed that apoE4 inhibits neurite outgrowth isoform specifically, and that this effect is associated with microtubular depolymerization.[12] Actin and tubulin, unlike synaptophysin, are not neuron specific. It is thus possible that local compartmentalized changes in the levels of actin and tubulin do occur, but that they are masked when assessed by immunoblot assays. This possibility is currently being investigated utilizing immunohistochemistry.

The hippocampal specificity of the inhibitory effects of apoE4 on the elevation of synaptophysin levels following environmental stimulation may be due either to differences in the response of hippocampal and cortical apoE receptors to apoE4, or to differential susceptibility of the cortex and hippocampus to the cellular processes which are induced by apoE4. Future studies of the levels and distributions of the different members of the apoE receptor family, and of the effects thereon of environmental stimulation, are needed in order to unravel the receptor(s) which mediate the isoform and brain area-specific synaptic effects of apoE4.

The finding that the cognitive impairments of apoE4 transgenic mice following environmental stimulation are associated with impaired hippocampal synaptic plasticity provides a novel mechanism by which the phenotypic expression of the apoE genotype can be mediated by environmental factors.

ACKNOWLEDGEMENTS

We thank Duke University and Glaxo Wellcome for kindly providing the transgenic mice, and Dr Orr from MabGenics GmBH for generously providing us with the antitubulin monoclonal antibody.

This work was supported in part by grants to D.M.M. from the Fund for Basic Research of the Israel Academy of Science and Humanities (grant no. 43/001); from the European Community (grant no. 2001/00972), and from the Jo and Inez Eichenbaum Foundation. D.M.M. is the incumbent of the Myriam Lebach Chair in Molecular Neurodegeneration.

REFERENCES

1. Corder EH, Saunders AM, Strittmatter WJ, et al. Gene dose of apolipoprotein E type 4 allele and the risk of Alzheimer's disease in late onset families. Science 1993; 261: 828–9

2. Saunders AM, Strittmatter WJ, Schmechel D, et al. Association of apolipoprotein E allele epsilon 4 with late-onset familial and sporadic Alzheimer's disease. Neurology 1993; 43: 1467–72

3. Roses AD. Alzheimer's disease: a model for gene mutations and susceptibility polymorphisms for complex psychiatric diseases. Am J Med Genet 1998; 81: 49–57.

4. Katzman R. Education and the prevalence of dementia and Alzheimer's disease. Neurology 1994; 43: 13–20

5. Kawas CH, Katzman R. Epidemiology of dementia and Alzheimer's disease. In Terry RD,

Bick KL, Sisodia SS, eds, Alzheimer's Disease, 2nd edn. Philadelphia: Lippincott, Williams & Wilkins, 1999: 95–116

6. Moceri VM, Kukull WA, Emanuel I, et al. Using census data and birth certificates to reconstruct the early life socio-economic environment and the relation to the development of Alzheimer's disease. Epidemiology 2001; 12: 383–9

7. Van Praag H, Kempermann G, Gage FH. Neural consequences of environmental enrichment. Nat Rev Neurosci 2000; 1: 191–8

8. Levi O, Jongen-Relo AL, Feldon J, et al. ApoE4 impairs hippocampal plasticity isoform-specifically and blocks the environmental stimulation of synaptogenesis and memory. Neurobiol Dis 2003; 13: 273–82

9. Avila J, Dominguez J, Diaz-Nido J. Regulation of microtubule dynamics by microtubule-associated protein expression and phos-phorylation during neuronal development. Int J Dev Biol 1994; 38: 13–25

10. Mandelkow E, Mandelkow EM. Microtubules and microtubule-associated proteins. Curr Opin Cell Biol. 1995; 7: 72–81

11. Wheal HV, Xchen Y, Mitchell J, et al. Molecular mechanisms that underlie structural and functional changes in postsynaptic membrane during synaptic plasticity. Prog Neurobiol 1998; 55: 611–40

12. Nathan BP, Bellosta S, Sanan DA, et al. Differential effects of apolipoproteins E3 and E4 on neuronal growth in vitro. Science 1994; 264: 850–2

13. Xu PT, Schmechel D, Rothrock-Christian T, et al. Human apolipoprotein E2, E3, and E4 isoform-specific transgenic mice: human-like pattern of glial and neuronal immunoreactivity in central nervous system not observed in wild-type mice. Neurobiol Dis 1996; 3: 229–45

Chapter 16

Cholesterol and the Aβ cascade: pathological implication of apolipoprotein E in Alzheimer's disease

K Yanagisawa

INTRODUCTION

From the time it was reported that the expression of one of the apolipoprotein E (apoE) alleles, ε4, is closely associated with the development of Alzheimer's disease (AD), it was suggested that cholesterol may be involved in the pathological processes of AD. This possibility has been strongly supported by evidence obtained from recent epidemiological[1,2] and biological studies.[3–9] On the other hand, one of the fundamental questions about the pathogenesis of AD is how soluble amyloid β-protein (Aβ) is converted to its aggregated form. In the case of familial AD, it is likely that deposition of AD in the brain is related to altered generation of Aβ. However, in the case of sporadic AD, a major form of the disease, no evidence has been reported that the generation of Aβ is changed. Based on these results, it would be interesting to investigate how pathological processes of Aβ aggregation could be modulated by cholesterol in the brain.

CHOLESTEROL-DEPENDENT ACCELERATION OF THE Aβ CASCADE

Aβ generation

It was previously reported that the processing of amyloid precursor protein (APP) was modulated by alteration in the cellular cholesterol concentration.[3,4] In 1998, Simons and co-investigators reported that the level of secreted Aβ from cultured cells was directly modulated by cellular cholesterol level: the suppression of *de novo* cholesterol synthesis by cells significantly induced a reduction in the level of Aβ generation.[5] With regard to the molecular mechanisms underlying cholesterol-dependent alteration in the levels of generated Aβ, several investigators suggested that the activities of α-, β- and γ-secretases are involved in the processing of APP.[3,4,6,8,9]

Aβ aggregation

Since no evidence has been provided that the generation of Aβ is altered in sporadic AD, it is reasonable to assume that Aβ aggregation in AD may be due to some, as yet unidentified, post-translational modifications of Aβ and/or altered clearance mechanisms. On this subject, we previously performed an immunochemical study to determine the mechanism(s) underlying the initiation of Aβ aggregation in the brain. We identified a unique Aβ species, which was characterized by its tight binding to GM1 ganglioside in brains exhibiting early pathological changes of AD.[10–12] Based on its unique molecular characteristics, we hypothesized that Aβ binds to GM1 ganglioside and adopts an altered conformation, and then acts as a seed for aggregation of soluble Aβ.[10–12] We further investigated the mechanism(s) underlying the binding of Aβ to GM1 ganglioside, and noted that an increase in the level of cholesterol in the membranes significantly accelerated the binding of Aβ to GM1 ganglioside.[13]

APOLIPOPROTEIN E-DEPENDENT MODULATION OF CHOLESTEROL DISTRIBUTION

Based on the evidence that one of the endogenous foci for Aβ aggregation, GM1 ganglioside-bound Aβ, is generated in a cholesterol-dependent manner, we attempted to examine the possibility that concentration and/or distribution of cholesterol in neuronal membranes may be altered by risk factors for the development of AD. We performed a lipid chemical analysis of human apoE knock-in mice (apoE3 and apoE4). In this experiment, we isolated subcellular fractions, including smooth and rough endoplasmic reticulum, and plasma membrane fractions.[14] Synaptic plasma membranes (SPM) were also isolated from mouse brains. From these materials, we determined the levels of lipids, including phospholipids and cholesterol (free and esterified). We also determined the transbilayer distribution of cholesterol in SPM by fluorescence-quenching assay using trinitro-benzene-sulfonic acid (TNBS) and dehydro-ergosterol (DHE). There were no significant differences in the levels of phospholipids and cholesterol in these fractions, including SPM, between wild-type, apoE3 knock-in, and apoE4 knock-in mice. However, in apoE4 knock-in mice, there was a significant increase and a concomitant decrease in cholesterol level in the exofacial and cytofacial leaflets of SPM, respectively.[14] These results suggest that apoE modulates the transbilayer distribution of cholesterol in the SPM in an isoform-dependent manner, leading to an increase in cholesterol level in the exofacial leaflet of SPM. Together with the results of our previous study, the increase in cholesterol level of the neuronal surface is likely to induce the formation of a GM1 ganglioside cluster,[13] which may be a receptor for soluble Aβ.

At this point, we are far from understanding the mechanism underlying the generation of asymmetry of cholesterol distribution in SPM; however, we recently observed that apoE potentially causes lipid efflux from cultured astrocytes and neurons in an isoform-dependent manner. The potency of apoE to cause lipid efflux was in the order of apoE2 > apoE3 > apoE4.[15] Thus, it may be possible to assume that an increase in cholesterol level in the exofacial leaflets of SPM in apoE4 knock-in mice is due to poor lipid efflux caused by apoE4. This possibility may be supported by the evidence that an increase in cholesterol level in the exofacial leaflet of SPM was previously confirmed in the brains of apoE knock-out mice.[16]

Alteration of transbilayer distribution of cholesterol with age

Previously, Igbavboa and co-investigators reported that increasing age altered transbilayer fluidity and cholesterol asymmetry in SPM of the mouse brain.[17] In that study, they noted that there was an approximately two-fold increase in exofacial leaflet cholesterol level in the oldest group compared with the youngest group. Aging is the strongest risk factor for the development of AD. Thus, together with the results of our study of apoE knock-in mice, it is suggested that an increase in cholesterol level in the exofacial leaflet of SPM, caused by alteration in the asymmetric distribution of cholesterol, may be critical for the initiation of Aβ aggregation through the generation of seed Aβ molecules (Figure 16.1).

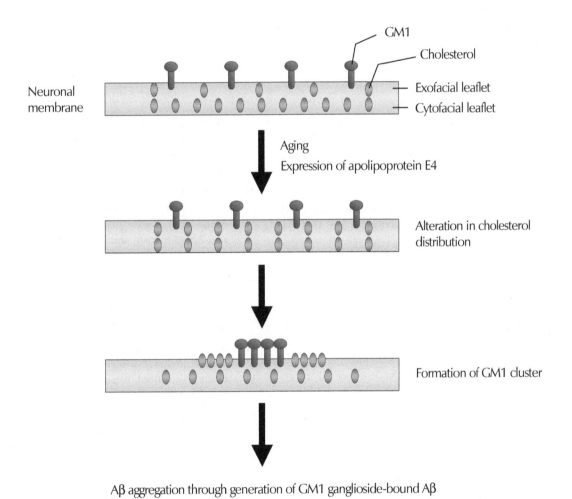

Figure 16.1 Hypothetical model of alteration of asymmetric distribution of cholesterol in the synaptic plasma membrane, and the formation of a GM1 cluster which could be a receptor for soluble amyloid β-protein (Aβ)

CONCLUSION

The generation of GM1 ganglioside-bound Aβ, one of the candidates for an endogenous focus for amyloid fibril formation in the AD brain, depends on the increase in cholesterol level in the neuronal membrane. ApoE4 knock-in mice showed a significant increase in cholesterol level in the exofacial leaflet of SPM. Based on these results, one could assume that one of the possible pathological implications of apoE in the development of AD may be an alteration of cholesterol distribution in neuronal membranes.

ACKNOWLEDGEMENTS

The author would like to thank Dr Fujita and his collegues of Mitsubishi Kagaku Institute for Life Science, Dr Matsuzaki of Kyoto University and Drs Wood and Igbavboa for providing human apoE knock-in mice, for the physicochemical study of GM1 ganglioside-bound Aβ and for the lipid chemical analysis of human apoE knock-in mice, respectively.

REFERENCES

1. Wolozin B, Kellman W, Ruosseau P, et al. Decreased prevalence of Alzheimer disease associated with 3-hydroxy-3-methylglutaryl coenzyme A reductase inhibitors. Arch Neurol 2000; 57: 1439–43

2. Jick H, Zornberg GL, Jick SS, et al. Statins and the risk of dementia. Lancet 2000; 356: 1627–31

3. Bodovitz S, Klein WL. Cholesterol modulates α-secretase cleavage of amyloid precursor protein. J Biol Chem 1996; 271: 4436–40

4. Racchi M, Baetta R, Salvietti N, et al. Secretory processing of amyloid precursor protein is inhibited by increase in cellular cholesterol content. Biochem J 1997; 322: 893–8

5. Simons M, Keller P, De Strooper B, et al. Cholesterol depletion inhibits the generation of β-amyloid in hippocampal neurons. Proc Natl Acad Sci USA 1998; 95: 6460–4

6. Frears ER, Stephens DJ, Walters CE, et al. The role of cholesterol in the biosynthesis of β-amyloid. Neuroreport 1999; 10: 1699–705

7. Refolo LM, Malester B, LaFrancois J, et al. Hypercholesterolemia accelerates the Alzheimer's amyloid pathology in a transgenic mouse model. Neurobiol Dis 2000; 7: 321–31

8. Kojro E, Gimpl G, Lammich S, et al. Low cholesterol stimulates the nonamyloidogenic pathway by its effect on the α-secretase ADAM 10. Proc Natl Acad Sci USA 2001; 98: 5815–20

9. Fassbender K, Simons M, Bergmann C, et al. Simvastatin strongly reduces levels of Alzheimer's disease β-amyloid peptides Aβ 42 and Aβ 40 in vitro and in vivo. Proc Natl Acad Sci USA 2001; 98: 5856–61

10. Yanagisawa K, Odaka A, Suzuki N, Ihara Y. GM1 ganglioside-bound amyloid β-protein (Aβ): a possible form of preamyloid in Alzheimer's disease. Nat Med 1995; 1: 1062–6

11. Yanagisawa K, Ihara Y. GM1 ganglioside-bound amyloid β-protein in Alzheimer's disease brain. Neurobiol Aging 1998; 19 (Suppl 1): S65–7

12. Yanagisawa K, McLaurin J, Michikawa M, et al. Amyloid β-protein (Aβ) associated wih lipid molecules: immunoreactivity distinct from that of soluble Aβ. FEBS Lett 1997; 420: 43–6

13. Kakio A, Nishimoto SI, Yanagisawa K, et al. Cholesterol-dependent formation of GM1 ganglioside-bound amyloid β-protein, an endogenous seed for Alzheimer amyloid. J Biol Chem 2001; 276: 24985–90

14. Hayashi H, Igbavboa U, Hamanaka H, et al. Cholesterol is increased in the exofacial leaflet of synaptic plasma membranes of human apolipoprotein E4 knock-in mice. Neuroreport 2002; 13: 383–6

15. Michikawa M, Fan QW, Isobe I, Yanagisawa K. Apolipoprotein E exhibits isoform-specific promotion of lipid efflux from astrocytes and neurons in culture. J Neurochem 2000; 74: 1008–16

16. Igbavboa U, Avdulov NA, Chochina SV, Wood WG. Transbilayer distribution of cholesterol is modified in brain synaptic plasma membranes of knockout mice deficient in the low-density lipoprotein receptor, apolipoprotein E, or both proteins. J Neurochem 1997; 69: 1661–7

17. Igbavboa U, Avdulov NA, Schroeder F, Wood WG. Increasing age alters transbilayer fluidity and cholesterol asymmetry in synaptic plasma membranes of mice. J Neurochem 1996; 66: 1717–25

Chapter 17

Brain inflammation and psychogeriatric diseases

H Akiyama, H Uchikado

BRAIN INFLAMMATION AND NEURONS

The long-held concept of the immune privilege of the brain has been revised significantly in the past 15 years. The blood–brain barrier (BBB) exists, but isolation from the periphery by the BBB is not as complete as it was thought to be and plays a limited role in the immune privilege. Recent evidence suggests that the brain parenchyma has unique mechanisms for regulating immune and inflammatory responses. For example, expression of CD200,[1] intercellular adhesion molecule (ICAM)-5/telencephalin[2] and transforming growth factor (TGF)-β[3] may contribute to the maintenance of the anti-inflammatory environment of the brain. Despite these mechanisms, low-grade inflammation occurs in association with brain lesions such as Alzheimer's disease,[4] cerebrovascular diseases and head trauma, with the full complexity of peripheral inflammatory responses. Studies on these non-immunological diseases have revealed that the brain has its own innate immune system and shares a variety of cytokines and other bioactive molecules with the peripheral immune system.

In the brain, microglia and astrocytes are thought to be the major cell populations that are engaged in the inflammatory responses. In a classic view, neurons are regarded as cells that perform only passive roles in inflammation. Neurons may become bystander victims that fuel the inflammatory processes by providing cell debris, which has to be removed by phagocytic cells and triggers further activation of these cells. However, there is a growing body of evidence that neurons not only respond to a number of inflammatory mediators but also produce many pro- and anti-inflammatory molecules.[5] These include complement proteins and inflammatory cytokines, as well as cyclo-oxygenase (COX)-2, prostaglandin E_2 receptors and inducible nitric oxide synthase, iNOS. Figure 17.1 illustrates the expression of COX-2 by hippocampal pyramidal neurons in an Alzheimer's disease patient, complicated with prolonged convulsion at the agonal stage. Interestingly, the literature indicates that some inflammatory molecules are involved in the modulation of neuronal functions such as neurotransmission.[5–7]

The physiological relevance of inflammatory molecules in neuronal activity leads to the hypothesis that mild or moderate inflammation, which does not visibly destroy brain tissue, can interfere with brain functions. It has been known that very strong systemic inflammation, as in

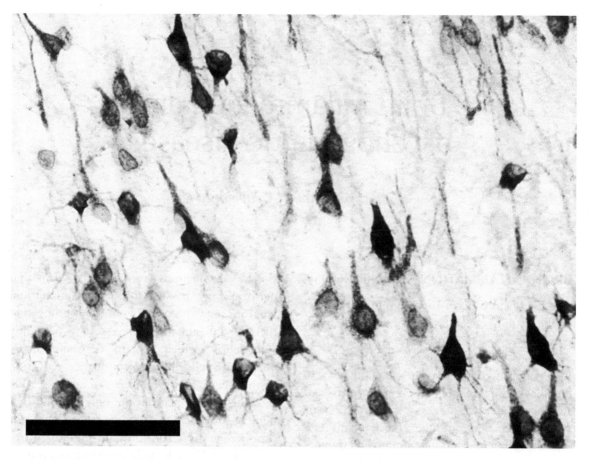

Figure 17.1 Cyclo-oxygenase-2 expression by hippocampal pyramidal neurons. An Alzheimer's disease case complicated with prolonged convulsion at the agonal stage. Scale bar, 100 μm

sepsis and toxic shock syndrome, are associated with central nervous system symptoms.[8,9] Clinical manifestations include delirium and other consciousness abnormalities, which are generally considered to be transient disorders. In these conditions, peripheral inflammation appears to disturb neural transmission in the absence of apparent encephalitic pathology. It has to be emphasized that, in elderly patients with such brain lesions as Alzheimer's disease or cerebrovascular diseases, even mild systemic inflammatory diseases frequently cause delirium.[6,10,11]

ACTIVATION OF VASCULAR CELLS BY SYSTEMIC INFLAMMATION

Vascular endothelial cells and perivascular cells are located at the interface between the peripheral blood and the brain parenchyma. These cells could therefore be involved in the transmission of inflammation from the periphery to the brain. The BBB may be effective in preventing large molecules such as complement and other inflammatory proteins from entering the brain. However, it may easily pass inflammatory signals through activation of these vascular cells.

We investigated activation of vascular endothelial cells and perivascular cells in the cerebral cortex of postmortem brain from patients with or without brain lesions. Many patients suffer from a variable degree of systemic inflammation at the agonal stage. In some cases, we used serum concentrations of an acute-phase reactant, C-reactive protein (CRP), as an index of systemic inflammation. Since the serum concentration of CRP at the agonal stage was available only in a limited number of patients, we estimated the degree of systemic inflammation by the intensity of immuno-histochemical staining of the residual blood in brain tissue for CRP. In cases where we were able to obtain from the clinical records the serum CRP concentration on the day of or a day before death, intensity of CRP immunoreactivity in brain tissue showed a good correlation with serum CRP concentration.

Activation of vascular endothelial cells was investigated with three markers: ICAM-1, CD40 and COX-2. ICAM-1 is a cell adhesion molecule that belongs to the immunoglobulin superfamily. In the periphery, ICAM-1 expression plays a principal role in leukocyte adhesion to vascular endothelial cells and subsequent infiltration into tissues at the site of inflammation.[12] In the brain, reactive astrocytes and vascular endothelial cells express ICAM-1.[13] Figure 17.2a illustrates low expression of ICAM-1 by vascular endothelial cells in a control case without systemic inflammation. In cases without significant brain lesions, ICAM-1 immuno-reactivity increased in parallel with the degree of systemic inflammation (Figure 17.2b). In neurological cases such as Alzheimer's disease, the correlation was less clear. A number of cases with brain lesions were high in vascular ICAM-1 expression even in the absence of systemic inflammation (Figure 17.2c).

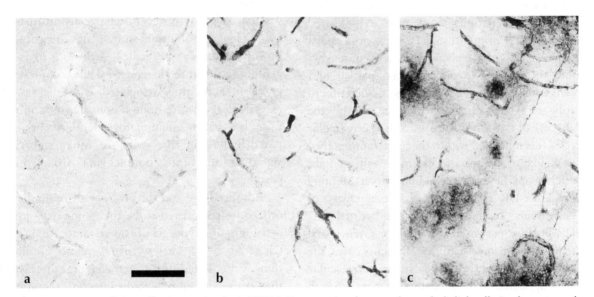

Figure 17.2 Intercellular adhesion molecule-1 (ICAM-1) expression by vascular endothelial cells in the temporal cortex. (a) A control case without systemic inflammation. Scale bar, 100 μm. a–c are at the same magnification. (b) A control case with strong systemic inflammation at the agonal stage. (c) A case with Alzheimer's disease without systemic inflammation. Patchy labeling of the brain parenchyma indicates ICAM-1 expression by reactive astrocytes around senile plaques. Note that vascular ICAM-1 expression is comparable with that in (b) even in the absence of systemic inflammation

The other two markers, CD40 and COX-2, showed similar changes. CD40 is a cell-surface molecule that is involved in immune and inflammatory processes and is overexpressed upon inflammation.[14,15] In the human brain, CD40 is expressed by reactive microglia and vascular endothelial cells.[16] COX is the rate-limiting enzyme in the conversion of arachidonic acid to prostanoids. COX-2 is the inducible isoform of COX and is expressed by neurons and vascular endothelial cells in the brain. The intensity of vascular staining for CD40 and COX-2 generally paralleled the degree of systemic inflammation in cases without brain lesions, although a number of cases with brain lesions showed increased expression of CD40 and COX-2 by vascular endothelial cells in the absence of systemic inflammation.

Activation of perivascular cells was investigated with immunostaining for HLA-DR and CD68. Perivascular cells constitute, with meningeal macrophages, a monocyte-derived phagocytic population.[17] Therefore, perivascular cells share phenotypes with parenchymal microglia. We distinguished perivascular cells from microglia by their close association to collagen IV positive vasculature and by the absence of ramified processes. Since perivascular cells are embedded within the basal lamina, they look like a part of the vascular wall on light microscopy. In postmortem brain tissue, staining for HLA-DR revealed a variable intensity of perivascular cell labeling. The number of HLA-DR-positive perivascular cells in a given visual field varied from case to case. In many cases, the occurrence of HLA-DR-positive perivascular cells appeared to be increased in parallel with the degree of systemic inflammation. In cases with brain lesions, the relationship was less clear. It seemed that expression of HLA-DR by perivascular cells was increased by both systemic inflammation and brain lesions. The occurrence

of CD68-positive perivascular cells showed similar changes; it was increased upon systemic inflammation. A number of neurological cases exhibited high CD68 expression by perivascular cells even in the absence of systemic inflammation.

INFLAMMATION AND DELIRIUM

Our results indicate that systemic inflammation activates vascular endothelial cells and .perivascular cells in the brain. Brain parenchymal lesions also activate these vascular cells. In the brains of patients with neurodegenerative diseases, activated microglia and astrocytes are capable of producing a great variety of pro-inflammatory mediators,[4] which may raise the inflammatory level of the brain parenchyma and activate the vascular cells. It seems that inflammatory stimuli in the peripheral blood and the brain parenchyma adjunctly activate the vascular cells. Activated vascular cells, in turn, could be a potential source of diffusible proinflammatory molecules such as prostaglandin E_2[18] and nitric oxide.[19] Thus, even low-grade inflammation associated with the pre-existing degenerative brain lesions may not only raise the basal inflammatory level of brain parenchyma but also enhance inflammatory signaling to brain parenchyma from the periphery.

Advanced age and the presence of brain disorders are considered to be the major risks for delirium, an acute confusional state that is triggered by a variety of systemic conditions.[10,11,20] The different extracerebral diseases that cause delirium include infection, trauma and major surgery, many of which are associated with systemic inflammation. We consider that the adjunctive pro-inflammatory effect of peripheral inflammation and parenchymal lesions to brain vasculature are a part of the mechanism that increases the risk of delirium in patients with brain disorders. While strong systemic inflammation can induce central nervous system symptoms by itself,[8,9] mild to moderate systemic inflammation may also cause similar symptoms if the patients have preexisting parenchymal lesions. Our results may therefore explain the vulnerability of neurological patients to delirium caused by inflammatory systemic conditions. Appropriate anti-inflammatory agents might, therefore, be a potential treatment of delirium in elderly neurological patients.

REFERENCES

1. Wright GJ, Jones M, Puklavec MJ, et al. The unusual distribution of the neuronal/lymphoid cell surface CD200 (OX2) glycoprotein is conserved in humans. Immunology 2001; 102: 173–9

2. Lindsberg PJ, Launes J, Tian M, et al. Release of soluble ICAM-5, a neuronal adhesion molecule, in acute encephalitis. Neurology 2002; 58: 446–51

3. Milner R, Campbell IL. The extracellular matrix and cytokines regulate microglial integrin expression and activation. J Immunol 2003; 170: 3850–8

4. Neuroinflammation Working Group: Akiyama H, Barger S, Barnum S, et al. Inflammation and Alzheimer's disease. Neurobiol Aging 2000; 21: 383–421

5. Akiyama H, Neurons. In: Rogers J, ed. Neuroinflammatory Mechanisms in Alzheimer's Disease. Basel: Birkhauser, 2001: 225–36

6. Eikelenboom P, Hoogendijk WJG, Jonker C, van Tilburg W. Immunological mechanisms and the spectrum of psychiatric syndrome in Alzheimer's disease. J Psychogeriat Res 2002; 36: 269–80

7. Kaufmann WE, Worley PF, Pegg J, et al. COX-2, a synaptically induced enzyme, is expressed by excitatory neurons at postsynaptic sites in rat cerebral cortex. Proc Natl Acad Sci USA 1996; 93: 2317–21

8. Rosene KA, Copass MK, Kastner LS, et al. Persistent neuropsychological sequelae of toxic shock syndrome. Ann Intern Med 1982; 96: 865–70

9. Young GB, Bolton CF, Austin TW, et al. The encephalopathy associated with septic illness. Clin Invest Med 1990; 13: 297–304

10. Eikelenboom P, Hoogendijk WJG. Do delirium and Alzheimer's dementia share specific pathogenetic mechanisms? Dementia Geriatr Cogn Disord 1999; 10: 319–24

11. Elie M, Cole MG, Primeau FJ, Bellavance F. Delirium risk factors in elderly hospitalized patients. J Gen Intern Med 1998; 13: 204–12

12. Carlos TM, Harlan JM. Membrane proteins involved in phagocyte adherence to endothelium. Immunol Rev 1990; 114: 5–28

13. Akiyama H, Kawamata T, Yamada T, et al. Expression of intercellular adhesion molecule (ICAM)-1 by a subset of astrocytes in Alzheimer and some other degenerative neurological disorders. Acta Neuropathol 1993; 85: 628–34

14. Alderson MR, Armitage RJ, Tough TW, et al. CD40 expression by human monocytes: regulation by cytokines and activation of monocytes by the ligand for CD40. J Exp Med 1993; 178: 669–74

15. Karmann K, Hughes CCW, Schechner J, et al. CD40 on human endothelial cells: inducibility by cytokines and functional regulation of

adhesion molecule expression. Proc Natl Acad Sci USA 1995; 92: 4342–6

16. Togo T, Akiyama H, Kondo H, et al. Expression of CD40 in the brain of Alzheimer's disease and other neurological diseases. Brain Res 2000; 885: 117–21

17. Gehrmann J, Matsumoto Y, Kreutzberg GW. Microglia: intrinsic immune effector cell of the brain. Brain Res Rev 1995; 20: 269–87

18. Ek M, Engblom D, Saha S, et al. Pathway across the blood-brain barrier. Nature 2001; 410: 430–1

19. Wong Ma-Li, Rettori V, AlShekhlee A, et al. Inducible nitric oxide synthase gene expression in the brain during systemic inflammation. Nature Med 1996; 2: 581–4

20. Lerner AJ, Hedera P, Koss E, Stuckey J, Friedland RP. Delirium in Alzheimer disease. Alzheimer Dis Assoc Disord 1997; 11: 16–20

Neuroinflammatory mechanisms are involved in the early steps of the pathological cascade in Alzheimer's disease

P Eikelenboom, JJM Hoozemans, JM Rozemuller, R Veerhuis, WA van Gool

OVERVIEW

Amyloid plaques in Alzheimer's disease (AD) brains are closely associated with a locally induced, non-immune-mediated, chronic inflammatory response. Clinicopathological and neuroradiological studies have shown that activation of microglia is a relatively early pathogenic event that precedes the process of neuropil destruction in AD. Recent epidemiological studies have suggested that increased serum levels of some acute-phase reactants are associated with an increased risk of AD and that polymorphisms of certain cytokines, most notably interleukin-1, are genetic risk factors of AD. Epidemiological studies have also shown that the use of classical non-steroidal anti-inflammatory drugs (NSAIDs) can prevent the risk of AD; however, clinical trials with anti-inflammatory drugs have failed to arrest disease progression. These findings indicate that anti-inflammatory drugs can be helpful in the prevention but not in the treatment of AD. Thus, pathological, genetic and pharmacoepidemiological studies suggest that inflammatory mechanisms are most likely to be involved in the early steps of the pathological cascade in AD.

Independent of the etiological agent, AD is characterized at the histopathological level by extracellular deposits of amyloid-β (Aβ) protein in senile plaques and abnormal accumulation of paired helical filaments (PHFs) in neurofibrillary tangles, dystrophic neurites and neuropil threads. The view that an altered metabolism of β-amyloid precursor protein (βAPP) with progressive deposition of its Aβ fragment should be considered as the key step in the molecular pathogenesis of AD is strongly supported by the findings that all the three causal genes (*APP*, *PS1*, *PS2*) increase the propensity of Aβ to aggregate and to form insoluble fibrils, thus accelerating the deposition of Aβ. These findings stimulated the controversial concept that AD may be a purely 'amyloid-driven' process, with the neurofibrillary tangles and neuropil threads as secondary phenomena that are closely related to the syndrome of dementia.[1] AD probably results from a complex sequence of steps involving multiple factors beyond the production of Aβ alone. Several lines of evidence have indicated that an inflammatory process contributes to the pathology of AD. First, a variety of inflammatory proteins are reported to be associated with the neuritic plaques. The finding that amyloid plaques are characterized by the presence of activated complement factors and clusters of activated microglia cells strongly suggests an inflammatory process. Second, some polymorphisms of cytokines and higher serum levels of certain acute-phase proteins are risk factors for AD. Third, data obtained from epidemiological studies suggest that anti-inflammatory drugs can prevent or retard the development of AD.

A CHRONIC INFLAMMATORY RESPONSE IN ALZHEIMER'S DISEASE BRAINS

The observations that plaques are characterized by the presence of activated complement factors and clusters of activated microglia in the absence of immunoglobulins and T-cell subsets have stimulated the view that amyloid plaques are closely associated with a locally induced, non-immune-mediated, chronic inflammatory response. The finding that fibrillar Aβ can bind complement factor C1 and, hence, stimulate the classical pathway of complement in an antibody fashion supports the concept that fibrillar Aβ itself can induce a local inflammatory response.[2] After the initial report of the presence of complement factors in senile plaques, a large number of mostly inflammation-related proteins were described to be associated with Aβ plaques.[3] These so-called Aβ-associated proteins include several complement factors, α_1-antichymotrypsin, intercellular adhesion molecule (ICAM)-1, α_2-macroglobulin, clusterin, apolipoprotein E, serum amyloid P component and heparan sulfate proteoglycan. *In vitro* studies have shown that these proteins are involved in Aβ fibrillogenesis, deposition and removal. Findings in transgenic human APP mice show that α_1-antichymotrypsin and apolipoprotein E lead to higher amyloid load, whereas inhibition of complement results in lower brain amyloid load. These observations support the idea that certain Aβ-associated

proteins play an important role in the dynamic balance between brain amyloid deposition and removal. The activated microglial cells in the cerebral cortex of AD patients are mainly found as clusters associated with congophilic deposits in senile plaques. Clinicopathological studies have revealed that these microglia/amyloid plaques were significantly increased in the cerebral cortex of AD patients at an early stage, while extensive tau pathology was found in the later stages of the disease.[4,5] Recent data, based on the use of positron emission tomography (PET) using the peripheral benzodiazepine ligand PK11195 as a marker for activated microglial cells, support the notion that activation of microglia is an early pathogenic event that precedes cerebral atrophy.[6] Neuropathological and neuroradiological studies have indicated that activation of microglia is a relatively early pathogenic event that precedes the process of neuropil destruction in AD patients. Similarly, it has been found that the onset of microglial activation coincides with the earliest changes in cerebral morphology in mouse scrapie models, many weeks before neuronal loss and subsequent clinical signs of disease.[7]

Although the role of inflammatory molecules in the pathological process of AD is not fully understood, current findings indicate that these molecules may be involved in a number of key steps in the proposed amyloid-driven cascade (Figure 18.1):[8]

1. It has been shown that interleukin (IL)-1 (possibly together with other cytokines) can regulate APP synthesis and Aβ production *in vitro*. Such a cytokine production *in vivo* may initiate a vicious cycle whereby Aβ deposits stimulate further cytokine production by activated microglia to even higher synthesis rates of APP and its Aβ fragments.

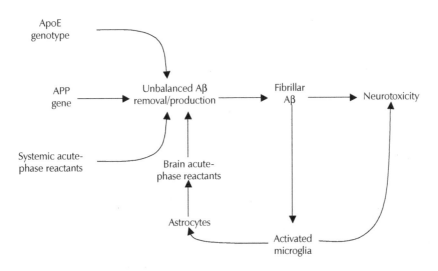

Figure 18.1 The role of inflammatory molecules in the pathological cascade of Alzheimer's disease

2. The Aβ-associated proteins (most of which are acute-phase proteins) are involved in regulation of the Aβ amyloidogenic process. There appears to be an imbalance in AD brains between those Aβ-associated proteins that stimulate fibril formation and deposition, and those Aβ-associated proteins that prevent it.

3. Once fibrils are deposited, Aβ can induce a microglia-mediated chronic inflammatory response. Activated microglial cells, particularly those in the vicinity of neuritic plaques, have been shown to be immunoreactive for IL-1, IL-6 and tumor necrosis factor-α (TNF-α). Activated microglial cells can produce and release potentially toxic products, including reactive oxygen species, proinflammatory cytokines, excitotoxins and proteases, which could damage the neighboring neurons. For this reason, activated microglial cells might contribute to neuronal degeneration.

Therefore, it is important to keep in mind that the involvement of numerous inflammatory proteins in the pathological cascade is not related to a single pathogenic event but to a number of subsequent steps. Moreover, the beneficial or detrimental effects of all these distinct steps are not well known. On the one hand, inflammatory activation by Aβ could be viewed as a potential contributor to AD neurodegenerative processes. Alternatively, inflammatory mechanisms, particularly complement-mediated mechanisms, may also play a necessary role in microglia-mediated Aβ removal. For this reason the role of inflammation as a double-edged sword in neurodegenerative disorders attracts much interest in AD research.[9]

ACUTE-PHASE RESPONSE IN ALZHEIMER'S DISEASE PATIENTS

Tissue injuries and infections, which represent a threat to the integrity of an organism, appear to require readjustments in the usual metabolic and physiological equilibria. In addition to the local tissue response, systemic changes occur which are referred to as 'acute-phase responses'. The acute-phase response can be considered as part of a complex generalized stress reaction in which the activation of the sympathetic nervous system coincides with endocrine changes, such as activation of the hypothalamic–pituitary–adrenal (HPA) axis. Abnormalities of the HPA system in AD patients include both basal cortisol hypersecretion and insufficient cortisol suppression following dexamethasone administration. Non-suppression of cortisol during the dexamethasone suppression test has been shown to occur in up to 50% of non-depressed AD patients.[10] With respect to the activation of the sympathetic nervous system, the surviving noradrenergic neurons in the locus coeruleus of AD patients show increased activity compared with those of non-demented controls.[11]

Another important systemic consequence of a local inflammatory response is a change in plasma concentrations of a group collectively known as acute-phase reactants. In serum from AD patients, a significant increase in the levels of several acute-phase reactants has been reported. Most notably, an increase of the acute-phase reactant α_1-antichymotrypsin has been described in several studies.[12] Moreover, although not conclusively established, increased levels of IL-6, and TNF-α, and decreased levels of albumin, have been reported in AD patients.[13]

These findings on the activation of the HPA axis and the sympathetic nervous system, together with changes in the serum levels of some acute-phase proteins, indicate that a systemic acute-phase response can be found in AD patients. The acute-phase response found in AD patients can perhaps be considered as a relatively late and non-specific disease phenomenon. However, recent epidemiological studies favor the conclusion that the acute-phase response in AD patients can be a crucial part of the pathophysiology of AD. In prospective case–cohort studies it has been found that high

serum levels of the acute-phase proteins α_1-antichymotrypsin, C-reactive protein and IL-6, and low serum levels of insulin-like growth factor-I, were each associated with an increased risk of AD.[14–16] These findings strongly indicate that non-demented patients with a profile of an acute-phase response in serum are at risk of developing AD. The acute-phase response is initiated and orchestrated by cytokines, most notably IL-1. Several studies have shown that specific polymorphisms of certain cytokines are associated with AD, suggesting that there seems to be a genetically determined role for cytokines, especially related to the IL-1 family, in modifying the risk of AD.[17,18]

ANTI-INFLAMMATORY DRUGS

The suggestion that the neuroinflammatory response is an interesting target for treatment with anti-inflammatory drugs was stimulated by epidemiological studies showing that the use of classical NSAIDs could prevent or retard AD.[19,20] During the past few years, four large randomized controlled trials with anti-inflammatory drugs have been performed, in which treatment lasted for 12–18 months. Studies on the effect of prednisone, hydro-chloroquine, naproxen (a non-cyclo-oxygenase (COX)-specific inhibitor), rofecoxib and celecoxib (COX-2-specific NSAIDs) in patients with early AD, all failed to document a benefit in favor of patients who were treated with the specific anti-inflammatory drug under study.[21,22] Taken together, it is clear that the best available evidence to date does not support the suggestion that AD patients benefit from treatment with anti-inflammatory drugs.

Thus, in respect to a potential beneficial effect of anti-inflammatory drugs in AD, there is a striking difference between the beneficial effects of NSAIDs in epidemiological studies and the negative results of clinical trials with anti-inflammatory drugs in AD patients. A possible explanation for this discrepancy is that the positive epidemiological findings are reported for the classical NSAIDs that are known to inhibit both COX-1 and COX-2, but that have also other modes of action that are independent of COX activity. Some of the widely used classical NSAIDs, such as indomethacin and ibuprofen, can activate peroxisome proliferator receptor γ (PPRAγ), a nuclear receptor that has been shown to inhibit the expression of a wide range of pro-inflammatory genes. In addition, these classical NSAIDs also have a direct lowering effect on Aβ(1-42) production, independent of COX activity. However, these COX-independent effects of classical NSAIDs require much higher doses than the dosage used in the epidemiological studies. The other explanation for the discrepancy between the epidemiological findings and the clinical trials is the timing of anti-inflammatory treatment.[22] Inhibition of the neuroinflammatory response at the time that clear symptoms of dementia are present might simply be too late to attenuate the detrimental effects of the inflammatory process. If that is the case, anti-inflammatory agents can be helpful in the prevention, but not in the treatment, of AD.

DISCUSSION

During the past decade the research agenda for unravelling the pathogenesis of AD was strongly dominated by findings in rare familial autosomal dominant variants of AD. The finding that all causal genes led to higher production of Aβ(1-42) has strongly stimulated the concept that faulty metabolism of βAPP

with increased production of its Aβ fragment must be considered as the crucial pathogenic event in all forms of AD. However, it is becoming increasingly clear that factors other than faulty metabolism of APP can initiate or stimulate the pathological cascade.

In this chapter we have reviewed the evidence from genetic, pathological and treatment studies, indicating that inflammation-related mechanisms are most likely to be involved in the early stages of the pathological process. The involvement of cytokines and acute-phase proteins in Aβ production, and in fibril formation, deposition and removal, indicate that inflammatory molecules are involved in early key events in the pathological cascade. In this respect the findings in transgenic mouse models are revealing. On the one hand, these models convincingly documented the important effects of APP or presenilin mutants, but, on the other hand, it was shown that cross-breeding of mice with variations in the expression of Aβ-associated proteins strongly influenced the rate and load of cerebral amyloid deposition. The critical pathogenic event in AD seems to be an imbalance between Aβ production and removal. In the familial autosomal dominant forms of AD the overproduction of Aβ(1-42) is the main factor responsible for this imbalance.

Recent studies reviewed in this chapter suggest a role for inflammatory molecules in the deposition and removal of Aβ. Multiple factors seem to be involved in the imbalance between cerebral Aβ production and removal. This could explain why AD is heterogeneous and multifactorial in its etiology, while the clinical picture and neuropathological end-stage characteristics are strikingly uniform, irrespective of the specific etiological factor in the several forms of AD.

REFERENCES

1. Selkoe DJ. Translating cell biology into therapeutic advances in Alzheimer's disease. Nature 1999; 399: A21–31

2. Rogers J, Cooper NL, Webster S, et al. Complement activation by β-amyloid in Alzheimer's disease. Proc Natl Acad Sci USA 1992; 89: 10016–20

3. Akiyama H, Barker S, Barnum S, et al. Inflammation and Alzheimer's disease. Neurobiol Aging 2000; 21: 383–421

4. Arends YM, Duyckaerts C, Rozemuller JM, et al. Microglia, amyloid and dementia in Alzheimer's disease. A correlative study. Neurobiol Aging 2000; 21: 39–47

5. Vehmas AK, Kawas CH, Stewart WF, et al. Immunoreactive cells in senile plaque and cognitive decline in Alzheimer's disease. Neurobiol Aging 2003; 24: 321–31

6. Cagnin A, Brooks DJ, Kennedy AM, et al. In-vivo measurement of microglia in dementia. Lancet 2001; 358: 461–7

7. Williams AE, Van Dam A-M, Eikelenboom P, et al. Immunocytochemical appearance of cyto-kines, prostaglandin E2 and lipocortin-1 in the CNS during the incubation period of murine scrapie correlates with progressive PrP accumulations. Brain Res 1997; 754: 171–80

8. Eikelenboom P, Bate C, Van Gool WA, et al. Neuroinflammation in Alzheimer's disease and prion disease. Glia 2002; 40: 232–9

9. Wyss-Coray T, Muckle L. Inflammation in neurodegenerative disease: a double-edged sword. Neuron 2002; 35: 419–32

10. Molchan SE, Hill JL, Mellow AM, et al. The dexamethasone supression test in Alzheimer's disease and major depression: relationship to dementia severity, depression and CSF monoamines. Int Psychogeriatr 1990; 2: 99–122

11. Hoogendijk WJG, Feenstra MGP, Botterblom MH, et al. Increased activity of surviving locus coeruleus neurons in Alzheimer's disease, Ann Neurol 1999; 45: 82–91

12. Licastro F, Parnetti L, Morini C, et al. Acute phase reactant alpha1-antichymotrypsin is increased in cerebrospinal fluid and serum of patients with probable Alzheimer's disease. Alzheimer Dis Assoc Disord 1995: 9; 112–18

13. Maes M, DeVos N, Waurets A, et al. Inflammatory markers in younger vs elderly normal volunteers and in patients with Alzheimer's disease. J Psychiatr Res 1999; 33: 397–405

14. Engelhart MJ. Inflammation, nutrition and the risk of Alzheimer's disease. The Rotterdam Study PhD thesis. Erasmus University, Rotterdam, 2002

15. Dik MG, Pluijm SM, Jonker C, et al. Insulin-like growth factor I (IGF-I) and cognitive decline in older persons. Neurobiol Aging 2003; 24: 533–81

16. Yaffe K, Lindquist MS, Pennix BW, et al. Inflammatory markers and cognition in well-functioning African-American and white elders. Neurology 2003; 51: 76–80

17. Nicoll JA, Mrak RE, Graham DI, et al. Association of interleukin-1 gene poly-morphisms with Alzheimer's disease. Ann Neurol 2000; 47: 365–8

18. Du Y, Dodel RC, Eastwood BJ, et al. Association of an interleukin-1α poly-morphisms with Alzheimer's disease. Neurology 2000; 55: 480–3

19. McGeer PL, Schultzer M, McGeer EG. Arthritis and anti-inflammatory agents as possible protective factors for Alzheimer's disease: a review of 17 epidemiological studies. Neurology 1996; 47: 425–32

20. In 't Veld BA, Ruitenberg A, Hofman A, et al. Nonsteroidal antiinflammatory drugs and the risk of Alzheimer's disease. N Engl J Med 2001; 345: 1515–21

21. Aisen PS, The potential of anti-inflammatory drugs for the treatment of Alzheimer's disease, Lancet Neurol 2002; 1: 279–84

22. Van Gool WA, Aisen PS, Eikelenboom P. Anti-inflammatory therapy in Alzheimer's disease: is hope still alive? J Neurol 2003; 250: 788–92

Chapter 19

Vascular nitric oxide: a key molecule in Alzheimer's disease pathogenesis

JC de la Torre

INTRODUCTION

There is general agreement that nitric oxide (NO) pathways are important in Alzheimer's disease (AD). The degree of that importance and the specific actions exerted by those pathways prior to and during the development of AD is the object of intense investigation.[1–5]

NO is a multi-functional messenger molecule involved in vascular regulation, immune reactions, inflammation and neuro-transmission.[6,7] NO is produced from the oxidation of L-arginine by a family of enzymes called NO synthases (NOS).[8] The synthases occur in three isoforms: endothelial (eNOS), neuronal (nNOS) and inducible (iNOS). The first two are constitutively expressed and Ca^{2+} dependent, whereas iNOS is Ca^{2+} independent.[9] The main function of eNOS is the regulation of cerebral blood flow homeostasis and vascular tone.[10,11] Neuronal NOS produces NO as a neurotransmitter in the central nervous system[12,13] and the cytokine-inducible isoform iNOS is involved in the immune response.[14]

This chapter discusses some of the actions of vascular NO, and how knowledge of its actions may help explain key elements in the etio-pathology of AD.

VASCULAR NITRIC OXIDE ACTIONS

The main source of vascular NO in mammals is from eNOS contained within the endothelial cells. The loss or uncoupling of eNOS impairs cerebrovascular function in part by promoting vasoconstriction, platelet aggregation, smooth muscle cell proliferation, leukocyte adhesion and greater endothelial–immune cell interaction.[15–17] Vascular NO production from the endothelium is regulated by eNOS enzyme activity and/or NOS gene expression (Figure 19.1).

Besides the key role that vascular NO plays in vascular tone, blood pressure and vascular homeostasis, it also acts to inhibit platelet and leukocyte adhesion to the endothelium, a process that may down-regulate proin-flammatory events.[18,19]

Vascular NO, therefore, acts as an antiatherogenic, antithrombotic and anti-ischemic molecule by reducing oxidative stress, by preventing platelet aggregation and by stimulating angiogenesis via vascular endo-thelial growth factor (VEGF) while reducing shear stress on the vessel wall (Figure 19.1).[7,9,20]

Inhibition of eNOS has been reported to reduce cerebral blood flow (CBF) and to promote brain tissue damage after experimental focal cerebral ischemia.[21] It is not known what

Normal endothelial cell synthesis of NO

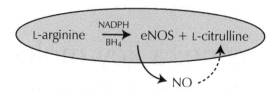

- ➢ EC shape changes
- ↙ mitochondria
- ↙ eNOS–NO
- ↙ Glut 1
- ↗ TNF-α
- ➢ NF-κβ translation to nucleus and transcription inflam genes
- ↗ ET-1
- ➢ VSMC migration & fibrous plaque
- ➢ HIF-1α release
- ↗ VCAM
- ↗ Aβ angiopathy
- ↗ free radicals: H_2O_2 (SO·)
- ↙ VEGF

  low shear stress

Chronic brain hypoperfusion

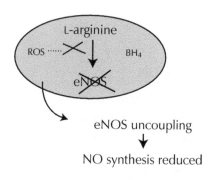

eNOS uncoupling
↓
NO synthesis reduced

Figure 19.1 Normal synthesis of vascular nitric oxide (NO) from L-arginine by the action of eNOS and specific cofactors NADPH and BH$_4$ in endothelium (top). In chronic brain hypoperfusion (bottom), formation of reactive oxygen species (ROS) at the injury site may induce a deficiency in BH$_4$ (a rate-limiting step in endothelial NO synthase (eNOS) synthesis), resulting in eNOS uncoupling and reduced release of vascular NO. Reduced vascular NO is reported to involve many of the changes listed in the inset including: endothelial cell (EC) shape changes, mitochondrial stress, reduced eNOS, impaired glucose transporter 1 (Glut 1) (thus lowering glucose delivery to brain cells), tumor necrosis factor-α (TNF-α) activation, neutral factor-kappa B (NF-κB) translocation from cytosol to nucleus, to activation of transcription inflammatory (inflam) genes, release of the powerful vasoconstrictor endothelin-1 (ET-1), migration of vascular smooth muscle cells (VSMC) leading to formation of vessel wall plaques, activation of hypoxic inducible factor-1α (HIF-1α), increase of vascular adhesion molecules (VCAM), increased Aβ peptide angiopathy, excess free radical formation including hydrogen peroxide (H$_2$O$_2$) and superoxide anion (SO·), impairment of the angiogenic vascular endothelial growth factor (VEGF) and persistent shear stress on vessel walls

role, if any, vascular NO may play in chronic brain hypoperfusion, a blood flow deficit known to be present prior to the development of AD,[22–25] and, as we first proposed in 1993, its pathogenic trigger.[26]

One of the actions that vascular NO may have on memory mechanisms appears to involve cerebral perfusion homeostasis (Figure 19.2). In this scheme, chronic brain hypoperfusion resulting from blockade of the common carotid

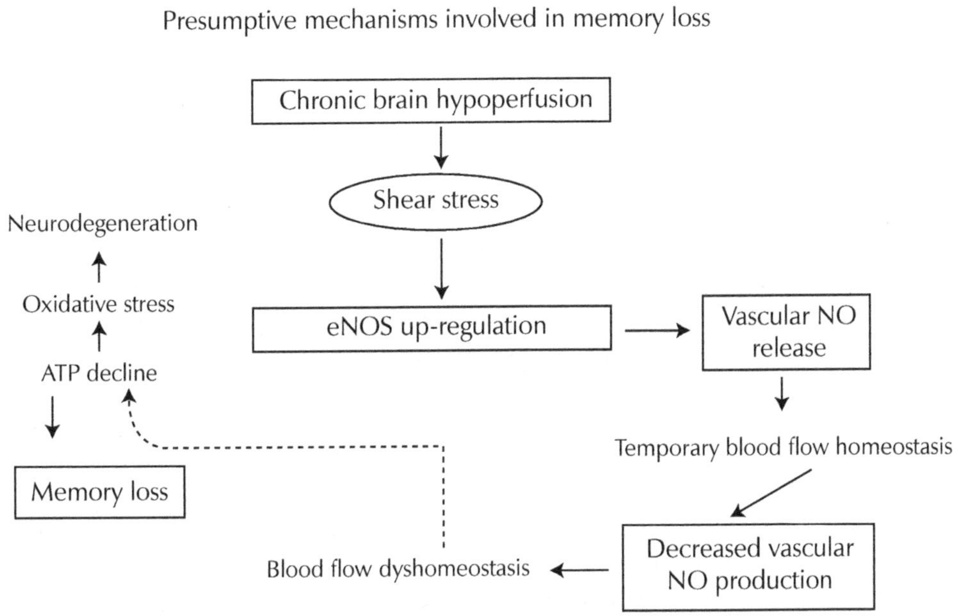

Presumptive mechanisms involved in memory loss

Figure 19.2 The cascading effect of chronic brain hypoperfusion (CBH) on memory mechanisms. CBH induces stimulation of shear stress which leads to up-regulation of vascular nitric oxide (NO) from endothelial cells in order to maintain vascular homeostasis. This action is a futile attempt to maintain cerebral perfusion homeostasis, but is temporary and dependent on NO endothelial store depletion. As shear stress continues unabated, reduced vascular NO cannot maintain optimal glucose–oxygen delivery to brain cells for conversion to ATP fuel. Neuronal hypometabolism ensues, particularly in memory-associated regions such as the hippocampus, resulting in short-term, and later, long-term memory failure. The endothelial-initiated chemical cascade may continue by involving oxidative stress mechanisms and evolution of neurodegeneration

arteries triggers persistent low shear stress, which can be especially harmful to ischemia-sensitive brain neurons such as those found in the CA1 hippocampus in rats and humans.[27,28]

Disturbed (or oscillating) shear stress, as opposed to laminar shear stress, temporarily stimulates rapid release of vascular NO by way of eNOS up-regulation in a futile attempt to maintain cerebral perfusion homeostasis. Continued oscillating shear stress, however, eventually depletes vascular NO production, resulting in loss of blood flow homeostasis and decline of glucose delivery needed for optimal brain-cell ATP synthesis. The outcome of this vicious cycle is persistent oxidative stress and commencement of neurodegenerative changes in

the hippocampus and, in time, other sensitive brain regions (Figure 19.2).

The bulk of evidence in support of the scheme represented in Figure 19.2 comes from experiments conducted in our own laboratories. In one experiment, aging rats were subjected to chronic brain hypoperfusion by bilateral common carotid artery occlusion for 2 and 8 weeks. We saw that, after 2 weeks of chronic brain hypoperfusion, NO levels in the hippocampus were 3.9 times higher in the group with chronic brain hypoperfusion than in non-occlusion controls.[29] At the 8-week time point, impairment of spatial memory ability was observed to be present but the 3.9-fold increase in NO levels observed at 2 weeks in the group with hypoferfusion had declined to just below baseline levels. These findings suggest that NO up-regulation, possibly from constant stimulation of low shear stress, preceded memory loss by at least 6 weeks. Moreover, the NO up-regulation was only temporary, since by week 8, NO levels were slightly below baseline. In addition to the spatial memory impairment seen 8 weeks after chronic brain hypoperfusion, measurement of Aβ1-40 in the hippocampus but not Aβ1-42 showed a significant increase in the hypoperfused rats only.[29]

Since Aβ1-40 is reported to be associated with memory loss more than Aβ1-42,[30] this finding was not especially surprising. What remains unresolved, however, is the significance of this Aβ1-40 increase at 8 weeks following chronic brain hypoperfusion. Is the increase due to higher expression of Aβ1-40 by ischemic brain cells, by a lowered degradation of this peptide's breakdown during hypoperfusion, or by some other mechanism? The answer requires further investigation. Although we could not distinguish between nNOS and eNOS in this experiment, owing to the nature of the nano-amperometric measurements, the NO up-regulation was presumed to be due to bursts of high vascular NO release in response to persistent low shear stress. The reason for this conclusion is that nNOS is expressed in the early phase of brain ischemia while eNOS levels generally rise in the later phase.[31] For example, nNOS up-regulation after acute focal cerebral ischemia peaks between 24 and 48 h and disappears by day 3, while eNOS expression peaks after 7 days and disappears by day 14.[31,32]

In our study, NO levels were still very high after 14 days, possibly because chronic and unrelenting ischemia (rather than acute focal ischemia) was maintained in our animals. In support of this notion, recent unpublished findings from our laboratory revealed that 8 weeks after chronic brain hypoperfusion, only

rats given an eNOS inhibitor (but not nNOS or iNOS inhibitors) markedly worsened their spatial memory ability (de la Torre et al., unpublished data). In the above experiment, when NO up-regulation could no longer maintain adequate cerebral perfusion, NO levels recorded from the hippocampal tissue dipped back to baseline. It is only speculative on our part that vascular NO levels might have significantly dropped below baseline had the observation period of hypoperfusion extended beyond 8 weeks.

These findings are particularly intriguing, since they reasonably explain part of the subcellular and molecular chronology that may trigger AD from risk factors that diminish cerebral blood flow, sometimes for decades.[33-36] Conceivably, the simplified scheme depicted in Figure 19.2 from our studies in rats could serve as a model of how chronic brain hypoperfusion can initiate eNOS activation, a condition that escalates from temporary normal cerebral perfusion to permanent disrupted blood flow homeostasis and with it, the start of memory failure in Alzheimer's dementia.

ENDOTHELIAL DYSFUNCTION AFFECTING VASCULAR NITRIC OXIDE REGULATION

Many studies have reaffirmed that endothelial dysfunction commonly occurs during aging in both animals and humans.[37-41] In some diseased states, this impairment originates in part from the formation of reactive oxygen and nitrogen species near the vascular endothelium to produce toxic peroxynitrite.[42-45] These toxic products can cause DNA strand breakage by activating the cell-death promoter poly(ADP ribose) polymerase.[46-49]

We know from our studies and those of others that dysregulation of vascular NO production can occur from chronic cerebral hypoperfusion as a result of various disease states during aging.[4,50–54] In our judgement, the process might unfold as follows: chronic cerebral hypoperfusion resulting from aging plus a vascular risk factor induces eNOS activation and dysregulation of NO release from the endothelium, primarily in the hippocampus and entorhinal cortex. This action results in increased vascular resistance and viscosity, causing microenvironmental hemorheological and hemodynamic disturbances.[4,26,35,36] This mechanotransduction effect on eNOS activity 'up-regulates' NO as a response to reset normal homeostasis and diminish the damage caused by hypoperfusion. Unable to achieve homeostasis, basal NO levels diminish and, consequently, are unable to: regulate normal vascular perfusion; block granulocyte adherence in blood vessels; and prevent proinflammatory reactions intra-neuronally. Additionally, low basal levels of NO are unable to maintain endothelial cell conformation, resulting in endothelial cell shape distortions.[4] Such a phenomenon may explain basement membrane thickening commonly found regionally in Alzheimer's brain capillaries.[55–57]

Vascular NO dysregulation can result in multiple pathological conditions involving oxidative stress, Aβ peptide accumulation, inflammatory reactions, reduced ATP synthesis, atherosclerosis and synaptic transmission failure (Figure 19.1). What is important to note is that the collective studies implicating vascular NO in

these activities support the idea that capillary endothelial cell function and release of NO play a critical role in the hemodynamic, humoral and inflammatory signals to which it is constantly exposed by circulating blood cells. Furthermore, such activities[7,11,21] are part of the AD pathological complex.[4,34,35]

AD, therefore, may develop as an endotheliopathy driven by chronic brain hypoperfusion, resulting from the presence of one or several vascular risk factors in the presence of advancing age.[33–36] For this and other reasons, we believe that AD should be classified as a vasocognopathy, a term we have coined to provide better explaination of the nature of this dementia.[58,59]

These findings and those that others have shown about vascular NO support the concept that this molecule may be a key element in the initiation of subcellular pathology, leading to cognitive disability and eventual dementia. Confirmation of our preliminary findings would mean that vascular NO release could become an important primary target in the search for a means to arrest or reverse cognitive dysfunction, which begins with spatial memory impairment and proceeds to total mental chaos.

ACKNOWLEDGEMENTS

This research was supported by an Investigator-Initiated Research Grant from the Alzheimer's Association.

REFERENCES

1. de la Monte SM, Bloch KD. Aberrant expression of the constitutive endothelial nitric oxide synthase gene in Alzheimer disease. Mol Chem Neuropathol 1997; 30: 139–59

2. Akama KT, Albanese C, Pestell RG, Van Eldik LJ. Amyloid beta-peptide stimulates nitric oxide production in astrocytes through an NFkappaB-dependent mechanism. Proc Natl Acad Sci USA 1998; 95: 5795–800

3. de la Monte, SM, de la Torre JC. Basic cellular and molecular mechanisms in dementia. In Duckett S, de la Torre JC, eds. Pathology of the Aging Human Nervous System. Oxford University Press, 2001; 123–55

4. de la Torre JC, Stefano GB. Evidence that Alzheimer's disease is a microvascular disorder: the role of constitutive nitric oxide. Brain Res Rev 2000; 34: 119–36

5. Cacabelos R, Fernández-Novoa L, Valter Lombardi V, et al. Cerebrovascular risk factors in Alzheimer disease: brain hemodynamics and pharmacogenomic implications. Neurol Res 2003; 25: 567–80

6. Mayer B, Hemmens B. Biosynthesis and action of nitric oxide in mammalian cells. Trends Biochem Sci 1998; 23: 87

7. Maxwell AJ. Mechanisms of dysfunction of the nitric oxide pathway in vascular diseases. Nitric Oxide Biol Chem 2002; 6: 101–24

8. Moncada S, Higgs A. The L-arginine–nitric oxide pathway. N Engl J Med 1993; 329: 2002–12

9. Moncada S, Palmer RM, Higgs EA. Nitric oxide: physiology, pathophysiology, and pharmacology. Pharmacol Rev 1991; 43: 109

10. Palmer RMJ, Ferrige AG, Moncada S. Nitric oxide release accounts for the biological activity of endothelium derived relaxing factor. Nature 1987; 327: 524–6

11. Li H, Wallerath T, Forstermann U. Physiological mechanisms regulating the expression of endothelial-type NO synthase. Nitric Oxide 2002; 7: 132–47

12. Bredt DS, Snyder SH. Isolation of nitric oxide synthetase, a calmodulin-requiring enzyme. Proc Natl Acad Sci USA 1990; 87: 682–5

13. Bredt DS, Snyder SH. Nitric oxide: a physiologic messenger molecule. Annu Rev Biochem 1994; 63: 175–95

14. Stuehr DJ, Cho HJ, Kwon NS, et al. Purification and characterization of the cytokine-induced macrophage nitric oxide synthase: an FAD- and FMN-containing flavoprotein. Proc Natl Acad Sci USA 1991; 88: 7773–7

15. Radomski, MW, Palmer RM, Moncada S. An L-arginine/nitric oxide pathway present in human platelets regulates aggregation. Proc Natl Acad Sci USA 1990; 87: 5193–7

16. Huang PL, Huang Z, Mashimo H, et al. Hypertension in mice lacking the gene for endothelial nitric oxide synthase. Nature (London) 1995; 377: 239–42

17. Furchgott, RF, Zawadzki, JV. The obligatory role of endothelial cells in the relaxation of arterial smooth muscle by acetylcholine. Nature (London) 1980; 288: 373–6

18. Kubes P, Granger DN. Nitric oxide modulates microvascular permeability. Am J Physiol 1992; 262: H611–15

19. Kubes P, Kanwar S, Niu XF. Nitric oxide synthesis inhibition induces leukocyte adhesion via superoxide and mast cells. FASEB J 1993; 7: 1293–9

20. Napoli C, Ignarro LJ. Nitric oxide and atherosclerosis. Nitric Oxide 2001; 5: 88–97

21. Huang Z, Huang PL, Panahian N, et al. Effects of cerebral ischemia in mice deficient in neuronal nitric oxide synthase. Science 1994; 265: 1883–5

22. Johnson KA, Albert MS. Perfusion abnormalities in prodromal Alzheimer's disease. Neurobiol Aging 2000; 21: 289–92

23. Kogure D, Matsuda H, Ohnishi T, et al. Longitudinal evaluation of early Alzheimer's

disease using brain perfusion SPECT. J Nucl Med 2000; 41: 1155–62

24. Okamura N, Shinkawa M, Arai H, et al. Prediction of progression in patients with mild cognitive impairment using IMP-SPECT. Nippon Ronen Igakkai Zasshi 2000; 37: 974–8

25. Rodriguez G, Vitali P, Calvini P, et al. Hippocampal perfusion in mild cognitive impairment. Psychiatry Res 2000; 100: 65–74

26. de la Torre JC, Mussivand T. Can disturbed brain microcirculation cause Alzheimer's disease? Neurol Res 1993; 15: 146–53

27. de la Torre JC, Fortin T, Park G, et al. Brain blood flow restoration rescues chronically damaged rat CA1 neurons. Brain Res 1993; 623: 6–15

28. West MJ, Coleman PD, Flood DG, Troncoso JC. Differences in the pattern of hippocampal neuronal loss in normal ageing and Alzheimer's disease. Lancet 1994; 344: 769–72

29. de la Torre JC, Pappas BA, Emmerling M, et al. Hippocampal nitric oxide upregulation precedes memory loss and $A\beta_{1-40}$ accumulation after chronic brain hypoperfusion in rats. Neurol Res 2003; 25: 635–41

30. Malin DH, Crothers MK, Lake JR, et al. Hippocampal injections of amyloid beta-peptide 1-40 impair subsequent one-trial/day reward learning. Neurobiol Learn Mem 2001; 76: 125–37

31. Niwa M, Inao S, Takayasu M, et al. Time course of expression of three nitric oxide synthase isoforms after transient middle cerebral artery occlusion in rats. Neurol Med Chir (Tokyo) 2001; 41: 63–72

32. Leker RR, Teichner A, Ovadia H, et al. Expression of endothelial nitric oxide synthase in the ischemic penumbra: relationship to expression of neuronal nitric oxide synthase and vascular endothelial growth factor. Brain Res 2001; 909: 1–7

33. de la Torre JC. Alzheimer's disease: how does it start? J Alzheimer's Dis 2002; 4: 497–12

34. de la Torre JC. Alzheimer's disease as a vascular disorder: nosological evidence. Stroke 2002; 33: 1152–62

35. de la Torre JC. Critically-attained threshold of cerebral hypoperfusion: the CATCH hypothesis of Alzheimer's pathogenesis. Neurobiol Aging 2000; 21: 331–42

36. de la Torre JC. Hemodynamic consequences of deformed microvessels in the brain in Alzheimer's disease. Ann NY Acad Sci 1997; 826: 75–91

37. Hatake K, Kakishita E, Wakabashi I, et al. Effect of aging on endothelium-dependent vascular relaxation of isolated human basilar artery to thrombin and bradykinin. Stroke 1990; 21: 1039–43

38. Higashi Y, Oshima T, Ozono R, et al. Aging and severity of hypertension attenuate endothelium-dependent renal vascular relaxation in humans. Hypertension 1997; 30: 252–8

39. Imaoka Y, Osani T, Kamada T, et al. Nitric oxide-dependent vasodilator mechanism is not impaired by hypertension but is diminished with aging in the rat aorta. J Cardiovasc Pharmacol 1999; 33: 756–61

40. Küng CF, Lüscher TF. Different mechanisms of endothelial dysfunction with aging and hypertension in rat aorta. Hypertension 1995; 25: 194–200

41. Taddei S, Virdis A, Mattei P, et al. Aging and endothelial function in normotensive subjects and patients with essential hypertension. Circulation 1995; 91: 1981–7

42. Halliwell B. What nitrates tyrosine? Is nitro-tyrosine specific as a biomarker of peroxynitrite formation in vivo? FEBS Lett 1997; 411: 157–60

43. Hamilton CA, Brosnan MJ, McIntyre M, et al. Superoxide excess in hypertension and aging: a common cause of endothelial dysfunction. Hypertension 2001; 37: 529–34

44. Inoue M, Inoue K. Role of free radicals in and around vascular endothelial cells in the mechanism of aging. Ann NY Acad Sci 1996; 786: 224–32

45. Liaudet L, Soriano FG, Szabo E, et al. Protection against hemorrhagic shock in mice genetically deficient in poly (ADP-ribose) polymerase. Proc Natl Acad Sci USA, 2000; 97: 10203–8

46. Pacher P, Liaudet L, Soriano FG, et al. The role of poly(ADP-ribose) polymerase in the development of cardiovascular dysfunction in diabetes mellitus. Diabetes 2002; 51, 514–21

47. Pacher P, Mabley J, Soriano F, et al. Endothelial dysfunction in aging animals: the role of poly(ADP-ribose) polymerase activation. Br J Pharmacol 2002; 135: 1347–50

48. Szabo C, Cuzzocrea S, Zingarelli B, et al. Endothelial dysfunction in a rat model of endotoxic shock. Importance of the activation of poly (ADP-ribose) synthetase by peroxynitrite. J Clin Invest 1997; 100: 723–35

49. Szabo C, Zingarelli B, O'Connor M, Salzman A. DNA strand breakage, activation of poly(ADP-ribose) synthetase, and cellular energy depletion are involved in the cytotoxicity of macrophages and smooth muscle cells exposed to peroxynitrite. Proc Natl Acad Sci USA 1996; 93: 1753–8

50. Temiz C, Tun K, Ugur HC, et al. L-arginine in focal cerebral ischemia. Neurol Res 2003; 25: 465–70

52. Yamakawa H, Jezova M, Ando H, Saavedra JM. Normalization of endothelial and inducible nitric oxide synthase expression in brain microvessels of spontaneously hypertensive rats by angiotensin II AT1 receptor inhibition. J Cereb Blood Flow Metab 2003; 23: 371–80

52. Uetsuka S, Fujisawa H, Yasuda H, et al. Severe cerebral blood flow reduction inhibits nitric oxide synthesis. J Neurotrauma 2002; 19: 1105–16

53. Veltkamp R, Rajapakse N, Robins G, et al. Transient focal ischemia increases endothelial nitric oxide synthase in cerebral blood vessels. Stroke 2002; 33: 2704–10

54. Zvan B, Zaletel M, Pogacnik T, Kiauta T. Testing of cerebral endothelium function with L-arginine after stroke. Int Angiol 2002; 21: 256–9

55. Bué L, Hof PR, Bouras C, et al. Pathological alterations of the cerebral microvasculature in Alzheimer's disease and related demented disorders. Acta Neuropathol 1994; 87: 469–80

56. Fisher VW, Siddigi A, Yusufaly Y. Altered angioarchitecture in selected areas of brains with Alzheimer's disease. Acta Neuropathol 1990; 79: 672–9

57. Mancardi GL, Perdelli F, Leonardi A, Bugiani O. Thickening of the basement membrane of cortical capillaries in Alzheime's disease. Acta Neuropathol 1980; 49: 79–83

58. de la Torre JC. Alzheimer's disease is a vasocognopathy. Abstr Soc Neurosci 2004; in press

59. de la Torre JC. Alzheimer's disease is a vasocognopathy: a new term to describe its nature. Neurol Res 2004; 26: 517–24

Chapter 20

Alzheimer pathology and endoplasmic reticulum stress

T Kudo, T Katayama, K Imaizumi, D Kanayama, J Hitomi,
M Okochi, M Tohyama, M Takeda

INTRODUCTION

Alzheimer's disease (AD) is a progressive neurodegenerative disorder, characterized pathologically by cerebral neuritic plaques of amyloid-β peptide (Aβ) and neurofibrillary tangles of phosphorylated tau. Some early-onset cases of autosomal-dominant familial AD are caused by mutations in the amyloid precursor protein (*APP*) gene located on chromosome 21, presenilin-1 (*PS1*) located on chromosome 14 and presenilin-2 (*PS2*) located on chromosome 1. Of these three loci, mutations in *PS1* are the most prevalent in cases of familial AD. It has been reported that PS1 is located in subcellular compartments and appears to be present in particularly high levels in the endoplasmic reticulum (ER), the intermediate compartment and the *cis*-Golgi region.[1–3] This led us to study the relationship between ER function and PS1.

The ER performs the synthesis, post-translational modification and proper folding of proteins. A variety of conditions, for instance the disturbance of calcium homeostasis, nutrient deprivation, or the overexpression of relatively insoluble proteins, cause stress to the ER, resulting in the accumulation of unfolding or misfolding proteins in the ER. Because incompletely folded molecules are threatening to

living cells, efficient quality control systems have been evolved to prevent these substandard entities from moving along the secretory pathway. Eukaryotic cells have three different mechanisms for dealing with an accumulation of unfolded proteins in the ER, known as the unfolded protein response (UPR): transcriptional induction, translational attenuation and degradation. In response to the accumulation of unfolded proteins in the ER, eukaryotic cells induce molecular chaperones, such as BiP/GRP78 and GRP94, which assist or facilitate normal folding of unfolded or misfolded proteins.[4] Because continuous delivery of newly synthesized proteins is burdensome to the ER under ER stress, the second strategy of cells against ER stress is the generalized suppression of translation mediated by the serine/threonine kinase PERK. PERK phosphorylates the translational initiation factor eIF2α, causing translational attenuation.[5,6] Third, ER stress activates an ER-associated degradation (ERAD) system, by which misfolded proteins are transported out of the ER to the cytoplasm and then are ubiquitinated and degraded by the 26S proteasome[7]. By these three protective responses, cells can overcome ER stress, which potentially leads to apoptosis. It has been revealed that cells deficient in the UPR are more vulnerable to ER stress-induced apoptosis.[8-10]

We initially investigated the involvement of familial AD-linked PS1 mutants in the UPR. Our data showed that a PS1 mutant altered UPR signaling and indicated that this alteration may contribute to the pathogenic mechanism in the brains of familial AD patients. According to the so-called amyloid hypothesis, Aβ accumulation is the pivotal event in sporadic AD cases as well as in familial AD. Therefore, we studied the relationship between Aβ accumulation and the UPR. We found that, in neurons exposed to Aβ, the UPR was stimulated to activate ER-resident caspases. We also found that, in the neurons whose UPR was disturbed, Aβ production was elevated. This brief review focuses on our work examining the pathology of AD and ER stress interaction.

FAMILIAL ALZHEIMER'S DISEASE-LINKED PS1 MUTANTS ATTENUATE THE UNFOLDED PROTEIN RESPONSE

To date, three ER-resident transmembrane molecules, PERK, IRE1 and ATF6, which sense the accumulation of unfolded proteins to induce the UPR, have been identified. We investigated how *PS1* mutants involve these molecules in dysfunction.

ER stress-induced oligomerization and autophosphorylation of IRE (inositol requiring), typeI transmembrane proteins in the ER, results in activation of the endonuclease domains that are postulated to initiate splicing of mRNA encoding a putative transcription factor. It leads to enhanced transcription of ER chaperone genes, such as BiP/GRP78 and GRP94.[4,11,12] Under tunicamycin treatment (3 mg/ml, for 6 h), which prevents protein glycosylation and causes ER stress, the induction of GRP78 mRNA expression was significantly inhibited in permanent cell lines expressing mutant PS1 (the ΔE9 variant) compared with those transfected with wild-type PS1 or empty vector. To confirm that familial AD-linked mutants generally cause inhibition of GRP78 mRNA induction, other familial AD-linked PS1 mutants, such as A246E, M146V and I213T, were studied with transiently transfected cells. These mutations also suppressed the induction of GRP78 mRNA. IRE1 leads to downstream signaling by a process that depends on oligomerization and autophosphorylation of its kinase domain.[4,11,12] Therefore, we studied the effects of mutations in PS1 on autophosphorylation of IRE1. SK-N-SH cells stably transfected with wild-type PS1, mutant PS1, or empty vector were stimulated with thapsigargin (1 μmol/l) and Western blotting of IRE1 was performed. When cells were treated with 1 μmol/l thapsigargin, within 15 min, the bands of IRE1 were completely shifted (phosphorylated-IRE1) in cells expressing wild-type PS1. In contrast, no shifts of IRE1-immunoreactive bands were seen in mutant PS1-expressing cells that were treated with the same dose of thapsigargin within 30 min. These results indicate that familial AD-linked PS1 mutants attenuate the autophosphorylation of IRE1 to impair the signaling for GRP78 induction.

PERK is a type I transmembrane protein kinase localized in the ER. ER stress-induced oligomerization and autophosphorylation of PERK results in phosphorylation of the subunit of eukaryotic translation initiation factor 2 (eIF2α) at serine 51. The phosphorylation of eIF2α interferes with the formation of a 43S initiation complex, resulting in inhibition of translation initiation.[6] Activation of PERK during ER stress correlates with the autophosphorylation of those cytoplasmic kinase domains. At first, to examine the effects of PS1 mutants on the activation of PERK, Western blotting was perfomed using lysate from N2a cells expressing either wild-type PS1 or mutant PS1, stimulated for 5–60 min by 1 µmol/l thapsigargin. Phosphorylation of PERK retarded their mobility on sodium dodecyl sulfate (SDS)-polyacrylamide gels, and thus serves as a convenient marker for their activation status. In N2a cells expressing mock or wild-type PS1, the bands of PERK were completely shifted within 15 min after treatment with thapsigargin. In contrast, in cells expressing PS1 mutants, the mobility shifts were not observed 15–30 min after the treatment. These results indicate that familial AD-linked PS1 mutants disturb the autophosphorylation of PERK during ER stress. Because disturbed function of PERK is known to cause the downregulation of phosphorylation of eIF2α, we examined the levels of phosphorylated-eIF2α after ER stress in N2a cells expressing PS1 mutations. Western blotting using antiphosphorylated eIF2α antibody showed that phosphorylation of eIF2α was inhibited in cells expressing mutant PS1. Thus, activation of PERK and the resultant phosphorylation of eIF2α were disturbed by the expression of the PS1 mutation.

ATF6 is a type II transmembrane protein localized in the ER and is activated by ER stress-induced proteolysis. Upon ER stress, the bZIP-containing N-terminal fragment facing the cytoplasm is liberated from the ER membrane to translocate into the nucleus. It results in activation of ER chaperone gene transcription, which facilitates protein folding.[13] Under ER stress, the translocation of ATF6 fragments into the nucleus was investigated by immunohistochemistry in cells with either wild-type PS1 or mutant PS1. In wild-type fibroblasts, the N-terminal fragments of ATF6 were quickly translocated into the nucleus by ER stress. In contrast, in homozygous PS1 knock-in fibroblasts, the translocation was delayed. The disturbance of the ATF6 pathway in homozygous PS1 knock-in fibroblasts was also

confirmed by Western blotting. In wild-type fibroblasts, the appearance of a 50-kDa ATF6 fragment was detected quickly by ER stress, whereas it was delayed in homozygous fibroblasts. Therefore, the familial AD-linked PS1 mutation also attenuates the signaling pathway through ATF6.

Our data thus showed that PS1 mutants alter the function of three transducers of the UPR, and indicated that this alteration may contribute to the pathogenic mechanism in the brains of familial AD patients.

Aβ INDUCES NEURONAL APOPTOSIS VIA ENDOPLASMIC RETICULUM STRESS

To study the mechanism of Aβ-induced cell death, we exposed primary culture of mouse cortical neurons or SK-N-SH cell lines to Aβ or control peptide, for 12–48 h, and assessed the effect on neuron survival, as measured by lactate dehydrogenase (LDH) release. The fibrillar form of Aβ peptide (Aβ1-40), which was incubated at 37°C for 4 days beforehand, and 25 µmol/l concentration of a smaller Aβ peptide (Aβ25-35), but not a control peptide with the amino acid sequence inverted (Aβ35-25), were found to induce the death of cortical neurons efficiently. The Aβ25-35 peptide is a fragment of Aβ that has previously been shown to mimic the effects of the Aβ1-40.[14]

To test the hypothesis that Aβ-induced apoptosis of neurons might involve the UPR, we asked whether the treatment of these neurons with Aβ leads to activation of components of the UPR. By Western blotting with the anti-phospho-eIF2α antibodies, it is possible to detect the active form of eIF2α. Exposure of primary culture neurons or neuronal cell lines to Aβ25-35 or fibrillar Aβ1-40 enhanced the phosphorylation of eIF2α in a time-dependent manner. Western blotting with antibody that recognizes eIF2α regardless of its state of phosphorylation indicated that the overall levels of this protein were not affected by the addition of Aβ to neurons. Stress-induced activation of PERK stimulates phosphorylation of PERK itself, which can be evaluated by a mobility shift of its band upon SDS-polyacrylamide gel electrophoresis (PAGE) gel. In primary culture neurons or neuronal cell lines exposed to Aβ25-35, PERK completely underwent a shift in its mobility within 6 h. In contrast, in cells exposed to Aβ35-25, PERK was only partially phosphorylated, even 12 h after treatment. Northern blotting showed that GRP78 mRNA was induced in a time-dependent manner by Aβ25-35 exposure, but not by Aβ35-25.

To investigate the hypothesis that Aβ stimulates UPR to activate ER-resident caspase, we analyzed the cleavage of pro-caspase-12 in response to Aβ exposure. As described previously,[15] treatment of primary culture of mouse cortical neurons with Aβ25-35 induced the cleavage of procaspase-12 within 6 h. In contrast, procaspase-12 was not cleaved when cells were exposed to Aβ35-25. To confirm whether caspase-12 is required for Aβ-induced cell death, N2a cells that expressed endogenous caspase-12 were transfected with siRNA to caspase-12 or to green fluorescent protein (GFP; as control). The quantity of caspase-12 was decreased by incubation for 60 h after transfection with siRNA directed against caspase-12, but not with siRNA to GFP. The 3-(4,5-dimethlthiazol-2yl)-5-(3-carboxymethoxy-phenyl)-2-(4-sulfophenyl)-2H-tetrazolium, inner salt (MTS) assay showed that about 35% of untransfected cells were killed by treatment with Aβ25-35 for 48 h. The extent of cell death was unaffected by transfection with siRNA to GFP. In contrast, about 20% of the cells died after being transfected with caspase-12 siRNA and exposed to Aβ25-35. This result indicates that

cells with decreased expression of caspase-12 become more resistant to Aβ-induced cell death.

These data suggest that the UPR and the activation of caspase-12 by exposure of Aβ may be the main process of Aβ-induced neuronal death.

DYSFUNCTION OF THE UNFOLDED PROTEIN RESPONSE ALTERS Aβ PRODUCTION

To investigate the relationship between the UPR and Aβ production, we established N2a with a dominant negative Ire1. This Ire1 derivative, ΔIre1, has a truncated cytoplasmic region and therefore lacks the kinase and RNase L domains. We subsequently confirmed that cells expressing ΔIre1 showed down-regulation of GRP78 induction, and significantly increased vulnerability to ER stress. The N2a transformants of ΔIre1 showed that secreted Aβx-40 and Aβx-42 were significantly increased 1.3-fold compared with the cells expressing the mock substrate. The ratio of Aβx-42/Aβx-40 plus Aβx-42 was not changed in these cells. These data suggest that dysfunction of the UPR may alter Aβ production.

DISCUSSION

Our study showed that familial AD-linked mutant PS1 disturbs a variety of essential molecules. However, it remains unclear why mutant PS1 inhibits the activation of ER stress transducers. Our immunoprecipitation study indicated that full-length wild-type and mutant PS1 may specifically interact with IRE1 on the membrane of the ER. Recently, it was proposed that the activation of signaling-mediated ER stress transducers could be triggered by dissociation of GRP78/BiP from stress transducers.[16]

The dissociation causes the oligomerization of stress transducers to induce its autophosphorylation and the resultant activation of downstream signaling. If PS1 mutants form malfolded structures, GRP78/BiP may constitutively bind to PS1 molecules to promote its folding. The complex formation of mutant PS1, ER transducers and GRP78/BiP may inhibit the dissociation of GRP78/BiP from transducers under ER stress conditions.

PS1 mutations, which attenuate the UPR, alter the processing of APP and cause increased production of the more amyloidogenic Aβ peptide, Aβ1-42. According to the so-called amyloid hypothesis, Aβ accumulation is the pivotal event in sporadic AD cases as well as in familial AD. Therefore, we studied the relationship between Aβ accumulation and the UPR. The accumulation of Aβ in the brains of AD patients has been implicated as a cause of the neuronal loss that occurs in AD. However, the mechanisms by which Aβ induces neuronal death are not well understood. We provided evidence that Aβ induces the activation of the UPR followed by activation of ER-resident caspase. However, it is unclear why extracellular Aβ induces an intracellular UPR. Aβ has been shown to bind to a variety of proteins, including the Aβ precursor protein[17] and the receptor for advanced glycation end-products.[18] Whether one or several of these Aβ-binding proteins mediates Aβ induction of UPR activation is not known. One possibility is that one or several Aβ receptors promote apoptosis via the ER pathway, whereas other Aβ-binding proteins contribute to Aβ-mediated apoptosis through a distinct signaling pathway.

Furthermore, we investigated how dysfunction of the UPR alters Aβ production. To disturb IRE1, cell lines with ΔIre1 was employed. The cells showed down-regulation of GRP78 induction and significantly increased vulnerability to ER stress. The ER and ER–Golgi intermediate compartment may be important sites for generation of Aβ (1-42).[19] Interestingly, under ER stress, unfolded proteins are retrieved to the ER by retrograde transport, to prevent them from moving to the cell surface.[20] In view of the alteration in the UPR systems in cells expressing ΔIre1, it is possible that altered levels of Aβ (1-42) in these cells might be the result of retention of the unfolded APP in the ER due to the impaired protein-folding system. It was reported that amounts of secreted Aβ have been shown to be reduced by transfection with GRP78.[21] This result is consistent with our speculation that Aβ production may be associated with the UPR system.

In summary, our results indicate a new mechanism by which PS1 mutations may affect the UPR system. In neurons exposed to Aβ, the UPR is stimulated to activate ER-resident caspases. In neurons whose UPR is disturbed, Aβ production is altered. Therefore, experimental manipulations of the UPR might allow the development of therapeutic strategies for AD.

REFERENCES

1. Walter J, Capell A, Grunberg J, et al. The Alzheimer's disease-associated presenilins are differentially phosphorylated proteins located predominantly with the endoplasmic reticulum. Mol Med 1996; 2: 673–91

2. Culvenor JG, Maher F, Evin G, et al. Alzheimer's disease-associated presenilin 1 in neuronal cells: evidence for localization to the endoplasmic reticulum-Golgi intermediate compartment. J Neurosci Res 1997; 49: 719–31

3. Annaert WG, Levesque L, Craessaerts K, et al. Presenilin 1 controls γ-secretase processing of amyloid precursor protein in pre-golgi compartments of hippocampal neurons. J Cell Biol 1999; 147: 277–94

4. Sidrauski C, Chapman R, Walter P. The unfolded protein response: an intracellular signalling pathway with many surprising features. Trends Cell Biol 1998; 8: 245–9

5. Shi Y, Vattem KM, Sood R, et al. Identification and characterization of pancreatic eukaryotic initiation factor 2 α-subunit kinase, PEK, involved in translational control. Mol Cell Biol 1998; 18: 7499–509

6. Harding HP, Zhang Y, Ron D. Protein translation and folding are coupled by an endoplasmic-reticulum-resident kinase. Nature 1999; 397: 271–4

7. Bonifacino JS, Weissman AM. Ubiquitin and the control of protein fate in the secretory and endocytic pathway. Annu Rev Cell Dev Biol 1998; 14: 19–57

8. Liu H, Bowes RC 3rd, van de Water B, et al. Endoplasmic reticulum chaperones GRP78 and calreticulin prevent oxidative stress, Ca^{2+} disturbances, and cell death in renal epithelial cells. J Biol Chem 1997; 272: 21751–9

9. Harding HP, Zhang Y, Bertolotti A. PERK is essential for translational regulation and cell survival during the unfolded protein response. Mol Cell 2000; 5: 897–904

10. Imai Y, Soda M, Takahashi R. Parkin suppresses unfolded protein stress-induced cell death through its E3 ubiquitin-protein ligase activity. J Biol Chem 2000; 275: 35661–4

11. Tirasophon W, Ajith AW, Kaufman R. A stress response pathway from the endoplasmic reticulum to the nucleus requires a novel bifunctional protein kinase/endoribonuclease (Ire1p) in mammalian cells. Genes Dev 1998; 12: 1812–24

12. Wang XZ, Harding HP, Zhang Y, et al. Cloning of mammalian Ire1 reveals diversity in the ER stress responses. EMBO J 1998; 17: 5708–17

13. Haze K, Yoshida H, Yanagi H, et al. Mammalian transcription factor ATF6 is synthesized as a transmembrane protein and activated by proteolysis in response to endoplasmic reticulum stress. Mol Biol Cell 1999; 10: 3787–99

14. Imaizumi K, Morihara T, Mori Y, et al. The cell death-promoting gene DP-5, which interacts with the BCL2 family, is induced during neuronal apoptosis following exposure to amyloid β protein, J Biol Chem 1999; 274: 7975–81

15. Nakagawa T, Zhu H, Morishima N, et al. Caspase-12 mediates endoplasmic-reticulum-specific apoptosis and cytotoxicity by β-amyloid. Nature 2000; 403: 98–103

16. Bertolotti A, Zhang Y, Hendershot LM, et al. Dynamic interaction of Bip and ER stress transducers in the unfolded-protein response, Nat Cell Biol 2000; 2: 326–32

17. Lorenzo A, Yuan M, Zhang Z, et al. Amyloid beta interacts with the amyloid precursor protein: a potential toxic mechanism in Alzheimer's disease. Nat Neurosci 2000; 3: 460–4

18. Yan SD, Chen X, Fu J, et al. RAGE and amyloid-beta peptide neurotoxicity in Alzheimer's disease. Nature 1996; 382: 685–91

19. Cook DG, Forman MS, Sung JC, et al. Alzheimer's Abeta(142) is generated in the endoplasmic reticulum/intermediate compartment of NT2N cells. Nature Med 1997; 3: 1021–3

20. Hammond C, Helenius A. Quality control in the secretory pathway: retention of a misfolded viral membrane glycoprotein involves cycling between the ER, intermediate compartment, and Golgi apparatus. J Cell Biol 1994; 126: 41–52

21. Yang Y, Turner RS, Gaut JR. The chaperone BiP/GRP78 binds to amyloid precursor protein and decreases Aβ40 and Aβ42 secretion. J Biol Chem 1998; 273: 25552–5

Molecular mechanism of amyloid β-peptide-induced impairment of neurotransmission and memory in relation to oxidative stress

K Yamada, H-C Kim, T Nabeshima

INTRODUCTION

Alzheimer's disease (AD) is a neurodegenerative disorder characterized by the presence of senile plaques and neurofibrillary tangles in the brain, accompanied by a progressive loss of synapses and neurons. Histopathological analysis has demonstrated that the core of the senile plaques consists of an extracellular thioflavin S and Congo red-positive fibrous protein, which has been identified as amyloid β-peptide (Aβ).[1] The loss of neurons and synapses leads to cognitive impairment and the development of dementia. Among the various neurotransmitter systems affected, the cholinergic system is the one, at least partly, responsible for cognitive deficits.[2]

MEMORY IMPAIRMENT INDUCED BY CONTINUOUS INTRACEREBROVENTRICULAR INFUSION OF Aβ

Aβ possesses neurotoxicity *in vitro* and *in vivo*. We have used a technique of continuous intracerebroventricular infusion of Aβ with a mini-osmotic pump.[3,4] The infusion of Aβ1-40 caused a significant impairment of spatial memory in a water maze and a deficit of passive avoidance performance, which was accompanied by a slight but significant reduction of choline acetyltransferase (ChAT) activity in the hippocampus.[5] Accumulation of Aβ1-40 in the hippocampus and cerebral cortex was evident immunohistochemically following a 14-day period of infusion. No neuronal death or atrophy was observed in the brain following the continuous infusion of Aβ1-40, while the activation of glial cells was evident in the hippocampus.[6]

Memory impairment was induced by various neurotoxic Aβ fragments, including Aβ1-40, Aβ1-42 and Aβ25-35, while a non-neurotoxic reverse fragment, Aβ40-1, had no effect.[3,4] Moreover, continuous infusion of neurotoxic Aβ fragments resulted in a temporal increase in the BDNF mRNA expression in the hippocampus, whereas neither Aβ40-1 nor Aβ1-16 had any effect, suggesting that the induction of BDNF mRNA constitutes an intrinsic neuroprotective mechanism against the neurotoxicity of Aβ.[7]

Long-term potentiation (LTP) in the hippocampus following a brief high-frequency stimulation is considered a synaptic correlate of memory. To explore the effects of Aβ in learning and memory further, we examined whether continuous infusion of Aβ in rats affected the development and maintenance of LTP in the hippocampus. The enhanced response after tetanic stimulation was maintained for more than 45 min in the hippocampal slices from vehicle-infused control rats, whereas it declined rapidly to nearly the baseline levels in the Aβ1-40-treated group.[8] Thus, both behavioral and electrophysiological studies indicate that continuous infusion of Aβ causes learning and memory impairment.

IMPAIRMENT OF CHOLINERGIC NEUROTRANSMISSION INDUCED BY Aβ

Since the cholinergic hypothesis of AD was proposed, the question of whether Aβ impairs cholinergic neurotransmission is compelling. To assess the cholinergic neurotransmission in Aβ-infused rats, we used a microdialysis technique to examine acetylcholine (ACh) release under nicotine stimulation.[9,10] The amplitude of the nicotine-evoked ACh release was no different between naive rats and rats receiving either vehicle or the non-toxic reverse fragment Aβ40-1, whereas neurotoxic Aβ fragments, including Aβ1-42, Aβ1-40 and Aβ25-35, resulted in a marked decrease in nicotine-stimulated ACh release compared with Aβ40-1-infused control rats.[9,10] These findings suggest that only neurotoxic fragments of Aβ impaired nicotine-evoked ACh release and cognitive function.

We examined whether continuous infusion of Aβ affected the nicotinic ACh receptor (nAChR) system. Our preliminary data demonstrated that Aβ1-42 infusion decreased the affinity of nAChRs labeled with [³H]cytisine in the hippocampus. Since [³H]cytisine binds selectively to an α4β2 subtype of nAChRs and no evidence has been found indicating that Aβ1-42 directly affects the [³H]cytisine binding site, the direct binding of Aβ to the α4β2 subtype can be ruled out. Aβ may alter the affinity of the α4β2 sub-

type via an intracellular mechanism, and the decreased affinity of this subtype may be involved in the learning and memory impairment in Aβ-infused rats. It is possible that the effect may be mediated by an altered intracellular mechanism involving the protein kinases, which can regulate the surface expression of nAChRs. In this regard, we demonstrated the down-regulation of protein kinase C in the hippocampus of Aβ1-40-infused rats.[11]

ROLE OF OXIDATIVE STRESS IN Aβ-INDUCED BRAIN DYSFUNCTION

We have previously demonstrated that the potent antioxidants idebenone and α-tocopherol prevent learning and memory impairment in rats that received a continuous intracerebroventricular infusion of Aβ1-40, suggesting a role of oxidative stress in Aβ-induced learning and memory impairment.[12] To test the involvement of oxidative stress further in Aβ-induced learning and memory impairment, we examined the changes in endogenous antioxidant systems such as mitochondrial manganese (Mn)-superoxide dismutase, glutathione, glutathione peroxidase and glutathione-S-transferase following the continuous infusion of Aβ for 2 weeks.[13] The infusion of Aβ1-42 resulted in a significant reduction of the immunoreactivities of these antioxidant substances in such brain areas as the hippocampus, parietal cortex, piriform cortex, substantia nigra and thalamus, although the same treatment with Aβ40-1 had no effect. The alterations induced by Aβ1-42 were not uniform, but rather specific for each immunoreactive substance in a brain region-dependent manner. These results demonstrate a cytological effect of oxidative stress induced by Aβ1-42 infusion. Furthermore, these findings indicate a heterogeneous susceptibility to the oxidative stress produced by Aβ.[13]

ROLE OF NITRIC OXIDE IN Aβ-INDUCED BRAIN DYSFUNCTION

Nitric oxide (NO) synthesized by NO synthase (NOS) is a free radical gas that acts as an intercellular signaling molecule, but it also acts as a neurotoxin at high concentrations. In AD patients, the expression of inducible NOS (iNOS) in a subset of pyramidal neurons of the hippocampus and in tangle-bearing neurons has been reported.[14]

To examine whether Aβ induces iNOS expression in the brain and whether iNOS is involved in Aβ-induced brain dysfunction, rats were infused with Aβ1-40 and the iNOS expression was examined at different time points after Aβ infusion. Continuous infusion of Aβ1-40 induced a time-dependent increase in the expression of iNOS mRNA and the protein in the hippocampus, which was accompanied by a marked increase in the tissue contents of NO metabolites (nitrite and nitrate). The expression of iNOS protein was found in both microglia and astrocytes, indicating that Aβ activates non-neuronal cells.[10] We also examined the effects of iNOS inhibitors on cholinergic dysfunction and memory deficit in Aβ-infused rats, to clarify the pathophysiological significance of the Aβ-induced iNOS induction. Inhibition of NO production by iNOS inhibitors, such as aminoguanidine (AG) and S-methylisothiourea, prevented the Aβ-induced impairment of nicotine-evoked ACh release, as well as spatial memory deficit in a radial arm maze. In contrast to iNOS inhibitors, the neuronal NOS inhibitor 7-nitroindazole failed to ameliorate the impairment of nicotine-evoked ACh release induced by Aβ. These results suggest that Aβ-induced iNOS induction is attributable to cholinergic dysfunction and memory impairment in Aβ-infused rats.[10]

PROTEIN TYROSINE NITRATION INDUCED BY Aβ

Continuous Aβ infusion results in an impairment of ACh and dopamine release *in vivo* without an apparent cholinergic cell loss,[4,9,10] indicating that an impairment of the neurotransmitter release mechanism may be involved, rather than indicating a direct neurotoxic effect on cholinergic fibers. We examined whether overproduction of NO induced by Aβ led to the formation of peroxynitrite and subsequent nitration of synaptic proteins, thus affecting the signal transduction pathways of cellular regulation and release.[15] Immunohistochemical staining with specific nitrotyrosine antibodies showed an abundance of nitrotyrosine-immunoreactive cells in the hippocampus of Aβ-infused rats. Immunoprecipitation and Western blot analyses revealed that synaptophysin, a synaptic protein, was the main target of tyrosine nitration. Daily treatment with the iNOS inhibitor AG, or the peroxynitrite scavenger uric acid, prevented the tyrosine nitration of synaptophysin as well as the impairment of nicotine-evoked ACh release induced by Aβ. These findings suggest that iNOS induction and the consequent tyrosine nitration of synaptophysin are related to the Aβ-induced impairment of ACh release. Furthermore, it is suggested that agents that inhibit NO production and protein tyrosine nitration (iNOS inhibitors, NO scavengers and other antioxidants) would have potential therapeutic effects in AD.

ACKNOWLEDGEMENTS

This study was supported, in part, by Grants-in-Aid for Science Research (No. 14370031) from the Ministry of Education, Culture, Sports, Science and Technology of Japan, and by an SRF Grant for Biomedical Research.

REFERENCES

1. Selkoe DJ. Cell biology of amyloid β-protein precursor and the mechanism of Alzheimer's disease. Annu Rev Cell Biol 1994; 10: 373–403

2. Coyle JT, Price DL, DeLong MR. Alzheimer's disease: a disorder of central cholinergic innervation. Science 1983; 219: 1184–90

3. Yamada K, Nabeshima T. Animal models of Alzheimer's disease and evaluation of anti-dementia drugs. Pharmacol Ther 2000; 88: 93–113

4. Tran MH, Yamada K, Nabeshima T. Amyloid β-peptide induces cholinergic dysfunction and cognitive deficits: a minireview. Peptides 2002; 23: 1271–83

5. Nitta A, Itoh A, Hasegawa T, Nabeshima T. β-Amyloid protein-induced Alzheimer's disease animal model. Neurosci Lett 1994; 170: 63–6

6. Nitta A, Fukuta T, Hasegawa T, Nabeshima T. Continuous infusion of β-amyloid protein into the rat cerebral ventricle induces learning impairment and neuronal and morphological degeneration. Jpn J Pharmacol 1997; 73: 51–7

7. Tang YP, Yamada K, Kanou Y, et al. Spatiotemporal expression of BDNF in the hippocampus induced by the continuous intracerebroventricular infusion of β-amyloid in rats. Mol Brain Res 2000; 80: 188–97

8. Itoh A, Akaike T, Sokabe M, et al. Impairment of long-term potentiation in hippocampal slices of β-amyloid-infused rats. Eur J Pharmacol 1999; 382: 167–75

9. Itoh A, Nitta A, Nadai M, et al. Dysfunction of cholinergic and dopaminergic neuronal systems in β-amyloid protein-infused rats. J Neurochem 1996; 66: 1113–17

10. Tran MH, Yamada K, Olariu A, et al. Amyloid β-peptide induces nitric oxide production in rat hippocampus: association with cholinergic dysfunction and amelioration by inducible nitric oxide inhibitors. FASEB J 2001; 15: 1407–9

11. Olariu A, Yamada K, Mamiya T, et al. Memory impairment induced by chronic intracerebroventricular infusion of beta-amyloid (1-40) involves downregulation of protein kinase C. Brain Res 2002; 957: 278–86

12. Yamada K, Tanaka T, Han D, et al. Protective effects of idebenone and α-tocopherol on β-amyloid-(1-42) induced learning and memory deficits in rats: implication of oxidative stress in β-amyloid-induced neurotoxicity in vivo. Eur J Neurosci 1999; 11: 83–90

13. Kim HC, Yamada K, Nitta A, et al. Immunocytochemical evidence that amyloid β (1-42) impairs endogenous antioxidant systems in vivo. Neuroscience 2003; 119: 399–419

14. Vodovotz Y, Lucia MS, Flanders KC, et al. Inducible nitric oxide synthase in tangle-bearing neurons of patients with Alzheimer's disease. J Exp Med 1996; 184: 1425–33

15. Tran MH, Yamada K, Nakajima A, et al. Tyrosine nitration of a synaptic protein synaptophysin contributes to amyloid β-peptide-induced cholinergic dysfunction. Mol Psychiatr 2003; 8: 407–12

Regulating factors for microglial activation: implication for Alzheimer's disease and brain damage

VRM Lombardi, L Fernández-Novoa, I Etcheverría, S Seoane, R Cacabelos

INTRODUCTION

Although the origin of microglia is still controversial, several lines of evidence suggest that they are bone marrow-derived, monocyte–macrophage lineage cells that enter the brain during embryonic development, and differentiate into ramified resting microglia through a series of morphological transformations. Much has been learned about these cells in recent years, and perhaps the most consistent and important observation made in many different laboratories is that microglia are the first non-neuronal cells that respond to central nervous system (CNS) injury. Microglia have been called 'sensors of pathology' because of their ability to react quickly to virtually all kinds of acute CNS injury.[1–4] These cells are primary immune effector cells of the CNS and their functions include phagocytosis (they phagocytose latex beads *in vitro*, and are considered to remove remnants such as phagocytic cells during neurogenesis), antigen presentation (they express class I major histocompatibility complex (MHC) antigens and are induced to express MHC class II antigens), and production and release of cytokines (interleukin (IL)-1β, IL-6, tumor necrosis factor (TNF)-α, IL-12, IL-18), eicosanoids, complement components and excitatory amino acids such as glutamate, oxidative radicals and nitric oxide.[5–7] The response of microglia to CNS injury is called microglial activation, and this process involves at least five distinct characteristics of the microglial cell: its morphology; its mitotic activity; its surface phenotype; its gene up-regulation; and its secretory activity.

Therefore, microglia are considered to play similar roles to those of macrophages in the CNS, functioning as scavenger cells, inflammatory cells, antigen-presenting cells and immunoregulatory cells. In addition, microglia may function as effector cells that induce demyelination or neuronal degeneration, and may also play a major part in the development of gliosis via secreting cytokines or some other soluble factors.[8] In this chapter, we focus on the immunoregulatory functions, including antigen presentation and cytokine production, of primary microglial cell cultures derived from newborn rats.

MATERIALS AND METHODS

Cortical neuron-enriched cultures

Cortical neuron-glia seeded at 5×10^5/well in 24-well plates were treated with 5–10 µmol/l cytosine β-D-arabinofuranoside at 48 h. Two days later the cytosine β-D-arabinofuranoside was removed and cultures were maintained in DMEM/F-12 complete medium.

Microglia-enriched cultures

Microglial cells were obtained from the mixed brain cell culture of newborn Sprague–Dawley rats following a protocol described previously.[10] Briefly, brain tissues were triturated after removal of the meninges and blood vessels. Cells (5×10^7) were seeded in culture flasks. After a confluent monolayer of glial cells had been obtained, microglia were shaken and replated at 1×10^5/well on top of neuron-enriched cultures. Twenty-four hours later, the cells were treated with vehicle, Aβ and extracts.

Extract preparation

The plant materials were collected in the Vigo area, Spain. Rhizome of *Polypodium leucotomos* (PLE1), *Polypodium cambricum* L. spp. (PLE2) and *Polypodium vulgare* L. (PLE3) were dried at 40°C for 8 h and pretreated by means of the following method: the rhizome, after all of the villosite was removed, was stirred on a magnetic-stirrer for 10 min with sodium hypochlorite solution 5%, isopropyl alcohol 70% and sterile distilled water in three timed cycles. To test the biological activity, the dried crude extracts were dissolved in dimethyl sulfoxide (DMSO, Saint Louis, MO) to a final concentration of 50 µg/ml.

Cellular assay of antioxidant activity

2′,7′-Dichlorofluorescein diacetate (DCFH-DA), a peroxide-sensitive dye, was used for the evaluation of oxidative stress in primary microglial cell cultures.

MHC class-I and class-II antigen expression

The expression of antigens of the MHC, in both non-adherent microglia from mixed glial cultures[10] and adherent microglia in purified cultures, and after serum sample incubation, was investigated by two-color flow cytometric analysis using OX-6 and OX-18 anti-MHC class II and class I antibodies. Microglial cells were identified with fluorescein-conjugated RCA-I,[11] gated and measured.

Statistical analysis

Unless indicated otherwise, all experiments were repeated at least three times. The morphological data were tested by Student's t test. The data of viability were analyzed using the χ^2 test. The other data were evaluated by an analysis of variance, followed by the Fisher test.

RESULTS AND DISCUSSION

The pathological hallmark of Alzheimer's disease (AD) is the presence of numerous senile plaques, of which β-amyloid peptide (Aβ) is a major component throughout the hippocampus and cerebral cortex. The excessive deposition of Aβ is linked to neurodegenerative changes in neurons.[6,12,13] Several reports have shown that Aβ causes little cytotoxicity by itself, but is indirectly neurotoxic by activating microglia to release various proinflammatory factors which, in turn, kill neurons.[14,15]

Despite numerous studies on Aβ-induced neurotoxicity, it is still unclear whether or not Aβ-induced neurotoxicity can be mediated through the activation of microglia. We addressed this question by comparing the neurotoxic effects of Aβ on neuron–microglia cultures prepared from the hippocampus and cortex of newborn rats, and by using cell cultures from the cortical region in this study, because senile plaques are most abundant in the cortices of patients with AD. Dose–response studies showed that Aβ reduced the percentage of neuron survival in neuron-enriched cultures (Figure 22.1a). It is significant that in

neuron–glial cultures, the dose–response curves shifted to the left; the ED$_{50}$ shifted from 1.5 to 0.5 μmol/l. These results indicate that the presence of microglia potentiated the toxic effect of Aβ.

Previous reports from our laboratory indicated that, among the various glia in the brain, microglia were the primary source of the proinflammatory factors which mediated lipopolysaccharide (LPS)-induced neurotoxicity in rat cortex–glia cultures.[9] To examine the possibility that microglia might mediate Aβ-induced neurotoxicity, we evaluated the activation of microglia by performing immunostaining with OX-6 and OX-18 antibodies, which detect surface expression of MHC class-I

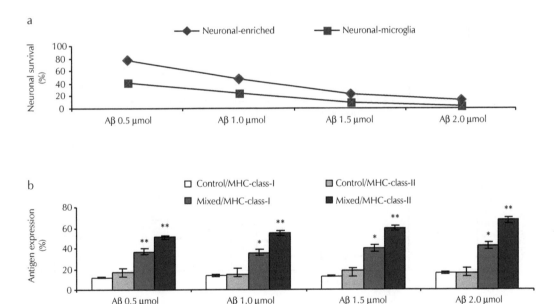

Figure 22.1 Microglia enhanced Aβ-induced neurotoxicity (a). Cortical-neuron–microglia cultures seeded in 24-well plates at 5×10^5 cells/well were treated with different concentrations of Aβ for 9 days. Data from 100 cells from each of three independent experiments show the percentage of neuronal survival. (b) The effects of different concentrations of Aβ on the constitutive and inducible expression of MHC class-I and MHC class-II molecules by microglia. The amount of antigen expression was measured by flow cytometry in the rat neuron–microglia mixed cultures. Spontaneous (vehicle) and Aβ-induced antigen expressions were measured in gated microglial populations. Each column represents the mean of five experiments and shows the percentage of antigen expression. *$p < 0.05$, **$p < 0.01$ versus controls, as determined using Student's t-test.

(continued)

and MHC class-II antigens, respectively. Primary cortex–neuron–microglia cultures were treated with vehicle or Aβ for 48 h. Cells were detached and immunostained with fluorescent red and green antibodies, and analyzed by flow cytometry. As can be seen in Figure 22.1b, microglia were predominant in a resting state in the control cultures treated with vehicle (MHC class I, 12%; MHC class II, 17%). In contrast, cultures treated with Aβ at 0.5, 1.0, 1.5 or 2.0 μmol/l displayed the characteristics of activated microglia (MHC class I, up to 42%; MHC class II, up to 67%). These results demonstrate that, since it might be difficult to estimate either the exact nature and the amounts of the pro-

inflammatory agents that are generated *in vivo*, the alternative employment of tissue cultures to study the mechanisms of cellular damage relevant to inflammation might prove to be highly informative.

Brain cells are at particular risk from damage caused by free radicals. The brain has an extremely high rate of oxygen consumption, and neuronal membranes have a high content of polyunsaturated fatty acids that are susceptible to lipid peroxidation. In healthy cells, there is a well-balanced equilibrium between free radical generation and various enzymatic and non-enzymatic antioxidant defense systems.[16,17] In neuronal diseases, an imbalance leading to free

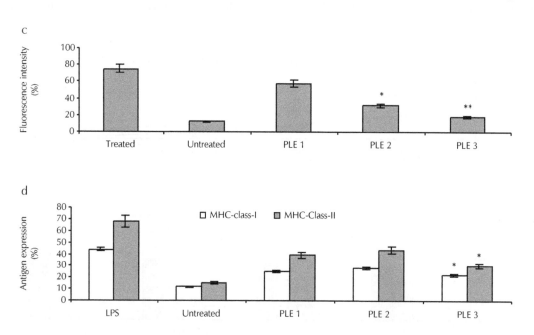

Figure 22.1 *continued*   (c) The antioxidant effects of *Polypodium leucotomos* (PLE1), *Polypodium cambricum* L. spp. (PLE2) and *Polypodium vulgare* L. (PLE3). This activity was measured by incubating primary microglial cultures with hydrogen peroxide and 50 μg/ml of each extract and the amounts of intracellular hydrogen peroxide were detected by a fluorescence activated cell sorter (FACScan) flow cytometer (Becton Dickinson). At least 10 000 cells were analyzed for each test, and the observed fluorescence reflects the intracellular hydrogen peroxide level. Each column represents the mean of five experiments and shows the mean of fluorescence intensity. *$p < 0.05$, versus treated control cultures, as determined using Student's *t* test. (d) The effects of PLE1, PLE2 and PLE3 treatment on the expression of MHC class-I and MHC class-II molecules by microglia. Each column represents the mean of five experiments and shows the percentage of antigen expression. *$p < 0.05$, versus lipopolysaccharide-positive controls, as determined using Student's *t* test. LPS, lipopolysaccharide

radical accumulation occurs, and free radicals have been implicated in several neurodegenerative diseases including Parkinson's disease (PD) and AD.

To examine whether extracts obtained from *Polypodium leucotomos* (PLE1), *Polypodium cambricum* L. spp. (PLE2) and *Polypodium vulgare* L. (PLE3) could inhibit the oxygen stress, primary microglial cells were preincubated with various dosages of extracts followed by treatment with hydrogen peroxide (H_2O_2). The intracellular H_2O_2 level was determined by using DCFH-DA and detected by flow cytometry. A 50-fold increase in fluorescence intensity was observed in microglial cells treated with $40\,\mu mol/l$ H_2O_2 for $20\,min$, as compared to untreated controls (Figure 1c, compare curves a and b). Under the same experimental conditions the H_2O_2 level was reduced to 58%, 32% and 18% in microglial cells treated with $50\,\mu g/ml$ of PLE1, PLE2 and PLE3 extracts, respectively. It is clear that the intracellular reactive oxygen species (ROS) in microglial cells were reduced after co-incubation with the extracts of all *Polypodium* species.

According to the above results, the crude extracts of *Polypodium* species, especially the *Polypodium vulgare* L. ethanolic extract, showed excellent antioxidant activity *in vitro*. To evaluate the immunoregulatory properties further of *Polypodium* extracts on primary microglial cells, a flow cytometric technique was employed. Figure 22.1d shows that this represents a powerful method for screening of new antioxidant and immunoregulatory molecules. An increased expression of both MHC class-I and class-II antigens, which could in turn reflect the active and phagocytic state of microglia, can be observed after incubation with LPS with respect to unstimulated cells. All *Polypodium* species (PL1–PL3), tested at a concentration of $50\,\mu g/ml$ were able to down-regulate the expression of both MHC class-I and class-II antigens.

What specific signals drive microglia to a reactive state? In culture systems, phagocytic signals, cytokines, including γ-interferon, and a variety of other immunoactivators (lectins, LPS and phorbol esters) as scavenger receptor ligands have been used to elicit microglial secretion, changes in shape, appearance of surface markers, or chemotactic responses.[18] Immunomodulators have also been implicated as microglial activators *in vivo*, where it has been found that systemic injections of TNF-α elicit microglial MHC class-II receptors. Perhaps systemic immune responses, which generate cytokine release, initiate a reactive state within the brain. Granulocyte–macrophage colony-stimulating factor (GM-CSF) has been found to expand microglial populations after infusions into brain tissues, and a GM-CSF-like factor has been recovered from the injured brain.[8] Microglial sensitivity to immunoregulatory signals represents, therefore, an important link between immune and neural tissues.

CONCLUSIONS

Reactive microglia appear in almost every type of CNS disorder, including infection, trauma, stroke, degeneration and demyelination. These inflammatory cells are the major source of CNS-derived cytokines, help to regulate wound healing in neural tissues and serve as an important link between systemic immune responses and the CNS. Moreover, microglia produce a wide spectrum of cytotoxic agents, and under special conditions neurotrophic factors, some of which demonstrate potent regulatory effects. In conclusion, inflammatory cell production of neuron-killing factors is a significant pathogenic mechanism common to a variety of CNS insults. Inhibition of inflammatory cell-derived toxins may help to preserve neurons near sites of tissue injury and, thus, improve recovery and function. Special attention has to be paid to the neurotrophic capabilities of microglia, as observed in the neuronal apoptosis protection experiments carried out in this study.

Furthermore, the administration of novel compounds from natural products might be useful as preventive strategies under certain conditions in cases where CNS damage involves microglia-associated inflammatory and/or degenerative processes.

REFERENCES

1. Aloisi F. Immune function of microglia. Glia 2001; 36: 165–9

2. Becher B, Prat A, Antel JP. Brain-immune connection: immuno-regulatory properties of CNS-resident cells. Glia 2000; 15: 293–304

3. Gebicke-Haerter PJ. Microglia in neurodegeneration: molecular aspects. Microsc Res Tech 2001; 54: 47–58

4. Gonzalez-Scarano F, Baltuch G. Microglia as mediators of inflammatory and degenerative diseases. Annu Rev Neurosci 1999; 22: 19–40

5. Cheng Y, Chen M, Wixom P, Sun AY. Extracellular ATP may induce neuronal degeneration by a free radical mechanism. Ann NY Acad Sci 1994; 738: 431–5

6. Cowell RM, Xu H, Galasso JM, Silverstein FS. Hypoxic–ischemic injury induces macrophage inflammatory protein-1alpha expression in immature rat brain. Stroke 2002; 33: 795–801

7. Eskes C, Honegger P, Juillerat-Jeanneret L, Monnet-Tschudi F. Microglial reaction induced by noncytotoxic methylmercury treatment leads to neuroprotection via interactions with astrocytes and IL-6 release. Glia 2002; 37: 43–52

8. Guo L, Sawkar A, Zasadzki M, et al. Similar activation of glial cultures from different rat brain regions by neuroinflammatory stimuli and downregulation of the activation by a new class of small molecule ligands. Neurobiol Aging 2001; 22: 975–81

9. Maneiro E, Lombardi VRM, Cacabelos R. Rat cell cultures: experimental models to study neurodegenerative disorders and new pharmacological compounds. Meth Find Exp Clin Pharmacol 1996; 18: 615–45

10. Varon S. Neurons and glia in neural cultures. Exp Neurol 1975; 48: 93–104

11. Haucke C, Korr H. RCA-I lectin histochemistry after trypsinization enables the identification of microglial cells in thin paraffin sections of the mouse brain. J Neurosci Methods 1993; 50: 273–7

12. Barber SA, Bruett L, Douglass BR, et al. Visna virus-induced activation of MAPK is required for virus replication and correlates with virus-induced neuropathology. J Virol 2002; 76: 817–28

13. Streit WJ, Conde JR, Harriso JK. Chemokines and Alzheimer's disease. Neurobiol Aging 2001; 22: 885–93

14. Campanella M, Sciorati C, Tarozzo G, Beltramo M. Flow cytometric analysis of inflammatory cells in ischemic rat brain. Stroke 2002; 33: 586–92

15. German DC, Liang CL, Song T, et al. Neurodegeneration in the Niemann-Pick C mouse: glial involvement. Neuroscience 2002; 109: 437–50

16. Gutteridge J, Halliwell B. Iron toxicity and oxygen radicals. Baillière's Clin Haematol 1989; 2: 195–256

17. Ames BN, Shigenaga MK, Hagen TM. Oxidants, antioxidants, and the degenerative disease of aging. Proc Natl Acad Sci USA 1993; 90: 7915–22

18. Lee WH, Kim SH, Jeong EM, et al. A novel chemokine, leukotactin-1, induces chemotaxis, proatherogenic cytokines, and tissue factor expression in atherosclerosis. Atherosclerosis 2002; 161: 255–61

Cerebrospinal fluid phosphorylated tau protein at serine 199 is a useful diagnostic biomarker in Alzheimer's disease and mild cognitive impairment

K Urakami, H Arai, N Itoh, K Ishiguro, H Oono, M Taniguchi, K Wada-Isoe,
Y Wakutani, S Kuzuhara, H Sasaki, K Nakashima, K Imahori

INTRODUCTION

Our recent studies of biological markers in Alzheimer's disease (AD) have focused specifically on analysis of cerebrospinal fluid (CSF) tau protein levels and amyloid β-protein ending at amino acid 42.[1–4] Although CSF total tau (t-tau) level in AD was significantly higher than in controls, there were overlaps between AD and non-AD dementias.[1–3] One possible explanation is that the enzyme-linked immunosorbent assay (ELISA) kit we used detects not only phosphorylated but also normal tau. Therefore, we

developed the sandwich ELISA system for phosphorylated tau at serine 199 (p-tau 199) in CSF[5] and examined 236 cases with AD, 206 cases with non-AD demented and non-demented disease controls, and 95 age-matched normal controls.[6]

SUBJECTS AND METHODS

Table 23.1 shows a summary of the patients' demographic data. We surveyed a total of 537 CSF samples. We also examined CSF p-tau 199

Table 23.1 Summary of patients' demographic data

	No. of patients	*Age* (years)	*Gender* (M/F)
Alzheimer's disease (AD)	235*	71 ± 9	66/172
Normal control	95	57 ± 16	51/44
Neurological disease control	122	59 ± 13	70/52
Frontotemporal dementia (FTD)	16*	63 ± 12	9/7
Progressive supranuclear palsy	21	63 ± 7	10/11
Corticobasal degeneration	15	64 ± 4	8/7
Dementia with Lewy body (DLB)	13*	63 ± 10	8/5
Vascular dementia	23	71 ± 6	16/7
Meningoencephalitis	18	51 ± 21	7/11
Creutzfeldt–Jakob disease (CJD)	11*	71 ± 6	6/5

* Two patients with AD, one patient with FTD, one patient with DLB and four patients with CJD were confirmed by autopsy

levels in a population with mild cognitive impairment (MCI). The MCI group was later subdivided into two different categories. One category was that which eventually later progressed to AD (progressive MCI). The other category was that which later did not progress to AD (non-progressive MCI). Memory complainers were patients who complained about memory disturbance, but were not demented. These constituted the control group. CSF samples were taken into polypropylene tubes by lumbar puncture after informed consent was obtained from each patient and/or family members. Bloody or traumatic CSF samples were excluded from this study. After centrifugation at 1500 rpm for 10 min, the aliquots were stored at −80°C until analysis. CSF levels of

p-tau 199 were measured by a sensitive sandwich ELISA.[5,6] CSF level of t-tau protein was measured using the sandwich ELISA assay provided by the Innogenetics Company, Belgium.[7]

RESULTS

CSF p-tau 199 levels in the AD group were significantly elevated ($p < 0.001$) compared to those in all the other non-AD groups, including patients with acute neurological conditions such as meningoencephalitis and Creutzfeldt–Jakob disease (CJD) (Figure 23.1). On the other hand, CSF t-tau levels were occasionally very high in the meningoencephalitis and CJD groups,

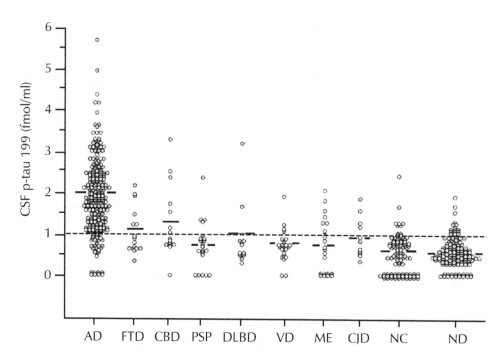

Figure 23.1 The results of cerebrospinal fluid (CSF) phosphorylated tau at serine 199 (p-tau 199) levels, among groups with Alzheimer's disease (AD), frontotemporal dementia (FTD), corticobasal degeneration (CBD), progressive supranuclear palsy (PSP), dementia with Lewy body disease (DLBD), vascular dementia (VD), meningoencephalitis (ME), Creutzfeldt–Jakob disease (CJD), normal controls (NC) and neurological disease controls (ND)

although most CSF t-tau levels were significantly increased in the AD group compared to normal control groups (Figure 23.2).

A receiver operating characteristics (ROC) curve analysis demonstrated that CSF p-tau 199

was more amenable than CSF t-tau to differentiating between AD and non-AD subjects (Table 23.2).

The results of CSF p-tau 199 levels in the progressive MCI group were significantly

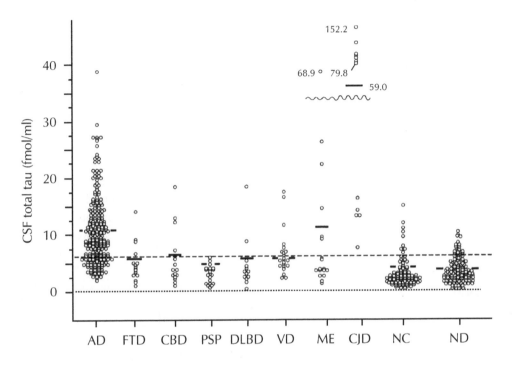

Figure 23.2 The results of cerebrospinal fluid (CSF) total tau levels, among groups with Alzheimer's disease (AD), frontotemporal dementia (FTD), corticobasal degeneration (CBD), progressive supranuclear palsy (PSP), dementia with Lewy body disease (DLBD), vascular dementia (VD), meningoencephalitis (ME), Creutzfeldt–Jakob disease (CJD), normal controls (NC) and neurological disease controls (ND)

Table 23.2 Receiver operating curve analysis

	Cut-off level (fmol/ml)	Sensitivity (%)	Specificity (%)
Alzheimer's disease vs. neurological disease controls and normal controls			
Total tau	4.8	82.7	82.0
p-tau 199	0.96	87.3	87.4
Alzheimer's disease vs. others			
Total tau	6.0	77.1	77.6
p-tau 199	1.05	85.2	85.0

p-tau 199, phosphorylated tau at serine 199

elevated ($p < 0.001$) compared to those in the non-progressive MCI and the control groups (Figure 23.3). We thus propose that CSF p-tau 199 may also be useful for the diagnosis of MCI as it is for AD.

DISCUSSION

In the present study, we examined CSF p-tau 199 levels in a total of 570 living ($n = 562$) or autopsy-confirmed ($n = 8$) subjects with AD and other dementing disorders that resemble AD, as well as normal and neurological diseased controls. A combination of HT-7 (phosphorylation-independent monoclonal antibody; Innogenetics) and the anti-p-tau 199 antibody anti-PS199 allowed us to detect and quantitate

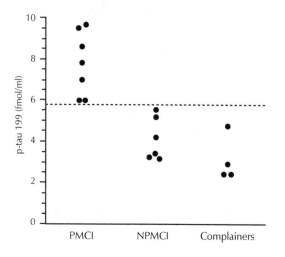

Figure 23.3 The results of cerebrospinal fluid (CSF) phosphorylated tau at serine 199 (p-tau 199) in mild cognitive impairment (MCI). PMCI, progressive MCI (Alzheimer's disease; AD); NPMCI, non-progressive MCI (non-AD). With a cut-off of 5.8 fmol/ml, sensitivity for PMCI 100% (7/7), and specificity for NPMCI 100% (6/6)

CSF levels of the p-tau 199 by a newly constructed sandwich ELISA.[5,6] We reported p-tau 199 to be elevated in AD using different diagnostic antibodies that uniquely recognize specific phosphorylation epitopes of tau. We also monitored the CSF t-tau levels side by side in the same patients to assess and compare the sensitivity and specificity by ROC. Here, it should be noted that CSF p-tau 199 is not only the first biomarker that exceeds (over 85%) both sensitivity and specificity as a sole biomarker of AD, but also meets many other recommended criteria as an ideal biomarker.[8] The improvement of the diagnostic accuracy using CSF p-tau 199 seems to be accomplished not only by enhancing the lowest detection limit but also by eliminating a subset of non-AD patients with high CSF t-tau levels. Indeed, it is noteworthy that a subset of CJD patients with extremely high CSF t-tau levels showed only a mild elevation or an elevation under the cut-off level of CSF p-tau 199.

Nonetheless, our study suggests that there might be a limitation even in the use of the p-tau assay for a clear-cut distinction to be made between AD and certain tauopathies. In fact, the CSF p-tau 199 levels were over the cut-off value in approximately 30% (16/52) of the non-AD tauopathy group (Figure 23.2). Additional studies reported that pathological tau isoforms purified from tauopathy brains were occasionally hyperphosphorylayed at serine 199.[9,10] Therefore, the CSF p-tau 199 testing may be less accurate in distinguishing AD from other types of degenerative dementia or tauopathies. New and/or modified biomarkers would be necessary to differentiate AD from tauopathies in the future.[11,12]

A substantial proportion of subjects with MCI later developed clinical AD.[13] At autopsy, subjects with MCI showed a broad spectrum of morphological brain changes including typical AD pathological characteristics. Therefore, MCI partly represents a predementia stage of AD. To maximize the benefit of therapeutic strategies, it is important to identify AD at the stage of MCI. Biochemical markers will be required to establish the diagnosis of MCI.[14] This study showed that CSF p-tau 199 levels in the progressive MCI group were significantly elevated compared to those in the non-progressive MCI and the control groups. We found that CSF p-tau 199 increased in an early stage of AD, the so-called MCI state, and confirmed that CSF p-tau 199 may be useful for the diagnosis of MCI as well as AD.

CONCLUSION

Our results suggest that CSF p-tau 199 is useful for an early diagnosis of AD.

REFERENCES

1. Isoe K, Urakami K, Shimomura T, et al. Tau proteins in cerebrospinal fluid from patients with Alzheimer's disease: a longitudinal study. Dementia 1996; 7: 175–6

2. Kanai M, Matsubara E, Isoe K, et al. Longitudinal study of cerebrospinal fluid levels of tau, Aβ1-40 and Aβ1-42(43) in Alzheimer's disease: a study in Japan. Ann Neurol 1998; 44: 17–26

3. Andreasen N, Minthon L, Davidsson P, et al. Evaluation of CSF-tau and CSF-A beta42 as diagnostic markers for Alzheimer disease in clinical practice. Arch Neurol 2001; 58: 373–9

4. Takeda M, Tanaka T, Arai H, et al. Basic and clinical studies on the measurement of beta-amyloid (1-42) in cerebrospinal fluid as a diagnostic marker for Alzheimer's disease and related disorders: multicenter study in Japan. Psychogeriatrics 2001; 1: 56–63

5. Ishiguro K, Ohno H, Arai H, et al. Phosphorylated tau in human cerebrospinal fluid is a diagnositic marker for Alzheimer's disease. Neurosci Lett 1999; 270: 91–4

6. Itoh N, Arai H, Urakami K, et al. Large-scale, multicenter study of cerebrospinal fluid tau protein phosphorylated at serine 199 for the antemortem diagnosis of Alzheimer's disease. Ann Neurol 2001; 50: 150–6

7. Vandermeeren M, Mercken M, Vanmechelen E, et al. Detection of tau proteins in normal and Alzheimer's disease cerebrospinal fluid with a sensitive sandwich enzyme-immunosorbent assay. J Neurochem 1993; 61: 1828–34

8. The Ronald and Nancy Reagan Research Institute of the Alzheimer's Association and the National Institute on Aging Working Group. Consensus Report of the Working Group on Molecular and Biochemical Markers in Alzheimer's Disease. Neurobiol Aging 1998; 19: 109–16

9. Delacourte A, Seargent N, Wattez A, et al. Vulnerable neuronal subsets in Alzheimer's and Pick's disease are distinguished by their tau isoform distribution and phosphorylation. Ann Neurol 1998; 43: 193–204

10. Seargent N, Wattez A, Delacourte A. Neurofibrillary degeneration in progressive supranuclear palsy and corticobasal degeneration: tau pathologies with exclusively 'exon 10' isoforms. J Neurochem 1999; 72: 1243–9

11. Urakami K, Mori M, Wada K, et al. A comparison of tau protein in cerebrospinal fluid

between corticobasal degeneration and progressive supranuclear palsy. Neurosci Lett 1998; 259: 1–3

12. Urakami K, Wada K, Arai H, et al. Diagnostic significance of tau proteins in cerebrospinal fluids from patients with corticobasal degeneration or progressive supranuclear palsy. J Neurol Sci 2001; 183: 95–8

13. Ritchie K, Touchon J. Mild cognitive impairment: conceptual basis and current nosological status. Lancet 2000; 355: 225–58

14. Riemenschneider M, Lautenschlager N, Wagenpfeil S, et al. Cerebrospinal fluid tau and beta-amyloid 42 proteins identify Alzheimer disease in subjects with mild cognitive impairment. Arch Neurol 2002; 59: 1729–34

Chapter 24

Stem cell strategies for Alzheimer's disease

K Sugaya

INTRODUCTION

Neuropathological conditions caused by the degeneration of neuronal cells have been considered incurable because of a long-held 'truism': neurons do not regenerate during adulthood. However, this statement has been challenged and we have found new evidence that neurons do indeed have the potential to be renewed after maturation. The discovery of multipotent neural stem cells (NSCs) in the adult brain[1,2] has brought revolutionary changes in the theory of neurogenesis, which currently posits that regeneration of neurons can occur throughout life, thus opening a door for the development of novel therapies to treat neurodegenerative diseases by neuronal regeneration using stem cell transplantation.

NSCs have been isolated from the embryonic and adult mammalian[3,4] and human[5] central nervous system (CNS) and propagated *in vitro* in a variety of culture systems.[6] The inability to grow NSCs *in vitro* in the absence of complex and undefined biological fluids (e.g. sera) has long been a major obstacle in understanding the biology of these cells. In our laboratory, human neural stem cells (HNSCs) have been cultured and expanded *in vitro* without differentiation, using a serum-free medium containing epi-

dermal growth factor (EGF) and basic fibroblast growth factor (bFGF).[7] Using a serum-free unsupplemented medium, HNSCs differentiated into βIII-tubulin-, glial fibrillary acidic protein (GFAP)- and O4-immunopositive cells, markers for neurons, astrocytes and oligodendrocytes, respectively.[7] These results suggest that HNSCs are capable of producing the endogenous factors necessary for their own differentiation and survival. Thus, it appears that HNSCs produce factors to differentiate and support themselves, which encouraged our investigation of the transplantation of HNSCs into aged animals. We found not only that HNSCs could survive for 30 days after xenotransplantation while retaining both multipotency and migratory capacity, but also that HNSC transplantation improved cognitive function in 24-month-old rats.

IMPROVEMENT OF COGNITIVE FUNCTION IN THE AGED RAT BY THE TRANSPLANTATION OF HUMAN NEURAL STEM CELLS

HNSCs, expanded without differentiation under the influence of mitogenic factors in supplemented serum-free media,[8] and labeled by the incorporation of bromodeoxyuridine (BrdU) into the nucleus DNA, were injected into the lateral ventricle of mature (6-month-old) and aged (24-month-old) rats. Cognitive function of the animals was assessed by the Morris water maze both before and 4 weeks after the transplantation of HNSCs. Before HNSC transplantation, some aged animals (aged memory-unimpaired animals) cognitively functioned in the range of mature animals, while others (aged memory-impaired animals) functioned entirely below the cognitive range of the mature animals. After HNSC transplantation, most aged animals had cognitive function in the range of the mature animals. Strikingly, one of the aged memory-impaired animals showed dramatic improvement in behavior, functioning even better than the mature animals. Statistical analysis showed that cognitive function was significantly improved in both mature and aged memory-impaired animals but not in aged memory-unimpaired animals after HNSC transplantation, which could have been due to the physical limitations of the aged animals. We also observed that the performance of three of the aged animals deteriorated in the water maze after HNSC transplantation. This observation needs further analysis, but it is possible that the physical strength of these animals deteriorated during the experimental period. These behavioral results show the beneficial effects of HNSC transplantation into the host brain in most animals tested.

After the second water maze task, postmortem brains were further analyzed by immunohistochemistry for human βIII-tubulin and human GFAP, markers for neurons and astrocytes, respectively. There was no sign of ventricular distortion and no evidence of tumor formation, and, further, no strong host antigraft immunoreactivity was observed. Intensely

and extensively stained with βIII-tubulin, neurons with BrdU-positive nuclei, were found in bilateral cingulate and parietal cortices and the hippocampus. The βIII-tubulin-positive neurons found in the cerebral cortex were typified by a dendrite pointing to the edge of the cortex. In the hippocampus, donor-derived neurons exhibited multiple morphologies varying in cellular size and shape, and one or more processes and branching. Thus, HNSCs may be the most promising candidate for neuroreplacement therapy. However, the ethical issues and risk of immunological rejection limit their value. The ideal biological source of cells for replacement therapies would be autologous transplantation of stem cells derived from the patient's own tissues.

NEURAL DIFFERENTIATION OF HUMAN MESENCHYMAL STEM CELLS

Bone marrow contains stem-like cells used not only for hematopoiesis but also for production of a variety of non-hematopoietic tissues. A subset of stromal cells in bone marrow, which has been referred to as mesenchymal stem cells (MeSCs), is capable of producing multiple mesenchymal cell lineages, including bone, cartilage, fat, tendons and other connective tissues.[9–12] Recent reports show that human MeSCs (HMeSCs) also have the ability to differentiate into a diverse family of cell types that may be unrelated to their phenotypic embryonic origin, including muscle and hepatocytes.[13–18] Although the potential therapeutic use of HMeSCs in the CNS has been discussed,[19,20] and several *in vivo* transplantation studies showed neural and glial differentiation of HMeSCs,[21–25] technologies to induce neural lineage from HMeSCs are not fully established.

In our previous study, we found that HNSCs spontaneously differentiated into brain cells; however, under basal media conditions HMeSCs never spontaneously differentiated into neural cells without the addition of certain factors. These results indicate that each stem cell contains specific information that would allow it to become a special type of cell; that is, cells are partially committed to differentiate in a tissue-specific manner. To investigate neural differentiation of HMeSCs *in vivo*, HMeSCs expanded without differentiation and labeled by the incorporation of BrdU into nuclear DNA were injected into the lateral ventricle of mature mice (C57/black). Four to six weeks after transplantation, mouse brains were analyzed by immunohistochemistry for human specific βIII-tubulin and GFAP, markers for neurons and astrocytes, respectively. Migration and differentiation patterns of the transplanted HMeSCs were quite similar to our previous results with HNSCs transplanted into rats. Intensely and extensively stained with βIII-tubulin neurons, BrdU-positive nuclei were found in the bilateral cingulate and parietal cortices, and in the hippocampus. The βIII-tubulin-positive neurons found in the cerebral cortex typically demonstrated a dendrite pointing to the edge of the cortex. In the hippocampus, donor-derived neurons exhibited multiple morphologies and varied in cellular size and shape, with one or more processes and branching. In our previous HNSC transplantation study, cells migrated to the target area in 4 weeks. The migration speed of HMeSCs seemed to be slower than that of HNSCs, because at 4 weeks after transplantation, HMeSCs were still migrating toward the pyramidal cell line of the hippocampus CA1 and it took 6 weeks for HMeSCs to reach the target area.

Recently, two different groups reported spontaneous fusion of stem cells.[26,27] In these reports, the authors found that stem cells acquired phenotypes from other cells by fusion, which may occur when these stem cells directly touch other cells after transplantation. To investigate the possibility of the neural differentiation of HMeSCs without fusion, we co-cultured BrdU-labeled HMeSCs with differentiated HNSCs. The HNSCs were differentiated under the basal medium condition: i.e. serum-free basal medium containing Earle's salt and L-glutamine for 5 days prior to co-culture. The HNSCs spontaneously differentiated into mixed cell populations, including neural precursors that formed a sphere in the middle of the culture, and coronary migrating immature and/or mature neurons and astrocytes. The HMeSCs were transferred onto a tissue-culture 0.4-μm membrane insert and placed on top of the differentiated HNSCs under the basal medium condition.

Immunocytochemical examination 7 days post-co-culture revealed that HMeSCs differentiated into βIII-tubulin immunopositive small bipolar and unipolar cells (approximately 40% of the total), and GFAP-immunopositive large flattened multipolar cells (approximately 60% of the total). Although the process of βIII-tubulin-immunopositive cells derived from HMeSCs was shorter than that found in differentiated HNSCs, the general cell morphology in both HNSCs and HMeSCs-differentiated cultures was similar. This result indicates that HMeSCs are capable of becoming neurons and astrocytes when co-cultured with differentiated NSCs. In this *in vitro* experiment, HMeSCs were cultured on the membrane insert and were kept totally separated from the HNSCs. Thus, the possibility of fusion between HMeSCs and HNSCs can be excluded.

These results indicate that the brain environment may produce factor(s) that allow the differentiation of not only NSCs but also MeSCs into neurons, and suggest that HMeSCs may serve as an alternative to HNSCs for potential therapeutic use in neuroreplacement.

AMYLOID β PROTEIN PRECURSOR FUNCTION IN STEM CELL BIOLOGY

The prevalence of the amyloid β (Aβ) neuro-toxicity theory in Alzheimer's disease (AD) pathology, and the absence of a phenotype in the amyloid β protein precursor (APP) knockout mouse, tend to limit our focus on the physiological functions of APP. Previous studies have shown that APP may be involved in neurite outgrowth,[28,29] cell proliferation,[30–32] neuronal migration[33] and neuronal differentiation.[34] APP expression is increased by brain injury[35,36] and amyloidogenic secretion increase in apoptotic cells.[37] APP may also be involved in cell survival.[38–40] Although these facts may indicate the involvement of APP in neuroplasticity, the physiological functions of APP are not clear.

We have found evidence that APP fragments are secreted from apoptotic HNSCs, and that these fragments may induce differentiation of other HNSCs *in vitro*. We have also observed that exogenously added secreted-type APP (sAPP) induces the differentiation of HNSCs, while an antibody recognizing the N-terminal of APP prevents the differentiation of HNSCs. These findings indicate that APP signaling is one of the regulatory systems involved in the differentiation of NSCs. We also found that HNSCs transplanted into the APP-knockout mouse brain could not migrate properly and failed to repair brain lesions, whereas HNSCs transplanted into the wild-type mouse successfully migrated into the proper position and differentiated into the correct kind of cells. This result is not only the first finding of a phenotypical change in APP-knockout mice, but also indicates a physiological role for APP in the regeneration of adult brain cells. Furthermore,

we found that the addition of a higher concentration of sAPP or the overexpression of APP by transgenes to HNSC cultures caused glial rather than neural differentiation of these cells. These findings indicate that the pathological alteration of APP metabolism in AD induces glial differentiation of neural stem cells and leads to the exhaustion of the stem cell population, which may be an important function in the ongoing neurogenesis of the adult brain.

It is not clear whether adult neurogenesis is essential for normal cognitive function in aging. Nonetheless, it is tempting to hypothesize that pathologically altered APP metabolism could impair NSC migration and differentiation into the proper ratio of neurons and glia in AD. Although the rate of endogenous neuro-regeneration in the adult brain may be minimal, in the long run, a defect in this process might significantly harm normal brain function. Incidentally, this possibility raises the question of whether Aβ immunization, which may also reduce APP fragments, is helpful for maintaining stem cell function in AD. It is the author's opinion that this is not helpful, owing to the fact that HNSCs transplanted into APP knockout mice do not migrate or effectively differentiate into neurons in the cerebral cortex. HNSCs may play an important role in neuroregeneration, and if APP is, indeed, involved in the regulation of HNSCs, destruction of the APP system may jeopardize the maintenance of brain function.

A possible scenario to reconstruct neuronal circuits under the guidance of NSCs could be that sAPP released from damaged or dying cells may preferentially induce glial differentiation of a specific population of NSCs. These NSC-derived glial cells can then produce factors that may support surrounding damaged cells[41] and promote neuronal migration and differentiation of other NSCs in the local area. This scenario fits in with our *in vitro* observations that initially apoptotic cell death-induced glial differentiation was followed by neuronal differentiation.[7] Thus, under normal physiological conditions, APP may be a key factor that is necessary to recover from brain damage. In the cases of familial AD and Down's syndrome, the increased levels of APP fragments produced in the brains of these patients may modify the biological equilibrium of HNSCs in such a way that a pathological shift toward premature differentiation of HNSCs will occur, thereby exhausting the HNSC population. Since the effective natural replacement of degenerating neurons in the adult brain during aging or the disease process may be important in maintaining normal brain function, exhaustion of the HNSC population would pose serious problems.

CONCLUSION

We have succeeded in developing neural and mesenchymal stem cell transplantation to produce neural cells in the brain. We have seen the improvement of cognitive function in a memory-impaired aged animal model following stem cell transplantation. Although these results may promise a bright future for stem cell strategies, we now have to consider the pathophysiological environments of individual diseases, which may affect stem cell biology, before clinical applications of neuroreplacement therapy could become a reality.

REFERENCES

1. Alvarez-Buylla A, Garcia-Verdugo JM. Neurogenesis in adult subventricular zone. J Neurosci 2002; 22: 629–34

2. Gould E, Reeves AJ, Fallah M, et al. Hippocampal neurogenesis in adult Old World primates. Proc Natl Acad Sci USA 1999; 96: 5263–7

3. Doetsch F, Caille I, Lim DA, et al. Subventricular zone astrocytes are neural stem cells in the adult mammalian brain. Cell 1999; 97: 703–16

4. Johansson CB, Svensson M, Wallstedt L, et al. Neural stem cells in the adult human brain. Exp Cell Res 1999; 253: 733–6

5. Johansson CB, Momma S, Clarke DL, et al. Identification of a neural stem cell in the adult mammalian central nervous system. Cell 1999; 96: 25–34

6. Svendsen CN, ter Borg MG, Armstrong RJ, et al. A new method for the rapid and long term growth of human neural precursor cells. J Neurosci Methods 1998; 85: 141–52

7. Brannen CL, Sugaya K. In vitro differentiation of multipotent human neural progenitors in serum-free medium. Neuroreport 2000; 11: 1123–8

8. Qu T, Brannen CL, Kim HM, Sugaya K. Human neural stem cells improve cognitive function of aged brain. Neuroreport 2001; 12: 1127–32

9. Majumdar MK, Thiede MA, Mosca JD, et al. Phenotypic and functional comparison of cultures of marrow-derived mesenchymal stem cells (MSCs) and stromal cells. J Cell Physiol 1998; 176: 57–66

10. Pereira RF, Halford KW, O'Hara MD, et al. Cultured adherent cells from marrow can serve as long-lasting precursor cells for bone, cartilage, and lung in irradiated mice. Proc Natl Acad Sci USA 1995; 92: 4857–61

11. Prockop DJ. Marrow stromal cells as stem cells for nonhematopoietic tissues. Science 1997; 276: 71–4

12. Pittenger MF, Mackay AM, Beck SC, et al. Multilineage potential of adult human mesenchymal stem cells. Science 1999; 284: 143–7

13. Ferrari G, Cusella-De Angelis G, Coletta M, et al. Muscle regeneration by bone marrow-derived myogenic progenitors. Science 1998; 279: 1528–30

14. Makino S, Fukuda K, Miyoshi S, et al. Cardiomyocytes can be generated from marrow stromal cells in vitro. J Clin Invest 1999; 103: 697–705

15. Petersen BE, Bowen WC, Patrene KD, et al. Bone marrow as a potential source of hepatic oval cells. Science 1999; 284: 1168–70

16. Mackenzie TC, Flake AW. Human mesenchymal stem cells persist, demonstrate site-specific multipotential differentiation, and are present in sites of wound healing and tissue regeneration after transplantation into fetal sheep. Blood Cells Mol Dis 2001; 27: 601–4

17. Imasawa T, Utsunomiya Y, Kawamura T, et al. The potential of bone marrow-derived cells to differentiate to glomerular mesangial cells. J Am Soc Nephrol 2001; 12: 1401–9

18. Liechty KW, MacKenzie TC, Shaaban AF, et al. Human mesenchymal stem cells engraft and demonstrate site-specific differentiation after in utero transplantation in sheep. Nat Med 2000; 6: 1282–6

19. Prockop DJ, Azizi SA, Phinney DG, et al. Potential use of marrow stromal cells as therapeutic vectors for diseases of the central nervous system. Prog Brain Res 2000; 128: 293–7

20. Bianco P, Riminucci M, Gronthos S, Robey PG. Bone marrow stromal stem cells: nature, biology, and potential applications. Stem Cells 2001; 19: 180–92

21. Schwarz EJ, Alexander GM, Prockop DJ, Azizi SA. Multipotential marrow stromal cells transduced to produce L-DOPA: engraftment in a rat model of Parkinson disease. Hum Gene Ther 1999; 10: 2539–49

22. Chopp M, Zhang XH, Li Y, et al. Spinal cord injury in rat: treatment with bone marrow stromal cell transplantation. Neuroreport 2000; 11: 3001–5

23. Chen J, Li Y, Chopp M. Intracerebral transplantation of bone marrow with BDNF after MCAo in rat. Neuropharmacology 2000; 39: 711–16

24. Li Y, Chopp M, Chen J, et al. Intrastriatal transplantation of bone marrow non-hematopoietic cells improves functional recovery after stroke in adult mice. J Cereb Blood Flow Metab 2000; 20: 1311–19

25. Kopen GC, Prockop DJ, Phinney DG. Marrow stromal cells migrate throughout forebrain and cerebellum, and they differentiate into astrocytes after injection into neonatal mouse brains. Proc Natl Acad Sci USA 1999; 96: 10711–16

26. Terada N, Hamazaki T, Oka M, et al. Bone marrow cells adopt the phenotype of other cells by spontaneous cell fusion. Nature 2002; 416: 542–5

27. Ying QL, Nichols J, Evans EP, Smith AG. Changing potency by spontaneous fusion. Nature 2002; 416: 545–8

28. Roch JM, Jin LW, Ninomiya H, et al. Biologically active domain of the secreted form of the amyloid beta/A4 protein precursor. Ann NY Acad Sci 1993; 695: 149–57

29. Salinero O, Moreno-Flores MT, Wandosell F. Increasing neurite outgrowth capacity of beta-amyloid precursor protein proteoglycan in Alzheimer's disease. J Neurosci Res 2000; 60: 87–97

30. Hayashi Y, Kashiwagi K, Ohta J, et al. Alzheimer amyloid protein precursor enhances proliferation of neural stem cells from fetal rat

brain. Biochem Biophys Res Commun 1994; 205: 936–43

31. Hoffmann J, Twiesselmann C, Kummer MP, et al. A possible role for the Alzheimer amyloid precursor protein in the regulation of epidermal basal cell proliferation. [In Process Citation]. Eur J Cell Biol 2000; 79: 905–14

32. Ohsawa I, Takamura C, Morimoto T, et al. Amino-terminal region of secreted form of amyloid precursor protein stimulates proliferation of neural stem cells. Eur J Neurosci 1999; 11: 1907–13

33. De Strooper B, Annaert W. Proteolytic processing and cell biological functions of the amyloid precursor protein. J Cell Sci 2000; 113: 1857–70

34. Ando K, Oishi M, Takeda S, et al. Role of phosphorylation of Alzheimer's amyloid precursor protein during neuronal differentiation. J Neurosci 1999; 19: 4421–7

35. Koszyca B, Blumbergs PC, Manavis J, et al. Widespread axonal injury in gunshot wounds to the head using amyloid precursor protein as a marker. J Neurotrauma 1998; 15: 675–83

36. Murakami N, Yamaki T, Iwamoto Y, et al. Experimental brain injury induces expression of amyloid precursor protein, which may be related to neuronal loss in the hippocampus. J Neurotrauma 1998; 15: 993–1003

37. Galli C, Piccini A, Ciotti MT, et al. Increased amyloidogenic secretion in cerebellar granule cells undergoing apoptosis. Proc Natl Acad Sci USA 1998; 95: 1247–52

38. Rohn TT, Ivins KJ, Bahr BA, et al. A monoclonal antibody to amyloid precursor protein induces neuronal apoptosis. J Neurochem 2000; 74: 2331–42

39. Wallace WC, Akar CA, Lyons WE, et al. Amyloid precursor protein requires the insulin signaling pathway for neurotrophic activity. Brain Res Mol Brain Res 1997; 52: 213–27

40. Wang C, Wurtman RJ, Lee RK. Amyloid precursor protein and membrane phospholipids in primary cortical neurons increase with development, or after exposure to nerve growth factor or Abeta(1-40). Brain Res 2000; 865: 157–67

41. Miyachi TK, Asai H, Tsuiki H, et al. Interleukin-1beta induces the expression of lipocortin 1 mRNA in cultured rat cortical astrocytes. Neurosci Res 2001; 40: 53–60

Chapter 25

Can mild cognitive impairment predict Alzheimer's disease?

H Soininen, S Tuomainen, C Pennanen, T Hänninen, M Kivipelto

INTRODUCTION

Mild cognitive impairment (MCI) has been considered to be associated with a 10-fold risk for developing dementia, most commonly Alzheimer's disease (AD). Different kinds of tests have been put forward as predictors for AD, such as neuropsychological tests, neuroimaging findings, genetic profile and biological markers. Neuropsychological tests, in particular tests of delayed recall, are sensitive at predicting who will suffer dementia. Promising results have also been obtained from magnetic resonance imaging (MRI) studies. Atrophy of the hippocampus and the entorhinal cortex is a sensitive indicator of early AD. A volume loss in the entorhinal cortex, in particular, has been suggested to predict AD in its preclinical stage. The apolipoprotein E ε4 allele is a significant contributor in predicting AD, especially when combined with neuropsychological and MRI volumetric data. With respect to biological markers, high cerebrospinal fluid (CSF) tau and low amyloid β (Aβ)1-42 levels have been reported in MCI, but the data are by no means unequivocal. The major problem encountered in MCI studies is the diversity of the criteria used to define the disorder. In a population-based setting the MCI category is heterogeneous. However, as will be shown in this chapter, it seems to be possible to identify among the MCI subjects those individuals who are at high risk for developing AD. In particular, amnestic MCI has been considered as a prodromal state for AD. This group represents a valid target for preventive measures as well as for pharmaceutical interventions.

MILD COGNITIVE IMPAIRMENT IS HETEROGENEOUS

Subjects with MCI are characterized by memory complaints, normal general cognitive functions, impaired memory for age, normal activities of daily living, and they are not demented.[1,2] MCI has been suggested as a term representing a boundary zone between normal aging and dementia, especially AD. The criteria used for MCI have varied in different clinical and epidemiological studies, and the heterogeneity in the use of the term has been recognized.[3] Petersen and co-investigators attempted to clarify the MCI classification by proposing the use of subclassifications for MCI, in particular introducing the term amnestic MCI as a prodromal state for AD. In a study on the natural history of MCI, it was shown that individuals with MCI exhibit an increased risk of death and incident AD, and they also experience a faster decline in certain cognitive domains such as in measures of episodic memory, semantic memory and perceptual speed as compared with persons without cognitive impairment.[4]

MCI has been considered to be associated with a 10-fold risk for developing dementia.[5] In follow-up studies, more than 50% of MCI subjects converted to dementia within 3–4 years. However, the annual frequency of conversion varies from 6 to 25% across different studies.[5] An important factor affecting the conversion rate in MCI is the source of subjects in a given study; population based versus memory-clinic based. Independently from the diagnostic criteria used to define MCI, some predictive factors for AD have been suggested. In this respect, neuropsychological tests, neuroimaging data, genetic findings and biological markers have been considered.

EPIDEMIOLOGY OF MILD COGNITIVE IMPAIRMENT

There are relatively few epidemiological data on the prevalence of MCI at the population level. Many studies have focused on clinical cohorts derived from memory clinics. The Kuopio MCI study was designed to investigate the prevalence, incidence and risk factors of MCI in an elderly population. A total of 806 subjects (60–76 years of age) from a population-based random sample of 1150 subjects living in the city of Kuopio in eastern Finland were evaluated initially in 1998; the follow-up of the cohort is ongoing.[6] Neuropsychological tests and a structured interview including the modified Clinical Dementia Rating (CDR) were used to apply diagnostic criteria of MCI as proposed by the Mayo Clinic Alzheimer's Disease Research

Center. Those subjects having a test score more than 1.5 SD below the age-appropriate mean in the memory tests and a CDR score of 0.5 but no dementia, were diagnosed as having MCI. A total of 43 subjects, 5.3% of the entire population, met the MCI criteria. MCI was more prevalent in older and less-educated subjects, but no difference was found between men and women.

The CDR appeared to be the most important part of the criteria. The memory tests had less impact on prevalence variables. The low prevalence of MCI indicates that in a population-based study design its criteria may identify a more homogeneous group of subjects at the lower end of the cognitive continuum in contrast with various other criteria of cognitive impairment in the elderly population. In another study[7] on the prevalence of MCI in the elderly eastern Finnish population, applying the MCI criteria of the Mayo Clinic Alzheimer's Disease Research Center in a population of 1449 subjects aged 65–79 years, 6.1% of the population (average age, 72 years) met the criteria for MCI.

PREDICTORS OF DEMENTIA

Many studies have shown that neuropsychological tests, in particular tests of delayed recall, are sensitive at predicting who will suffer dementia.[8] Memory test scores have high predictive value in studies with longer follow-up times (4–10 years), whereas in studies with shorter follow-up periods (1–3 years), tests of verbal and executive functions are also effective. This pattern is compatible with the progression of neuropathological changes occurring in AD, which first appear in the entorhinal cortex and later progress to the isocortical areas.

In addition, promising results have been obtained from MRI studies. Atrophy of the hippocampus and the entorhinal cortex is a sensitive indicator of early AD.[9,10] The volume loss in the entorhinal cortex in particular has been suggested to predict AD during its preclinical stage.[10] In a review of neuroimaging studies in MCI, 52 studies (33 cross-sectional, 25 providing longitudinal data) were evaluated.[11] Structural studies by using computed tomography (CT) or MRI highlighted atrophy of the medial temporal lobe structures and posterior cingular region, whereas functional studies emphasized the importance of hypometabolism in temporoparietal association regions, posterior cingulate and medial temporal lobe structures.

In the Kuopio MCI study, MRI volumetric analysis of the hippocampus and entorhinal cortex provided evidence that entorhinal atrophy precedes hippocampal atrophy in AD.[12] In subjects with MCI, the entorhinal volume loss (16%) was significantly greater than the hippocampal volume loss (8%) compared to controls, with intact cognitive performance. In AD patients compared to controls, volume losses were 36% for the entorhinal cortex and 37% for the hippocampus. The entorhinal volume loss predominated over the hippocampal volume loss in MCI, whereas more pronounced hippocampal volume loss appeared in mild AD.

The apolipoprotein E (apoE) ε4 allele is a well-established risk factor for AD. It is associated with earlier age of onset, more pronounced neuropathological disturbances and increased atrophy of the medial temporal lobe structures in AD. ApoE4 seems to be particularly harmful for memory functions in AD patients and non-demented elderly subjects.[13] ApoE4, in combination with neuropsychological and MRI volumetric data, has also been shown to be a significant contributor in predicting the risk of AD.[14,15]

There are also some potential biological markers. AD is associated with high CSF tau and low Aβ1-42 levels, and high plasma Aβ1-42 levels have been reported in familial AD cases even in the preclinical stage. The data concerning these biomarkers in MCI are controversial. A recent study reported that, at baseline, 35/44 of the MCI patients who converted to AD had high CSF total tau, 31/44 exhibited high CSF phosphorylated-tau, and 34/44 had low CSF-Aβ42 levels.[16]

CARDIOVASCULAR RISK FACTORS AND MILD COGNITIVE IMPAIRMENT

AD and MCI share many risk factors, and the frequency of risk factors in the MCI group is intermediate between that in AD and normal elderly subjects, suggesting that, in a population-based setting, the MCI category is heterogeneous. Vascular risk factors may be important in the development of cognitive impairment and AD.[17–20] However, the role of vascular risk factors in MCI has remained largely unexplored.

Kivipelto and co-investigators[7] evaluated the impact of midlife elevated serum cholesterol levels and blood pressure on the subsequent development of MCI in an elderly Finnish population, and applied the MCI criteria devised by the Mayo Clinic Alzheimer's Disease Research Center. Subjects were derived from random, population-based samples previously studied in the surveys carried out in 1972, 1977, 1982 and 1987. After an average follow-up of 21 years, 1449 subjects aged 65–79 years were re-examined in 1998. Eighty-two subjects of the population met the criteria for MCI. Midlife elevated serum cholesterol level (≥ 6.5 mmol/l) was a significant risk factor for MCI (OR 1.9; 95% CI 1.2–3.0, adjusted for age, body mass index, education, smoking and alcohol consumption). Furthermore, the effect of systolic blood pressure approached significance (OR 1.5; 95% CI 0.8–2.5, $p = 0.007$). Moreover, subjects with MCI more often had the diagnosis of hypertension at midlife than the controls, supporting the association between these conditions. These data point to a role for midlife vascular risk factors in the development of MCI in later life.

Data accumulating from different studies suggest that, among the MCI subjects, it is possible to identify a group that is at high risk for developing AD, in particular those subjects with amnestic MCI. The guidelines formulated by a subcommittee of the American Academy of Neurology[5] suggest that there are sufficient data to recommend the evaluation and clinical monitoring of persons with MCI, owing to their increased risk for dementia. For that purpose, screening instruments such as the Mini-Mental State Examination, as well as evaluation of the degree of cognitive impairment by neuropsychologic test batteries, are recommended. MCI subjects are a favorable target for preventive measures. Consequently, MCI is of major interest for pharmaceutical interventions.

REFERENCES

1. Flicker C, Ferris SH, Reisberg B. Mild cognitive impairment in the elderly: predictors of dementia. Neurology 1991; 41: 1006–9

2. Petersen RC, Smith GE, Waring SC, et al. Mild cognitive impairment. Clinical characterization and outcome. Arch Neurol 1999; 56: 303–8

3. Petersen RC, Doody R, Kurz A, et al. Current concepts in mild cognitive impairment. Arch Neurol 2001; 58: 1985–92

4. Bennett DA, Wilson RS, Schneider JA, et al. Natural history of mild cognitive impairment in older persons. Neurology 2002; 59: 198–205

5. Petersen RC, Stevens JC, Ganguli M, et al. Practice parameter: early detection of dementia: mild cognitive impairment (an evidence-based review). Report of the Quality Standards Subcommittee of the American Academy of Neurology. Neurology 2001; 56: 1133–42

6. Hänninen T, Hallikainen M, Tuomainen S, et al. Prevalence of mild cognitive impairment: a population-based study in elderly subjects. Acta Neurol Scand 2002; 106: 148–54

7. Kivipelto M, Helkala EL, Hänninen T, et al. Midlife vascular risk factors and late-life mild cognitive impairment. A population-based study. Neurology 2001; 56: 1683–9

8. Arnaiz E, Almkvist O. Neuropsychological features of mild cognitive impairment and preclinical Alzheimer's disease. Acta Neurol Scand Suppl 2003; 179: 34–41

9. Jack CR Jr, Petersen RC, Xu YC, et al. Prediction of AD with MRI-based hippocampal volume in mild cognitive impairment. Neurology 1999; 52: 1397–403

10. Killiany RJ, Hyman BT, Gomez-Isla T, et al. MRI measures of entorhinal cortex vs hippocampus in preclinical AD. Neurology 2002; 58: 1188–96

11. Wolf H, Jelic V, Gertz H-J, et al. A critical discussion of the role of neuroimaging in mild cognitive impairment. Acta Neurol Scand Suppl 2003; 179: 52–76

12. Pennanen C, Kivipelto M, Tuomainen S, et al. Hippocampus and entorhinal cortex in mild cognitive impairment and early AD. Neurol Aging 2004; 250: 303–10

13. Lehtovirta M, Laakso MP, Frisoni GB, Soininen H. How does the apolipoprotein E genotype modulate the brain in aging and in Alzheimer's disease? A review of neuroimaging studies. Neurobiol Aging 2000; 21: 293–300

14. Petersen RC, Smith GE, Ivnik RJ, et al. Apolipoprotein E status as a predictor of

development of Alzheimer's disease in memory-impaired individuals. J Am Med Assoc 1995; 273: 1274–8

15. Albert MS. Cognitive and neurobiologic markers of early Alzheimer disease. Proc Natl Acad Sci USA 1996; 93: 13547–51

16. Andreasen N, Vanmechelen E, Vanderstichele H, et al. Cerebrospinal fluid levels of total-tau, phospho-tau and A beta 42 predicts development of Alzheimer's disease in patients with mild cognitive impairment. Acta Neurol Scand Suppl 2003; 179: 47–51

17. Notkola I-L, Sulkava R, Pekkanen J, et al. Serum total cholesterol, apolipoprotein E ε4 allele, and Alzheimer's disease. Neuro-epidemiology 1998; 17: 14–20

18. Kilander L, Nyman H, Boberg M, et al. Hypertension is related to cognitive impairment. A 20-year follow-up of 999 men. Hypertension 1998; 31: 780–6

19. Launer LJ, Ross GB, Petrovitch H, et al. Midlife blood pressure and dementia: the Honolulu-Asia aging study. Neurobiol Aging 2000; 21: 49–55

20. Kivipelto M, Helkala EL, Laakso MP, et al. Midlife vascular risk factors and Alzheimer's disease in later life: longitudinal, population based study. Br Med J 2001; 322: 1447–51

Water quality and cholesterol-induced pathology: differential effects of the M-1 muscarinic receptor agonist AF267B on accumulation of Alzheimer-like amyloid β in rabbit brain

DL Sparks, J Lochhead, A Fisher, T Martin

INTRODUCTION

The clinical suspicion of Alzheimer's disease (AD) is confirmed only after neuropathological assessment for characteristic lesions of the disorder, to the exclusion of other conditions. Such hallmark features are senile plaques and neurofibrillary tangles (NFT). A sufficient number, set by convention, of both senile plaques and NFT are required by most neuropathologists to affix the diagnosis of AD.[1] The predominant component of the senile plaque is the amyloid β peptide (Aβ). A wealth of other compounds also occur in senile plaques, including cholesterol and its chaperone in the central nervous system (CNS) apolipoprotein E. The Aβ peptide is a by-product of a larger precursor protein, β-amyloid precursor protein (APP).

Genetic mutations of the APP gene have been associated with production and accumulation of Aβ as senile plaques in the brains of individuals with familial AD. Accumulation of Aβ is presumed to be a result of an induced overproduction, but reduced clearance is also a likely component. Investigators have capitalized on these observations in familial AD by isolating and inserting human genetic material containing such human APP mutations into the mouse genome. Memory deficits and accumulation of senile plaque-like deposits of Aβ occur with aging in these transgenic mouse models of AD. A role for reduced clearance as a reason for the accumulation of Aβ comes from recent antibody therapy studies. Introduction of Aβ antibodies into the blood, which need not enter the CNS proper, assist in the removal of the toxin from the brains of such transgenic mice.[2,3]

The effect of cholesterol on production and accumulation of Alzheimer-like Aβ in the brain has gained considerable prominence in recent years. The above-noted transgenic mouse models of AD have been shown to accumulate Aβ earlier or in greater abundance, or both, if the animals are administered cholesterol in the diet.[4–9] Culture studies have demonstrated that cholesterol is capable of shifting normal metabolism of APP to production of amyloidogenic peptides.[10–15] Analogous culture studies have shown that inhibition of the rate-limiting step of cholesterol synthesis with a statin overcomes the effect of exogenous administration of cholesterol and reduces the level of Aβ produced.[11,12,14,16,17] Similar to culture studies, it has been shown that co-administration of a cholesterol-lowering drug to cholesterol-fed AD transgenic mice reduces the levels of Aβ observed in the brain, and is often below levels observed with the transgene alone (control diet).[18]

Studies performed in New Zealand White rabbits showed that dietary cholesterol (2%) induced a pronounced accumulation of neuronal Aβ compared to the values in animals fed a normal chow diet.[19] It is of note that the APP, and thus Aβ, is identical in man and rabbit.[20,21] Further studies in the cholesterol-fed rabbit suggested that, at a minimum, the accumulation of Aβ in the brains of cholesterol-fed rabbits was dependent on the quality of the water the animals were administered.[22] Animals allowed tap water accumulated considerably more Aβ in the brain than animals allowed distilled water. Investigation of Aβ levels in the blood suggested that Aβ accumulated in the brain because of reduced clearance among cholesterol-fed rabbits administered tap water. We assessed the effect of the M1 muscarinic receptor agonist AF267B[23] on cholesterol-induced accumulation of neuronal Aβ, and determined whether drug efficacy might be dependent on the quality of water available.

METHODS

New Zealand White rabbits were fed normal diet and allowed distilled drinking water ($n = 12$; Arrowhead distilled drinking water) or local tap water ($n = 10$), or fed a 2% cholesterol diet and allowed distilled drinking water ($n = 17$) or local tap water ($n = 17$) for 10 weeks. Each of these animals was injected with isotonic saline on a daily basis. Two groups of cholesterol-fed animals were injected subcutaneously with AF267B (1.0 mg/kg body weight/daily): those allowed distilled water ($n = 5$) and those allowed tap water ($n = 5$). Two separate experiments were performed investigating any effect of AF267B. A full postmortem examination was performed on each animal. In this study, brains were investigated for altered severity of neuronal Aβ immunoreactivity induced by increased circulating cholesterol levels.

Adolescent male New Zealand White rabbits (3000–4000 g) were housed in the rabbit facility at the Sun Health Research Institute, operating under the guidelines of the United States Department of Agriculture, with a 12:12 light/dark cycle, at $67 \pm 7°F$ ($19 \pm 8°C$ and 45–50% humidity. Animals were randomly assigned to one of the six groups. Control and cholesterol diets were commercially obtained from Purina Mills, Inc. (Laboratory Rabbit Diet with and without 2% cholesterol). Dietary food intake was limited to one cup per day (8 oz) and *ad libitum* water consumption varied between 32 and 40 oz/day. Each of the animals in the six groups received daily injections of sterile isotonic saline, as part of a preclinical drug study not reported on herein.

Animals were sacrificed 10 weeks after initiating the experimental dietary (food and water) protocol. Animals were not given their daily injection of isotonic saline on the day of sacrifice; rather, they were administered intramuscularly a cocktail of ketamine and xylazine (45–75 mg/kg and 5–10 mg/kg, respectively).

After conclusion of the 10-week dietary experiments, the heart was exposed, a needle attached to a perfusion apparatus was inserted and secured in the left apex of the heart, the vena cava was incised and perfusion was initiated. Animals were perfused under pressure with 120 ml of 4% paraformaldehyde at a constant rate of 5 ml/min using a constant pressure pump.

The brain was removed and further fixed by immersion in 4% paraformaldehyde for 2 weeks before being sectioned for immunohistochemical assessment. Vibratome sections (50 µm) of hippocampus and hippocampal cortex of the brain were immunostained with β-amyloid antibody (10D5; provided by Dr Dale Schenk of Elan Pharmaceuticals) using published peroxidase–antiperoxidase immunohistochemical methods.[24] The number of Aβ immunoreactive neurons in five random 10× objective fields were counted in the inferior temporal hippocampal cortex. The mean number of immunoreactive neurons for each animal was averaged for the set of animals in each experimental group. The mean number of neurons showing Aβ immunoreactivity for each experimental group was compared by ANOVA, followed by appropriate t tests; significance was set at a value of $p < 0.05$.

RESULTS

As previously reported,[22] the number of Aβ immunoreactive neurons was increased (1.9–2.5-fold) among cholesterol-fed animals injected with saline compared to animals on a control diet, but the increase was less pronounced among those cholesterol-fed animals allowed distilled drinking water ($50.9 \pm 4.3/mm^2$) compared to those allowed tap water ($65.7 \pm 4.2/mm^2$). The 28% difference between cholesterol-fed animals on distilled and tap water achieved statistical significance. A clear,

and possibly more important, reduction of neuronal Aβ immunoreactivity intensity accompanied the reduction in affected neurons among the cholesterol-fed animals on distilled water.[22]

Daily administration of AF267B elicited a reduction in the number of Aβ immunoreactive neurons caused by dietary cholesterol among animals allowed tap water ($47.9 \pm 13.7/mm^2$). In contrast, this beneficial effect did not occur among animals on distilled water ($45.7 \pm 7.5/mm^2$) (Table 26.1). Variability in this pilot study precluded significance of the nearly 30% reduction in the number of affected neurons among animals on tap water. Furthermore, a reduction in the intensity of neuronal Aβ immunoreactivity with administration of AF257B occurred, but again, only among cholesterol-fed rabbits allowed tap water (Figure 26.1). This is generally consistent with previous findings,[22] where reduced intensity of Aβ immunoreactivity was produced by treatments causing reductions in the number of affected neurons.

DISCUSSION

Previous studies clearly established that production of Aβ induced by elevated

Table 26.1 Amyloid β immunoreactive neurons (mean ± SEM) from temporal cortex of New Zealand White rabbits fed either 2% cholesterol or control diet and allowed either bottled distilled drinking water or tap water *ad libitum*. Animals were administered saline or the M1 muscarinic receptor agonist AF267B

Water	n	10 weeks normal chow	n	10 weeks 2% cholesterol diet
Saline				
Tap	10	26.2 ± 4.8	17	65.7 ± 4.2[*]
Distilled	12	26.3 ± 4.6	17	50.9 ± 4.3[*]
AF267B				
Tap			5	47.9 ± 13.7[†]
Distilled			5	45.7 ± 7.5

[*] Significantly different from matched control chow-fed group
[†] Significantly different from matched saline-injected group

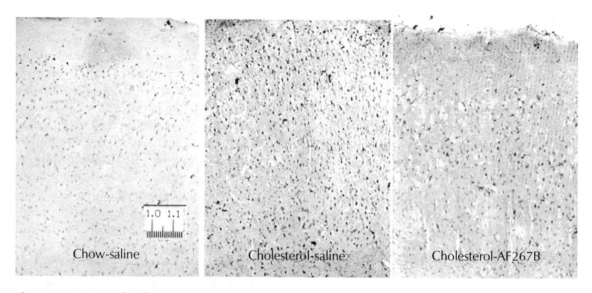

Figure 26.1 Amyloid β (Aβ) immunoreactivity in the cortex of New Zealand White rabbits fed chow or a cholesterol diet and administered either saline or M1 muscarinic receptor agonist AF267B (1 mg/kg body weight) by daily subcutaneous injection. AF267B reduced the cholesterol-induced neuronal accumulation of Aβ in only those animals on tap water (distilled water not shown). The scale is for all photomicrographs

circulating cholesterol can be either cleared to the blood or accumulated in neurons and eventually the neuropil as senile plaque-like structures.[22] The difference between clearance and accumulation of Aβ was disclosed by observing a difference in the CNS–circulation partition of Aβ depending on water quality. Among New Zealand White cholesterol-fed rabbits given distilled drinking water there were increases in the number of Aβ immunoreactive neurons, but with a minimal increase in the intensity of the immunoreactivity, and there was a nearly two-fold increase in blood Aβ levels. This was in contrast to cholesterol-fed animals on tap water, where there were more Aβ immunoreactive neurons, the intensity of the immunoreactivity was greatly enhanced, and there were only slight increases in blood levels of Aβ.

The difference in the intensity of the immunoreactivity is considered important, as there must be a relationship between the intensity of antibody immunoreactivity and concentration of its antigen, in this case Aβ. It seemed clear that some agent in tap water caused the inhibition of Aβ clearance from the brain either directly or through some cascade of influence. As this agent was not present in distilled water the natural clearance of Aβ from the brain to the blood occurred unhindered. In the case of increased Aβ production induced by dietary cholesterol the maximum clearance rate had been exceeded for Aβ efflux, leading to an increase in the number of affected neurons, but large increases of Aβ occurred in the blood of animals given distilled water. The existence of this system for Aβ clearance was suggested by disclosing a difference in the CNS–circulation partition between cholesterol-fed rabbits on distilled water compared to those on tap water. Additional support for this clearance system comes from studies showing the ability to manipulate the CNS–circulation partition of Aβ in a dose-related manner with a single trace metal ion added to distilled water.[25] Further support for this clearance comes herein via pharmacological manipulation of this Aβ brain-to-blood efflux system with the M1 muscarinic receptor agonist AF267B.

At first it was disconcerting to us that AF267B did not elicit an effect on Aβ accumulation in the brains of cholesterol-fed rabbits given distilled water. However, an important clue was revealed, because AF267B worked only in animals administered tap water. The drug overcomes the effect of the agent in tap water inhibiting clearance of Aβ, but has no effect in distilled water when there was no agent to disinhibit. Why AF267B is more effective against Aβ in the tap water group is not clear, and requires further studies. Several alternatives can be envisaged: AF267B displaces the tap water agent to restore a less compromised clearance of cholesterol-induced overproduction of Aβ; and/or the so-called tap water agent affected the affinity of AF267B towards the M1 muscarinic receptor. Notably copper cation, which occurs in the tap water used, increases the affinity of muscarinic receptors for agonists, unveiling a high-affinity agonistic site.[26]

In AD some unknown pathological process probably leads to the overload or breakdown of the Aβ clearance pathway, thus leading to Aβ accumulation in neurons and the neuropil as senile plaques. This reduced ability to clear Aβ from the AD brain may be exacerbated by the agent in tap water in a manner similar to that observed in the cholesterol-fed rabbit. It is of note that a major medical problem in the USA is the increased risk of disease due to increased circulating concentrations of cholesterol.

Based on the premise that aberrant production and accumulation of Aβ in the CNS is intimately linked to the etiology or progression of AD, M1 muscarinic receptor agonists as a class of drugs may hold promise in future treatment strategies. Overall, the data may suggest that activation of the M1 muscarinic receptor with agonist drugs could promote the clearance of Aβ in AD, and thus be of benefit in the treatment of the disorder. It is clear that only a proof-of-concept clinical trial will be able to assess whether M1 receptor agonists may be of value in the treatment of AD by reducing the Aβ load in the brain, observable as an increase of Aβ in the blood or as an excreted form.

ACKNOWLEDGEMENTS

This study was supported by the Arizona Disease Control Research Commission.

REFERENCES

1. NIA/Reagan work group. Consensus recommendations for the postmortem diagnosis of Alzheimer's disease. Neurobiol Aging 1997; 18: S1–2

2. DeMattos RB, Bales KR, Cummins DJ, et al. Peripheral anti-Abeta antibody alters CNS and plasma Abeta clearance and decreases brain Abeta burden in a mouse model of Alzheimer's disease. Proc Natl Acad Sci USA 2001; 98: 8850–5

3. DeMattos RB, Bales KR, Cummins DJ, et al. Brain to plasma amyloid-beta efflux: a measure of brain amyloid burden in a mouse model of Alzheimer's disease. Science 2002; 295: 2264–7

4. Durham RA, Parker CA, Emmerling MR, et al. Effect of age and diet on the expression of beta-amyloid 1-40 and 1-42 in the brains of apolipoprotein-E-deficient mice. Neurobiol Aging 1998; 19: S281

5. Shie FS, LeBoeuf RC, Leverenz JB, et al. Effects of cholesterol feeding on histopathologic hallmarks of Alzheimer's disease in β-amyloid precursor protein (APP) transgenic mice. Soc Neurosci 1999; 25: 1859

6. Li L, Zeigler S, Lindsey RJ, Fukuchi K. Effects of an atherogenic diet on amyloidosis in transgenic mice overexpressing the C-terminal portion of β-amyloid precursor protein. Soc Neurosci 1999; 25: 1859

7. Fishman CE, White SL, DeLong CA, et al. High fat diet potentiates β-amyloid deposition in the APP V717F transgenic mouse model of Alzheimer's disease. Soc Neurosci 1999; 25: 1859

8. Bales KR, Fishman C, DeLong C, et al. Diet-induced hyperlipidemia accelerates amyloid deposition in the APPv717f transgenic mouse model of Alzheimer's disease. Neurobiol Aging 2000; 21: S139

9. Refolo LM, Pappolla MA, Malester B, et al. Hypercholesterolemia accelerates Alzheimer's amyloid pathology in a transgenic mouse model. Neurobiol Dis 2000; 7: 321–31

10. Racchi M, Baetta R, Salvietti N, et al. Secretory processing of amyloid precursor protein is inhibited by increase in cellular cholesterol content. Biochem J 1997; 322: 893–8

11. Simons M, Keller P, De Strooper B, et al. Cholesterol depletion inhibits the generation of beta-amyloid in hippocampal neurons. Proc Natl Acad Sci USA 1998; 95: 6460–4

12. Frears ER, Stephens DJ, Walters CE, et al. The role of cholesterol in the biosynthesis of β-amyloid. NeuroReport 1999; 10: 1699–705

13. Galbete JL, Martin TR, Peressini E, et al. Cholesterol decreases secretion of the secreted form of amyloid precursor protein by interfering with glycosylation in the protein secretory pathway. Biochem J 2000; 348: 307–13

14. Austen BM, Frears ER, Davies H. Cholesterol upregulates production of Abeta 1-40 and 1-42 in transfected cells. Neurobiol Aging 2000; 21: S254

15. Beyreuther K. Physiological function of APP processing. Neurobiol Aging 2000; 21: S69

16. Bergmann C, Runz H, Jakala P, et al. Diversification of gamma-secretase versus beta-secretase inhibition by cholesterol depletion. Neurobiol Aging 2000; 21: S278

17. Fassbender K, Simons M, Bergmann C, et al. Simvastatin strongly reduces levels of Alzheimer's disease beta-amyloid peptides Abeta 42 and Abeta 40 in vitro and in vivo. Proc Natl Acad Sci USA 2001; 98: 5371–3

18. Refolo LM, Pappolla MA, LaFrancois J, et al. A cholesterol-lowering drug reduces beta-amyloid pathology in a transgenic mouse model of Alzheimer's disease. Neurobiol Dis 2001; 5: 890–9

19. Sparks DL, Scheff SW, Hunsaker III JC, et al. Induction of Alzheimer-like β-amyloid immunoreactivity in the brains of rabbits with dietary cholesterol. Exp Neurol 1994; 126: 88–94

20. Johnstone EM, Chaney MO, Norris FH, et al. Conservation of the sequence of the Alzheimer's disease amyloid peptide in dog, polar bear, and five other mammals by cross-species polymerase chain reaction analysis. Mol Brain Res 1991; 10: 299–305

21. Davidson JS, West RL, Kotikalapudi P, et al. Sequence and methylation in the beta/A4 region of the rabbits amyloid precursor protein gene. Biochem Biophys Res Comm 1992; 188: 905–11

22. Sparks DL, Lochhead J, Horstman D, et al. Water quality has a pronounced effect on cholesterol-induced accumulation of Alzheimer

amyloid beta (Aβ) in rabbit brain. J Alzheimer's Dis 2002; 4: 523–9

23. Fisher A, Brandeis R, Haring R, et al. Impact of muscarinic agonists for successful therapy of Alzheimer's disease. J Neural Transm 2002; 62: 189–202

24. Sparks DL, Hunsaker JC, Scheff SW, et al. Cortical senile plaques in coronary artery disease, aging and Alzheimer's disease. Neurobiol Aging 1990; 11: 601–7

25. Sparks DL, Schreurs BG. Trace amounts of copper in water induce β-amyloid plaques and learning deficits in a rabbit model of Alzheimer's disease. Proc Natl Acad Sci USA 2003; 100: 1065–9

26. Fisher A, Brandeis R, Karton I, et al. (Cis)-2-methyl-spiro(1,3-oxathiolane-5,3')quinuclidine, an M1 selective cholinergic agonist, attenuates cognitive dysfunctions in an animal model of Alzheimer's disease. J Pharmacol Exp Ther 1991; 257: 392–403

Chapter 27

Lack of effect of certoparin in P301L mutant tau pathology

M Walzer, M Hejna, S Lorens, J Lee

INTRODUCTION

Alzheimer's disease (AD) is a progressive neurodegenerative disease that will affect an estimated 22 million individuals by the year 2025. Current therapies treat only the symptoms but not the underlying etiology of the disease; therefore, new therapies that address the causes of AD are sorely needed. AD is characterized histopathologically by senile plaques, neurofibrillary tangles (NFTs), reactive astrocytosis and regionally specific cell loss. Senile plaques are an extracellular deposition of amyloid β (Aβ), a 40–42 amino acid peptide, while intracellular NFTs consist of paired helical filaments (PHFs) formed from microtubule-associated tau protein in a hyperphosphorylated[1] and/or conformationally altered state.[2] Many studies have shown an association between Aβ and tau pathology, including the fact that Aβ can stimulate tau phosphorylation through activation of GSK-3β,[3] MAPK,[4] src non-receptor family kinases,[5] ERK[6] and CDK5/p35[7] *in vitro*. In mutant amyloid precursor protein (APP) over-expressing mice there are phosphorylated tau-positive punctate dystrophic neurites in and around the Aβ-positive plaque, which are correlated with deregulation of Cdk5 and an increase in p25.[8] Mutant APP mice, when crossed with mutant tau mice, also show accelerated tau phosphorylation, sarcosyl insoluble tau formation, and NFT formation.[9] These data provide more evidence for the link between extracellular Aβ deposition and tau pathology.

Our laboratory has been studying compounds that prevent some of the Aβ-induced neuropathological features found in AD including tau pathology.[10] We have found that low-molecular-weight glycosaminoglycan (GAG) administration is capable of preventing Aβ-induced tau phosphorylational and conformational changes in a neuroblastoma cell line and also in Fischer 344 rats. These conformational changes in tau protein may represent early tau changes that precede PHF and NFT formation.[11] However, one drawback of the previously mentioned models is their lack of NFT formation, the pathological entity which has been linked to the progression and severity of AD.[12] Prevention of NFT formation in AD may provide a much needed treatment for the disease. Currently, only transgenic mice expressing mutant human tau protein show NFT formation.[13] Subsequent studies have shown that tau phosphorylation and NFT formation in these mice can be accelerated by an Aβ1-42 fibril injection.[14] In addition, the intracerebral Aβ1-42 injection produces tau phosphorylation and NFT formation in the hippocampus and amygdala, brain regions with little or no tau pathology in mutant P301L transgenic mice given the control Aβ42-1 peptide injection.[9] These areas are also affected early on in AD, thus making this animal model better able to recapitulate pathology and location of pathology found in AD. Furthermore, this research supports our previously studied Aβ microinjection F344 rat model, and gives us another *in vivo* model, one with greater relevance to AD neuropathology, in which to test the therapeutic properties of low-molecular-weight GAGs.

MATERIALS AND METHODS

Female JNPL3 mutant tau mice were obtained from Taconic (Germantown, NY, USA) at 2–3 months of age. JNPL3 mice express human P301L *Mtapt* cDNA containing exon 10 and lacking exons 2 and 3, thus encoding four-repeat tau without amino-terminal inserts (4RN0).[9] These mice express mutant human tau at levels roughly equivalent to endogenous mouse tau. Surgery was performed when the mice reached 7–9 months of age. Aβ1-42 and Aβ42-1 (BACHEM, Torrance, CA, USA) was supplied as a trifluoroacetic acid (TFA) salt with the peptide content of 92–93%. Aβ was reconstituted in sterile phosphate-buffered saline (PBS) at a final concentration of 250 μmol/l and shaken at 1000 rpm for 84 h at 37°C in an Eppendorf Thermomixer, to induce fibril formation, as previously described by Gotz and colleagues.[14] Certoparin (4600 Da) was provided by the Department of Pathology, Loyola University Chicago (Dr J. Fareed) and was made fresh daily and administered subcutaneously (5 mg/kg or 15 mg/kg) in saline, once a day, beginning 5 days prior to the Aβ injection. Surgery was performed as previously described.[14]

Distinct monoclonal phospho-specific tau antibodies R145D (K. Iqbal, 1 : 30, Ser-422) were used to detect phosphorylated tau epitopes as previously described.[14] Immunocytochemistry was performed using a nickel-intensified diamino-benzidine (DAB) procedure slightly modified from that previously reported for free-floating sections.[15] Brain tissue extraction was performed as previously described by Sahara and collaborators[16] with minor modifications. Chemiluminescence kits (Pierce) were employed, followed by exposure of samples to Hyperfilm (Amersham Inc.). Immunoblots were analyzed using NIH Image software (v. 1.61).

RESULTS

Previously, we found that certoparin treatment prevented Aβ-induced tau phosphorylation *in vitro* (M. Walzer, M. Hejna, S. Lorens, J. Lee, submitted for publication). Therefore, we stained brain sections from P301L mutant mice with the R145d monoclonal phosphospecific tau antibodies that recognize tau phosphorylation at Ser422 (R145d), an effect previously reported to occur only in mice that received the Aβ1-42 injection.[14] Some R145d neuronal staining was present in Aβ42-1-injected mice (Figure 27.1a) while no R145d neuronal staining was evident in uninjected non-transgenic mice (Figure 27.1b). R145d neuronal IR was increased in Aβ1-42-treated mice; however, this did not reach significance (Figure 27.1b). No effect of certoparin on R145d IR was seen in Aβ 1-42/certoparin-treated mice. R145d labeled phosphorylated tau throughout the neuron including its processes.

We prepared sarcosyl-insoluble fractions from the left brain hemisphere as described in Materials and methods. The sarcosyl insoluble P3 fraction was run on sodium dodecyl sulfate-

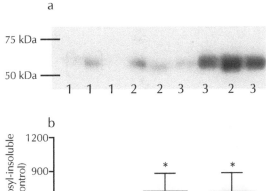

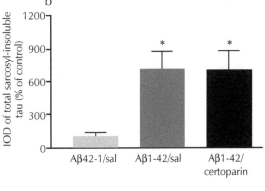

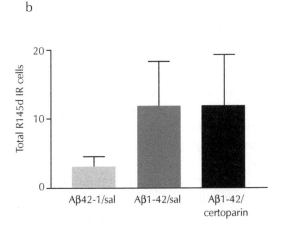

Figure 27.1 No effect of amyloid β (Aβ) or certoparin on R145d-positive cells in the amygdala of JNPL3 mice. R145d (Ser 422) IR in the amygdala of an (a) Aβ1-42/sal treated JNPL3. (b) Total R145d-positive cells were counted in five sections around the injection site on post-Aβ injection day 22. Data are means ± SEM. Certoparin (5 mg/kg per day). There was no statistically significant difference between groups (Kruskal–Wallis non-parametric test). $n = 3$–8 animals/group. Scale bar (a) = 50 μm

Figure 27.2 Amyloid β (Aβ) 1-42 increases total sarcosyl-insoluble tau in JNPL3 mutant tau mice: no effect of certoparin. (a) Immunoblot of sarcosyl-insoluble fraction with tau-13 antibody. Lanes coded: 1, Aβ42-1/veh; 2, Aβ1-42/veh; 3, Aβ1-42/certoparin (5 or 15 mg/kg per day) treatment. Mice were sacrificed 22 days after Aβ or veh injection. (b) IOD (% of control) of total sarcosyl-insoluble human tau from treated JNPL3 mice. $n = 3$–8 animals/group. Data are means ± SEM. *$p < 0.05$ compared to Aβ42-1/sal group (one-way ANOVA followed by a Tukey B post-hoc test)

polyacrylamide gel electrophoresis (SDS-PAGE) and total human tau was recognized with the monoclonal tau-13 antibody. We found that Aβ1-42 fibrils increased the amount of sarcosyl-insoluble tau, as evidenced by the increase in a 64-kDa tau species (Figure 27.2a). Unphosphorylated mutant 4R0N tau has previously

been shown to migrate much faster at 50 kDa, while the hyperphosphorylated 64-kDa tau band migrates more slowly.[16] Optical densitometry analysis revealed a significant ($p < 0.05$) six-fold increase in intensity of the 64-kDa band following Aβ1-42 injections (Figure 27.2b). However, neither 5 nor 15 mg/kg certoparin treatment had a significant effect on 64-kDa tau formation.

Figure 27.3 shows Bielschowsky-positive NFTs in the right amygdala of an Aβ1-42/veh-injected mouse (Figure 27.3a and b). Upon

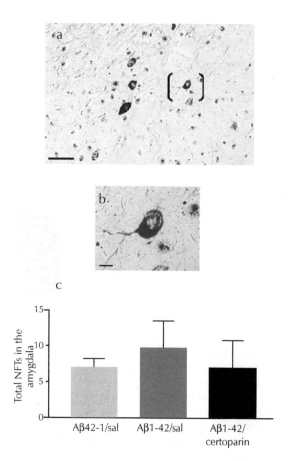

Figure 27.3 No significant effect of amyloid β (Aβ) or certoparin on neurofibrillary tangle (NFT) formation in JNPL3 mice. (a) Bielschowsky silver stain of NFTs in the amygdala of an Aβ1-42/sal treated JNPL3 mouse. (b) Higher magnification of the bracketed area. (c) Total NFTs (ten sections around the injection site) counted on post-Aβ injection day 22. Data are means + SEM (Certoparin 5 mg/kg per day). $n = 3$–8 animals/group. No statistically significant difference was evident between the groups. Scale bars (a) = 50 μm, (b) = 10 μm

analysis, there was an increase in the total number of NFTs in Aβ1-42-injected mice compared to Aβ42-1-injected mice (Figure 27.3c); however, this difference did not reach statistical significance. In addition, certoparin administration had no effect on NFT formation in the amygdala of Aβ42-1- or Aβ1-42-injected mice.

DISCUSSION

The association between Aβ and tau pathology has been extensively investigated *in vitro* for its possible mechanistic contribution to AD pathology. Recently, the link has received more prominence, as newly generated transgenic mouse models make it possible to study the association between Aβ deposition and tau pathology *in vivo*.[8,13] Inhibitors of amyloid aggregation and/or amyloid-induced cellular responses can now be investigated for their possible preventive effects on Aβ-induced tau pathology. These studies will provide more support for the direct association of Aβ deposition and tau pathology. Our current work has begun to address some of these issues by investigating the role of the low-molecular-weight heparin certoparin in the prevention of Aβ-induced tau pathology in P301L mutant tau mice.

Phosphorylated sarcosyl-insoluble tau and phosphorylated sarcosyl-soluble tau (data not shown) was elevated in mice receiving Aβ1-42 fibrils, suggesting that aggregated Aβ1-42 can induce tau phosphorylation. Aβ1-42 had no significant effect on total sarcosyl-soluble tau compared to Aβ42-1 treatment, suggesting a specific effect of Aβ1-42 on tau phosphorylation and insolubility, and not on total tau protein expression in these mice. In contrast to the sarcosyl-insoluble and soluble fractions, there was a lack of accelerated NFT formation in this experiment compared to the reported five-fold increase found by Gotz and colleagues.[14] The four most likely explanations for the differences may be a combination of the following: the different mouse strain used; a different time for injection; different effects of Aβ depending on the injection site; and small sample size. Regarding the sample size, although there were similar numbers of animals used in both our experiment and that of Gotz and collaborators,[14] the variability in our experiments was much higher that than reported by the Gotz team. This may be attributed to the intrinsic variability present in the JNPL3 mouse line compared to the pR5 mouse line. However, no reports have been published investigating these differences.

Certoparin administration has been shown to prevent Aβ-induced tau phosphorylation in differentiated SH SY-5Y cells (M. Walzer et al., submitted). In vivo, subcutaneous injections of certoparin also attenuated tau conformational changes induced by Aβ deposition in male F344 rats.[15] Based on these prior reports, we investigated whether certoparin treatment would be able to prevent tau phosphorylation, tau conformational changes and/or NFT formation accelerated by Aβ1-42 fibril deposition in P301L mutant tau mice. We did not see a significant effect of certoparin on any of these endpoints, although the further characterization of this Aβ injection model provides additional evidence for the involvement of Aβ deposition in tau pathology.

Together the presented data suggest that intracerebral Aβ1-42 fibril injections can accelerate tau phosphorylation and sarcosyl-insoluble 64-kDa tau formation in P301L mutant tau mice. Additionally, at the doses tested, certoparin treatment was unable significantly to prevent the effects of Aβ1-42 fibrils on P301L mutant human tau pathology. Together these studies further support the link between Aβ tau phosphorylation and insoluble tau formation, but they also demonstrate that preventive drugs, such as low-molecular-weight heparins, may need to be given very early in the disease processes.

REFERENCES

1. Goedert M, Spillantini MG, Cairns NJ, Crowther RA. Tau proteins of Alzheimer paired helical filaments: abnormal phosphorylation of all six brain isoforms. Neuron 1992; 8: 159–68

2. Lang E, Otvos L Jr. A serine to proline change in the Alzheimer's disease-associated epitope Tau 2 results in altered secondary structure, but phosphorylation overcomes the conformational gap. Biochem Biophys Res Commun 1992; 188: 162–9

3. Takashima A, Honda T, Yasutake K, et al. Activation of tau protein kinase I/glycogen synthase kinase-3beta by amyloid beta peptide (25-35) enhances phosphorylation of tau in hippocampal neurons. Neurosci Res 1998; 31: 317–23

4. Shea TB, Dergay AN, Ekinci FJ. Beta-amyloid induced hyperphosphorylation of tau in human neuroblastoma cells involves MAP kinase. Neurosci Res Commun 1998; 22: 45–9

5. Williamson R, Scales T, Clark BR, et al. Rapid tyrosine phosphorylation of neuronal proteins including tau and focal adhesion kinase in response to amyloid-beta peptide exposure: involvement of Src family protein kinases. J Neurosci 2001; 22: 10–20

6. Combs CK, Johnson DE, Cannady SB, et al. Identification of microglial signal transduction pathways mediating a neurotoxic response to amyloidogenic fragments of beta-amyloid and prion proteins. J Neurosci 1999; 19: 928–39

7. Town T, Zolton J, Shaffner R, et al. p35/Cdk5 pathway mediates soluble amyloid-beta peptide-induced tau phosphorylation in vitro. J Neurosci Res 2002; 69: 362–72

8. Otth C, Concha II, Arendt T, et al. AbetaPP induces cdk5-dependent tau hyperphosphorylation in transgenic mice Tg2576. J Alzheimer's Dis 2002; 4: 417–30

9. Lewis J, Dickson DW, Lin WL, et al. Enhanced neurofibrillary degeneration in transgenic mice expressing mutant tau and APP. Science 2001; 293: 1487–91

10. Dudas B, Cornelli U, Lee J, et al. Oral and subcutaneous (s.c.) administration of the glycosaminoglycan C3 attenuates amyloid beta (25-35)-induced abnormal tau protein immunoreactivity in rat brain. FASEB J 2000; 1434–8

11. Weaver CL, Espinoza M, Kress Y, Davies P. Conformational change as one of the earliest alterations of tau in Alzheimer's disease. Neurobiol Aging 2000; 21: 719–27

12. Alafuzoff I, Iqbal K, Friden H, et al. Histopathological criteria for progressive dementia disorders: clinical–pathological correlation and classification by multivariate data analysis. Acta Neuropathol 1987; 74: 209–25

13. Gotz J, Chen F, Barmettler R, Nitsch RM. Tau filament formation in transgenic mice expressing P301L tau. J Biol Chem 2001; 276: 529–34

14. Gotz J, Chen F, van Dorpe J, Nitsch RM. Formation of neurofibrillary tangles in P301l tau transgenic mice induced by Abeta 42 fibrils. Science 2001; 293: 1491–5

15. Walzer M, Lorens S, Hejna M, et al. Low molecular weight glycosaminoglycan blockade of beta-amyloid induced neuropathology. Eur J Pharmacol 2002; 445: 211–20

16. Sahara N, Lewis J, DeTure M, et al. Assembly of tau in transgenic animals expressing P301L tau: alteration of phosphorylation and solubility. J Neurochem 2002; 83: 1498–508

Chapter 28

Heparin-derived oligosaccharides as potential therapeutic agents in senile dementia and stroke

Q Ma, I Hanin, U Cornelli, J Lee, O Iqbal, J Fareed

INTRODUCTION (BRIEF HISTORY OF HEPARIN-DERIVED OLIGOSACCHARIDES)

The history of heparin-derived oligosaccharides began with heparin in 1916 when McLean discovered a substance derived from canine liver that prevented blood from clotting.[1] The new anticoagulant was named 'heparin', reflecting the compound's abundance in liver. Heparin was not practically applied by physicians until the early 1930s when large-scale isolation procedures on bovine lung and porcine intestinal mucosa were developed to make heparin available as a purified, plentiful and inexpensive supply safe for human use. An early documentation of the clinical trials of heparin was published in 1939 and the effectiveness of heparin treatment in the prevention of postoperative thrombosis was quickly established.[2] The use of heparin also became essential for cardiovascular surgery to maintain extracorporeal circulation of blood through the heart–lung machine. Even today, though challenged by low-molecular-weight heparins and synthetic anticoagulants, heparin plays a pivotal role in the treatment and prophylaxis of multiple thrombosis-related diseases, such as venous thromboembolism, myocardial infarction and unstable angina.[3]

Heparin owes its popularity and importance to the remarkable array of its polycomponent properties and, accordingly, various biological activities. Investigations have characterized heparin as a polysaccharide mixture, which is naturally present in the granules of mast cells of several tissues such as lung, skin, ileum, lymph nodes, thymus and liver. Most of the studies performed on the structure and function of heparin have concentrated on understanding its ability to inhibit blood coagulation. In the 1970s, the mechanism was first elucidated of the heparin–antithrombin interaction, which is responsible for the major anticoagulant activity of heparin.[4] Subsequently, it was discovered that heparin binds to and potentiates the activity of antithrombin through a unique pentasaccharide sequence[5]. Figure 28.1 illustrates the chemical structures of the natural pentasaccharide sequence, and of its synthetic analog. In recent years, the research focus on heparin has broadened to include a range of non-anticoagulant applications, such as anti-inflammatory properties in asthma, modulation of neovascularization and the control of tumor angiogenesis.

Low-molecular-weight heparins (LMWHs), also referred to as low-molecular-mass heparins,

Natural pentasaccharide present in heparin

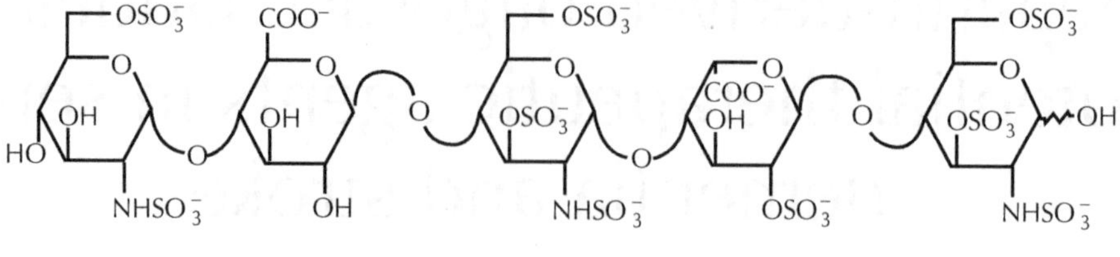

Pentasaccharide analog (SanOrg 32701)

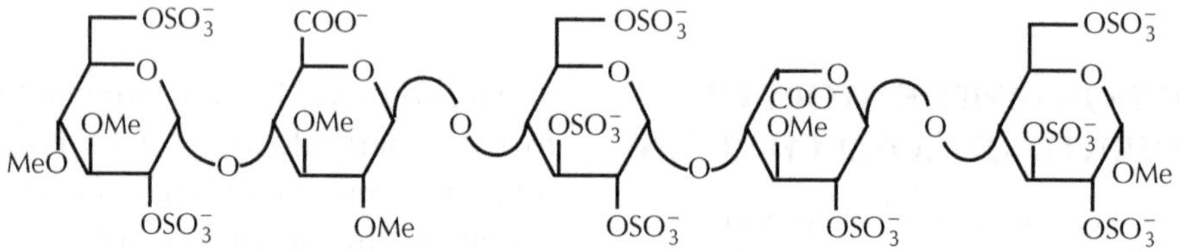

Figure 28.1 Chemical structures of the pentasaccharide sequences present in heparin and its synthetic derivative. The natural pentasaccharide binds to antithrombin with a high affinity. A synthetic form of pentasaccharide (SR 90107A / Org 31540) is the α-methyl glycoside of the natural pentasaccharide that reproduces exactly this unique sequence. SanOrg 32701 is the synthetic analog of the natural pentasaccharide with similar biological effects. (Adapted from reference 10)

are a group of heparin-derived fragments that emerged during the last quarter of the 20th century.[6] In the mid-1970s, several standard procedures were developed for controlled heparin depolymerization to prepare LMWHs. Figure 28.2 shows an illustration of the depolymerization of heparin to prepare LMWHs and heparin oligosaccharides. The discovery that heparin fragments maintained a similar antithrombotic activity while exhibiting reduced anticoagulant effects as compared to unfractionated heparin (UFH) prompted extensive research on the lower-molecular-weight fragments. Numerous preclinical and clinical trials examining the prevention and treatment of venous thromboembolism followed

in the 1980s and continue today. LMWHs are now being used widely as antithrombotic agents, either prophylactically after surgery, or therapeutically for deep vein thrombosis.[7] The first approval of a LMWH from the US Food and Drug Administration was granted in early 1993 for enoxaparin. Currently, there are four LMWHs, namely ardeparin, dalteparin, enoxaparin and tinzaparin, that are available for clinical use in the USA.

The extensive use of LMWHs has been prompted by three main advantages over heparin, namely reduced anticoagulant activity relative to antithrombotic activity, more favorable benefit–risk ratios (antithrombotic effects versus bleeding potential), and superior

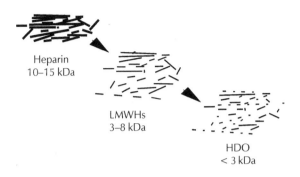

Heparin
10–15 kDa

LMWHs
3–8 kDa

HDO
< 3 kDa

Figure 28.2 The depolymerization of heparin to prepare low-molecular-weight-heparins (LMWHs) and heparin-derived oligosaccharides (HDO)

pharmacokinetic properties[8]. With an increased clinical importance of LMWHs, more attention has also been paid in recent years to their non-anticoagulant-related effects, such as their potential influence on lipid metabolism and anticancer activity.

Along with the development of LMWHs, the introduction of heparin-derived oligosaccharides has resulted from an improved understanding of the molecular basis of the coagulation cascade and non-anticoagulant effects associated with heparin.[5,9] Based upon the discovery of the specific binding sequence in heparin to antithrombin, the Choay group succeeded in synthesizing the first chemically defined heparin-derived oligosaccharide – pentasaccharide – as a potent antithrombotic agent in the 1980s.[5,10] The majority of heparin-derived oligosaccharides, however, are produced by chemical or enzymatic cleavage of heparin and, therefore, represent polysaccharide mixtures.[11] Even though recent investigations on heparin-derived oligosaccharides have focused on their anti-inflammatory and neuroprotective actions, which may lead to the development of heparin-derived oligosaccharides for the treatment of inflammatory bowel disease or Alzheimer's

disease (AD),[12] most of their biological functions and clinical implications are not fully known. The era of heparin-derived oligosaccharides is just beginning.

NON-ANTICOAGULANT EFFECTS OF HEPARINS

The non-anticoagulant actions of heparins primarily include anti-inflammatory effects and interactions with growth factors. These effects may provide rationales for expanded use of heparins as well as the further development of heparin oligosaccharides and heparin mimetics in the neurological areas.

Anti-inflammatory effects of heparins

Inflammation is a poorly defined concept. It is still described in terms of its process. It is initiated through immune recognition by T lymphocytes or antibodies, or by non-immune tissue injury. The effectors lead to multiple reactions through triggering, activation and extravasation of leukocytes and humoral cascade systems, which are collectively called inflammation. The physiological functions of this powerful response are to combat microbial invasion, to eliminate damaged tissue, and eventually to repair damaged tissue. The self-limiting control mechanisms normally lead to health. However, pathological inflammation is often the result of inadequate control within the immune system, leading to allergies or auto-immune diseases. Inflammation also contributes to morbidity in chronic infections (e.g. tuberculosis), chronic tissue injury (e.g. athero-sclerosis) or acute tissue injury (e.g. acute myocardial infarction).

The role for endogenous heparin in inflammation is suggested by the fact that heparin is stored in mast cell granules and is released by several inflammatory effectors.[13] It is also well known that shortly after administration of heparin to patients with deep vein thrombosis, amelioration of pain and swelling occurs, indicating an *in vivo* anti-inflammatory effect of heparin. Recent experimental studies have provided several mechanisms through which heparin may inhibit inflammatory reactions. These mechanisms include modulation of selectin–ligand inter-actions and integrin-dependent adhesion, interference of leukocyte extravasation and migration into tissues, inhibition of complement activation, interference with leukocyte chemotaxis and haptotaxis, and inhibition of platelet activation and aggregation.[14] In addition, it is becoming increasingly clear that coagulation augments inflammation and natural anticoagulants, in particular antithrombin, protein C, and tissue factor pathway inhibitor (TFPI), can limit the coagulation induced increases in inflammatory response.[15] Therefore, heparin may also exert its anti-inflammatory effects through interactions with these proteins. The main reason that heparin has not been used clinically for control of pathological inflammation is the high risk for bleeding.

Progress in the understanding of structure–activity relationships regarding anticoagulant effects and anti-inflammatory mechanisms of heparin have resulted in increased interest in heparin and its derivatives as a new treatment of inflammatory diseases. Two important findings have provided a basis for the development of heparin oligosaccharides in this area. First, heparin's inhibition of the inflammatory responses is independent of its anticoagulant activity.[16] Second, heparin oligosaccharides exhibit similar or even better anti-inflammatory effects in comparison to heparin.[17]

Since the anticoagulant activity of heparin can be distinguished from its anti-inflammatory properties, many efforts have also been made in the development of heparin oligosaccharides in the treatment of inflammation-associated diseases, such as asthma and ischemia-reperfusion injury. Using a sheep asthma model, Ahmed and co-investigators have demonstrated that inhaled heparin oligosaccharides can inhibit the antigen-induced airway responses and post-antigen airway hyper-responses that lead to asthma attack.[17] This anti-allergic activity of oligosaccharides is mediated by non-anticoagulant fractions and resides in chains with molecular weight of 2500 Da. In a model of cerebral ischemia in rodents, in which the animals are subjected to 1 h of ischemia and 48 h of reperfusion, the neural protective effects of UFH and LMWHs have been evaluated.[18] The treatment groups receiving UFH and enoxaparin showed a significant reduction in neutrophil accumulation, infarct size and neurological dysfunction 48 h after reperfusion. Although the authors concluded that neural protection was dependent upon the anti-leukocyte properties rather than the anticoagulant activity of heparins, the underlying mechanisms, in particular the structure–activity relationship, were not fully clear.

Heparins and fibroblast growth factors

The interactions between heparins and fibro-blast growth factors (FGFs) have been exten-sively studied for over two decades, and are still a subject of controversy. The potentiation of angiogenesis, i.e. growth of new blood vessels, by heparin was first reported by Folkman and colleagues, eventually leading to the discovery of modulatory effects of heparin on the mito-genicity and stability of FGFs.[19]

FGFs comprise a family of at least 17 structurally related proteins. The biological functions of FGFs are primarily associated with cell migration and differentiation, although they also include diverse cellular and developmental processes, such as limb, inner ear and brain development, wound healing, early embryogenesis, skeletal growth and differentiation.[20] Additionally, FGFs play an important role in the neuronal responses to central nervous system injury. It has been demonstrated that many of the neurons that transport FGFs are affected in neurodegenerative diseases such as AD and Parkinson's disease.[21] Hence, FGFs may be a potential neurotrophic factor for the slowing of cell death related to various neurodegenerative diseases.

The activity of FGFs is regulated at multiple levels. There are four fibroblast growth factor receptors (FGFRs), which are transmembrane tyrosine kinases displaying unique expression patterns and specific binding interactions. Additionally, glycosaminoglycans (GAGs) such as heparin or heparan sulfate are required for FGFs to bind to high-affinity receptors and constitute another level at which FGF biological activity may be modulated.

The mechanism by which heparin is involved in interacting with FGFs is largely unknown; several models have been proposed. The well-accepted 'dynamic' theory is that FGFs bind to heparan sulfate on the endothelial cell surface of the extracellular matrix (ECM), which acts as a reservoir for FGFs. Exogenous heparins compete with heparan sulfates for binding of FGFs, and may release these proteins from the ECM,[19] as well as promoting the activation of their receptors.[22] In humans, therapeutic dosages of heparin can cause an increase in plasma levels of FGFs.[23]

The molecular weight dependence of the heparin–FGF interaction is reviewed by D'Amore.[23] It has been proposed that heparin oligosaccharides inducing mitogenic activities of the FGFs must be: saccharides longer than the smallest oligosaccharides required to bind to the FGFs; and highly sulfated. Barzu et al. described the fractionation of heparin fragments on a column of immobilized FGFs; the smallest fragment that bound to the column was a hexasaccharide.[24] The bound fragments from 6 to 12 saccharides (hexa- to decasaccharide) were all capable of potentiating the mitogenic activity of FGF under appropriate conditions. However, in a recent study on the interaction between various heparin oligosaccharides and FGF_2, Ornitz et al. reported that several synthetic, unsulfated heparin di- and trisaccharides were capable of stimulating FGF_2-mediated DNA synthesis in a lymphoid cell line.[25] These results suggest that unique oligosaccharide structure rather than molecular weight is a more important determinant in the heparin–FGF interactions.

Despite the uncertainty about the interactions between heparin and FGFs, both heparin and FGFs are associated with Alzheimer's disease. In a recent study, it has been demonstrated that β-amyloid fibrils and FGF_2 have common binding sites on heparan sulfate. β-Amyloid fibrils and FGF_2 represent neurotoxic and neuroprotective pathways, respectively. Thus, heparin oligosaccharides might enhance the neuroprotective effects of FGF_2 by blocking the binding of β-amyloid fibrils with heparan sulfate.[26]

HEPARIN-DERIVED OLIGOSACCHARIDES AND ALZHEIMER'S DISEASE

Alzheimer's disease

Dementia is characterized by a decline in intellectual function severe enough to interfere with a person's normal daily activity and social relationships. AD is the most common form of dementing illness in the elderly and remains one of the major causes of death in the USA. It is currently estimated that approximately 4 million people in the USA have AD. This number is expected to rise to 14 million by the year 2040, as the elderly population continues to increase, with the so-called 'baby-boomers' aging. Thus, the potential impact of AD is enormous, and projected costs for health care could rise dramatically if AD cannot be prevented or managed better than it is today. Currently, the national cost of AD is placed at $50–100 billion per year.[27]

AD is characterized by three histopathological markers: amyloid deposition (senile plaques), neurofibrillary tangles (NFT) and neuronal cell loss in several cortical and subcortical regions. The main component of senile plaques is the β-amyloid peptide. This is derived from a large transmembrane protein, the amyloid precursor protein (APP), and is thought to play an important role in the pathogenesis of AD. Mutations in the APP gene located on chromosome 21 are associated with familial AD. The main component of the NFT is a paired helical filament, which consists largely of the microtubule associated protein, tau, in an abnormal state of hyperphosphorylation.[28]

Although the exact pathogenesis of AD remains to be fully defined, several pharmacological strategies for preventing and treating AD are under active investigation. These strategies include cholinesterase inhibition, M1 agonist administration, administration of nerve growth factor, estrogen replacement therapy, antioxidants and anti-inflammatory treatment.[29] More recently, new drug design has targeted molecular events involved in the pathogenesis of AD including β-amyloid and NFT formation.

Low-molecular-weight heparins and heparin-derived oligosaccharides have been proposed as promising agents in the management of AD, owing to their multiple interventions on the pathogenesis of AD. These interventions are summarized in the following sections, including potential competitive interactions with proteoglycans, vascular effects, interactions with serpins and anti-inflammatory actions.

Proteoglycans and vascular risk factors

Proteoglycan hypothesis

Heparan sulfate and related proteoglycans (PGs) have been implicated in the progressive development of polymerized amyloid-β (Aβ) deposits and other pathophysiological effects in AD.[30] This hypothesis is based on the fact that PGs and GAGs are found in a number of peripheral amyloidoses including reactive systemic amyloidoses, which are secondary to chronic inflammatory conditions. AD amyloid plaques, like any amyloidoses that produce β-pleated secondary structures, are associated with PGs. Studies have shown that the association between PGs and amyloid plaques in AD may be due to specific binding of the Aβ sequence and APP to PGs as well as to GAGs. In addition, because of the location of the binding of APP protein in relation to the heparan sulfate PGs, the enzyme (β secretase) that normally cleaves in the middle of the Aβ sequence is blocked, which promotes the aggregation of the Aβ peptide. Therefore, the inhibition of PG binding could theoretically lead to an increase in the amyloid fragments *in vivo* by allowing the β– and γ-secretases to cleave the APP molecule. On the other hand, GAGs, including heparins, which have been shown to block the binding of heparan sulfate PGs to the APP molecule, could theoretically be beneficial in preventing plaque deposition with aging.[12]

Moreover, PGs have been shown in both *in vitro* and *in vivo* models to increase the aggregation rate of Aβ into β-pleated fibrils.[30] Snow *et al.* have shown that, after Aβ along with heparan sulfate PG was infused into the lateral ventricles of the rat, there was an increased fibrillary Aβ deposition in the neuropil.[31] Interestingly, in the same study, when the Aβ and GAGs were infused together, no deposition was detected. However, they did not test whether the effects of heparan sulfate PG could be blocked by co-infusion with GAGs. PGs have also been shown to increase the polymerization of tau proteins into paired-helical filaments, which make up the NFTs of AD. Theoretically, GAGs could also decrease the polymerization of tau and block the formation of NFTs by competing with PGs.

Vascular risk factors

AD is a primary degenerative dementia and is not considered to be of vascular origin. Indeed, stroke and severe cerebrovascular diseases are generally exclusionary for the clinical diagnosis of AD. However, both epidemiological and neuropathological studies have recently suggested an association between AD and several vascular risk factors, such as thrombosis and atherosclerosis.

One of the milestone studies carried out to determine the risk factors associated with AD is the Rotterdam Study. More than 7000 elderly subjects have been studied since 1990 in a series of reports consisting of demented subjects and non-demented, age-matched controls. On the basis of the data gathered in this study, it was concluded that vascular risk factors and indicators of vascular disease, particularly in elderly subjects, have an association with AD.[32] The risk factors for AD reported in the Rotterdam Study include the following: diabetes mellitus, thrombosis, high fibrinogen concentrations, high serum homocysteine, atrial fibrillation, smoking and atherosclerosis. All these conditions have a vascular involvement and are known to reduce cerebral perfusion. Since heparins are extensively used in the modulation

of vascular functions, their effects on the brain and peripheral vasculatures may theoretically benefit AD patients.

Serine proteases and serine protease inhibitors

Serine proteases

The serine proteases are a family of enzymes that catalyze the hydrolysis of covalent peptide bonds of other proteins. This activity depends on a set of amino acid residues in the active site of the enzyme, one of which is always a serine, thus accounting for their name. In mammals, serine proteases perform many important functions, especially in digestion, blood clotting and the complement system.

Three protein-digesting enzymes secreted by the pancreas are serine proteases: chymotrypsin, trypsin and elastase. These three enzymes share similar tertiary as well as primary structures. In fact, the active serine residue is at the same position (Ser-195) in all three. Despite their similarities, they have different substrate specificities; that is, they cleave different peptide bonds during protein digestion. Most activated clotting factors and fibrinolytic proteins are serine proteases as well, such as factors VIIa, IXa, Xa, XIa, XIIa, prekallikrein, thrombin, plasmin and tissue plasminogen activator. An integral coagulation and fibrinolytic cascade is shown in Figure 28.3. Most of the serine proteases in these cascades present in their zymogenic form. When triggered, they are activated in a cascade fashion. In addition to protein-digesting enzymes and clotting factors, several proteins involved in the complement cascade are serine proteases, including C1r and C1s, and the C3 convertases C4b,2a and C3b,Bb, which possess potent pro-inflammatory effects.

Although the role of serine proteases in the pathogenesis of AD is not fully understood,

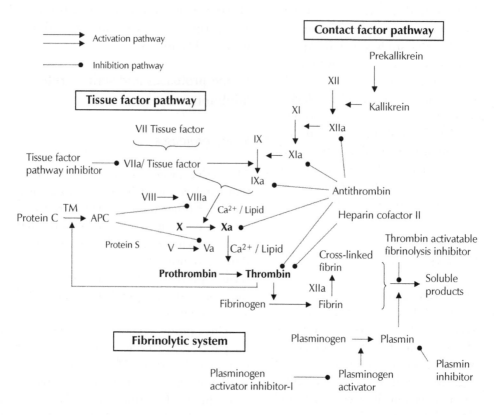

Figure 28.3 The blood coagulation cascade primarily consists of two pathways – the intrinsic (contact factor) and the extrinsic (tissue factor) – which converge at the step of activation of factor X (Adapted from reference 48). TM, thrombomodulin; APC, activated protein C

several reports have become available on the association of serine proteases and AD. Table 28.1 summarizes the recent studies on serine proteases and their association with AD.

Serine protease inhibitors and Alzheimer's disease

'Serpins' is an acronym given to a large family of serine protease inhibitors that share a complex, but well conserved, tertiary structure. Members of the family are diversely present in viruses, insects, plants and higher organisms, but not in bacteria or yeasts.[33] Serpins share about 30%

homology and have similar tertiary structure and inhibition mechanisms. Each serpin plays a role in inhibiting excessive action of its specific target proteases. The serpins combine with proteases to form inactive complexes, which are then cleared from the circulation. The serpins are, in fact, suicide substrates for their target proteases, in that they interact with the active sites on the proteases and are cleaved by proteases.

Although serpins regulate the activity of proteases involved in such diverse processes as coagulation, fibrinolysis, inflammation, cell migration and tumorigenesis, as depicted in

Table 28.1 Serine proteases involved in the pathogenesis of Alzheimer's disease

Serine proteases	Functions	Potential role in the pathogenesis of Alzheimer's disease	Reference
α_1-Trypsin	protein digestion	present in senile plaques	49
Factor IIa (thrombin)	coagulation protease	inducing APP secretion, cleaving APP into amyloidogenic fragments, increased in senile plaques	50
Factor Xa	coagulation protease	cleaving APP into amyloidogenic fragments	51
Factor XIa	coagulation protease	cleaving APP and modulating APP-mediated cell adhesion	52
Factor XIIa	coagulation protease	present in senile plaques	53
Kallikrein 8	coagulation protease	high mRNA levels in the hippocampus	54
Plasmin	fibrinolysis protease	cleaving APP, reduced in AD brains	55
uPA	fibrinolysis protease	present in senile plaques	56
tPA	fibrinolysis protease	present in senile plaques	56
C1q, C3, C4, C5 C6, C7, C8, C9	complement proteins	highly co-localized with Aβ deposits and NFT	57

APP, amyloid precursor protein; NFT, neurofibrillary tangles

Table 28.2 Serine protease inhibitors involved in the pathogenesis of Alzheimer's disease

Serpins	Functions	Expression in Alzheimer's disease	Reference
α_1-Antichymotrypsin	acute-phase protein in inflammation	increase in senile plaques	58
α_1-Antitrypsin	acute-phase protein in inflammation	increase in senile plaques	59
Antithrombin	destruction of released coagulation proteases, natural anticoagulant	increase in senile plaques	34
Plasminogen activator inhibitor	inhibition of plasminogen activator; regulation of fibrinolysis	increase in senile plaques	60
Protease nexin I	natural anticoagulant in the central nervous system	increase in senile plaques, decrease in the brain	61
Tissue factor pathway inhibitor	inhibition of tissue factor and factor Xa; natural anticoagulant	elevation in frontal cortex	35

Table 28.2, the physiological role of serpins remains largely unknown. For example, *in vitro* studies have demonstrated trypsin and plasmin as target proteases of antithrombin (AT), but the reaction of trypsin and plasmin with AT *in vivo* is too slow to be of any physiological importance. In addition, the expression of AT has been recently detected in the cerebral cortex and brain microvessels,[34] suggesting its role in the maintenance of neuronal integrity. Thus, the tissue

219

distribution patterns of serpins can provide clues about their physiological function.

Recently, a number of serpins have been linked with AD as summarized in Table 28.2, including AT, α_1-antichymotrypsin, α_1-antitrypsin, neuroserpin, protease nexin I and tissue factor pathway inhibitor.[35–37] The pathological mechanisms behind this assocation are not fully understood. Carrell and Lomas have proposed a 'serpinopathies' model to describe the pathogenesis of common neurodegenerative diseases using structural biology, in which point mutations of serpins eventually lead to conformational abnormalities, such as the amyloid aggregation, and AD.[37] On the other hand, Janciauskiene et al. reviewed various neuro-inflammatory factors involved in AD and proposed serpins as a part of anti-inflammatory mechanisms.[36] More interestingly, PGs and GAGs were also involved in neuroinflammation and AD, even though their functions, in particular interactions with serpins, were not clear.[36]

Tissue factor pathway inhibitor and Alzheimer's disease

TFPI is a member of the serpin superfamily (Figure 28.4). Like several other serpins, a strong expression and significantly elevated amount of TFPI in the frontal cortex in AD patients were demonstrated by Hollister et al.[35] using immunohistochemical localization. It is still unclear whether the increase in TFPI was due to a compensatory mechanism in which the functionality of TFPI decreases, or was the etiology in AD. Since TFPI is localized to microglia in both AD and non-AD individuals and to senile plaques, Hollister et al. suggested that TFPI might play a cell-specific role in protease regulation in the brain.[35]

TFPI is also involved in the regulation of atherosclerosis, which is one of the vascular risk factors of AD. Westrick et al. evaluated the effect

of heterozygous TFPI deficiency on the development of atherosclerosis and thrombosis in atherosclerosis-prone mice[38]. Compared with mice with a normal TFPI genotype, mice with a TFPI deficiency exhibited a greater athero-sclerotic burden and more tissue factor activity within the plaques involving the carotid and common iliac arteries. These observations indicated that TFPI protects from athero-sclerosis and is an important regulator of the thrombosis that occurs in the setting of atherosclerosis.

Heparin-derived oligosaccharides and Alzheimer's disease

Heparins are considered conventionally as cardiovascular medicines. The introduction of heparins in the treatment of AD was based on the hypothesis that heparins might improve the cerebral microcirculation through its anti-thrombotic effects. However, the hemorrhage potential and adverse effects of heparin such as heparin-induced thrombocytopenia (HIT) hindered its neurological applications. With the introduction of non-anticoagulant heparin oligosaccharides and a better understanding of the vascular risk factors associated with AD, the

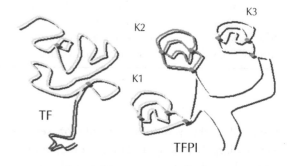

Figure 28.4 The secondary structures of tissue factor (TF) and tissue factor pathway inhibitor (TFPI)

re-evaluation of heparins as a potential therapy for Alzheimer's patients has been carried out in both preclinical and clinical studies.

In a study by Lorens et al.,[39] aged rats showed a significant partial reversal of age-related behavioral deficits following administration of a high-molecular-weight GAG polysulfate (Ateroid[TM]). Biochemical observations showed that Ateroid counteracted the age-related reduction in dopamine metabolites and also aided in the normalization of stress-induced corticosterone secretion seen in aged rats.[39] Conti et al.[40] prescribed Ateroid for primary dementia patients. These patients showed significant improvements in objective performance, psychology and social behavior over placebo groups[40]. Parnetti et al.[41] showed that prescribed doses of Ateroid could significantly improve certain biochemical abnormalities found in primary dementia[41]. In recent studies, Walzer et al. tested the neuroprotective effects of a LMWH certoparin in an animal model mimicking the pathology of AD. A significant decrease of tau toxicity by certoparin was observed among treated animals.[42] Using the same animal model, Dudas et al. demonstrated the protective effects of a heparin oligosaccharide mixture C3 on the brain after the injection of amyloid peptide into the amygdala.[43]

Despite the positive results obtained from these studies, the underlying mechanisms behind the effects of heparins on AD are not clear. Snow and Wight[30] proposed that heparin GAGs might interfere directly with endogenous PGs. In addition, heparins might also participate in the regulation of cerebral vascular functions by interactions with endogenous serpins, such as tissue factor pathway inhibitor. Since both PGs and serpins are associated with neuro-inflammation,[36] it is likely that the anti-inflammatory effects in the central nervous system contribute to the overall mechanism of heparins in AD.

HEPARIN AND STROKE

The benefit of heparin, LMWHs and heparinoids in acute ischemic stroke remains largely controversial, despite their widespread use for this indication. Some results from both preclinical and clinical studies are summarized in the following sections.

The neuroprotective effects of heparins have been well documented in animal models of stroke. Enoxaparin has been shown to reduce ischemic damage with a wide therapeutic window in a rat model of stroke induced by middle cerebral artery occlusion[44]. Enoxaparin and the other LMWHs have also been demonstrated to decrease infarct size and improve sensor–motor function in a rat model of focal cerebral ischemia.[45] These observations suggest that the anticoagulant properties of heparins explain their anti-ischemic effects. Furthermore, additional pharmacological effects of heparins, such as anti-inflammatory and neurotrophic effects, may act in synergy to explain their neuroprotective activity in stroke.[18]

Heparin, LMWHs and heparinoids have been studied in acute ischemic stroke with variable results. Of several recent controlled clinical trials, only one documented a net benefit of treatment.[46] The largest randomized clinical trial of heparin in acute stroke (the International Stroke Trial) showed that heparin was associated with significant excess in bleeding complications but no clinical benefit at 6 months. Analysis of the TOAST (Trial of ORG 10172 in Acute Stroke Treatment) study also showed an excess number of bleeding complications in the treatment group without corresponding benefit on stroke outcome at 3 months.[47] Therefore, although heparin, LMWHs and heparinoids continue to be used in the management of patients with acute ischemic stroke, their value in prevention and treatment of stroke warrants further investigation.

Several other clinical trials on such LMWHs such as certoparin (Novartis), tinzaparin (Leo/Pharmion), dalteparin (Pfizer) and reviparin (Abbott) have been conducted in stroke patients. None of these trials showed any statistically valid benefit from the use of these agents. However, there was a clear-cut reduction in the thromboembolic event rates in patients treated with various LMWHs for an extended period of time. This is to be expected, as bed-ridden patients have an increased prevalence of developing venous thrombosis. The dosage used with these LMWHs in the stroke trial was equal to, or higher than, the one used for treatment of thrombosis.

The pathogenesis of thrombotic stroke is rather complex and may involve several processes including the activation of platelets and coagulation. In the event of embolic stroke associated with atrial fibrillation, the LMWHs may be effective. However, in ischemic and thrombotic stroke, these drugs may have certain limitations. Regardless of these limitations and failures of current clinical trials to demonstrate positive results, the LMWHs may be useful as an adjunct therapy for thrombotic and embolic stroke.

6–120 hexose units. The LMWHs, on the other hand, comprise molecular components ranging from 0.5 to 10 kDA with 2–30 hexose units containing chains. The ultra-low-molecular-weight heparins even contain oligosaccharide components with much lower molecular weights which are mainly represented by tetra-, hexa-, octa-, deca- and dodecasaccharides, with an average molecular weight of 2–3 kDA. These agents are collectively called heparin-derived oligosaccharides (HDOs). Because of lower molecular weight these oligosaccharides exhibit much lower anticoagulant activity and are capable of passing through such barriers as the placental and blood–brain barriers. While these agents do not exhibit any anticoagulant activity, the HDOs are capable of modulating various cellular functions and inhibit adhesion processes directly or indirectly. The pharmacology of these agents is poorly understood. However, because of the polytherapeutic nature of these agents, the HDOs may be useful in the management of ischemic and thrombotic stroke, vascular dementia and acute coronary syndrome. These agents can be structurally modified to determine the structure–activity relationship, which may lead to the development of newer drugs for both cardiovascular and cerebral vascular disorders.

SUMMARY

Heparin is composed of various molecular components ranging from 2 to 50 kDA with

REFERENCES

1. McLean J. The discovery of heparin. Circulation 1959; 19: 75–78

2. Best CH. Preparation of heparin and its use in the first clinical cases. Circulation 1959; 19: 79

3. Fareed J, Hoppensteadt DA. Heparins in the new millennium: will unfractionated heparin survive? Epilogue. Semin Thromb Hemost 2000; 1 (Suppl 26): 87–8

4. Rosenberg RD, Lam L. Correlation between structure and function of heparin. Proc Natl Acad Sci USA 1979; 76: 1218–22

5. Choay J. Structure and activity of heparin and its fragments: an overview. Semin Thromb Hemost 1989; 15: 359–64

6. Fareed J, Hoppensteadt D, Jeske W, et al. Low molecular weight heparins: are they different? Can J Cardiol 1998; 14 (Suppl E): 28E–34E

7. Hirsh J, Warkentin TE, Shaughnessy SG, et al. Heparin and low-molecular-weight heparin: mechanisms of action, pharmacokinetics, dosing, monitoring, efficacy, and safety. Chest 2001; 119 (Suppl 1): 64S–94S

8. Weitz JI. Low-molecular-weight heparins. N Engl J Med 1997; 337: 688–98

9. Fareed J. Heparin, its fractions, fragments and derivatives. Some newer perspectives. Semin Thromb Hemost 1985; 11: 1–9

10. Walenga JM, Jeske WP, Bara L, et al. Biochemical and pharmacologic rationale for the development of a synthetic heparin pentasaccharide. Thromb Res 1997; 86: 1–36

11. Ma Q, Dudas B, Daud A, et al. Molecular and biochemical profiling of a heparin-derived oligosaccharide, C3. Thromb Res 2002; 105: 303–9

12. Cornelli U. The therapeutic approach to Alzheimer's disease. In Casu B, ed. Non-anticoagulant Action of Glycosaminoglycans. New York: Plenum Press, 1996: 249–79

13. Nelson RM, Cecconi O, Roberts WG, et al. Heparin oligosaccharides bind L- and P-selectin and inhibit acute inflammation. Blood 1993; 82: 3253–8

14. Tyrrell DJ, Horne AP, Holme KR, et al. Heparin in inflammation: potential therapeutic applications beyond anticoagulation. Adv Pharmacol 1999; 46: 151–208

15. Esmon CT. New mechanisms for vascular control of inflammation mediated by natural anticoagulant proteins. J Exp Med 2002; 196: 561–4

16. Koenig A, Norgard-Sumnicht K, Linhardt R, Varki A. Differential interactions of heparin and heparan sulfate glycosaminoglycans with the selectins. Implications for the use of unfractionated and low molecular weight heparins as therapeutic agents. J Clin Invest 1998; 101: 877–89

17. Ahmed T, Ungo J, Zhou M. Inhibition of allergic late airway responses by inhaled heparin-derived oligosaccharides. J Appl Physiol 2000; 88: 1721–9

18. Stutzmann JM, Mary V, Grosjean-Piot O, et al. Neuroprotective profile of enoxaparin, a low molecular weight heparin, in in vivo models of cerebral ischemia or traumatic brain injury in rats: a review. CNS Drug Rev 2002; 8: 1–30

19. Folkman J, Klagsbrun M, Sasse J, et al. A heparin-binding angiogenic protein – basic fibroblast growth factor – is stored within basement membrane. Am J Pathol 1988; 130: 393–400

20. Ortega S, Ittmann M, Tsang SH, et al. Neuronal defects and delayed wound healing in mice lacking fibroblast growth factor 2. Proc Natl Acad Sci USA 1998; 95: 5672–7

21. Mufson EJ, Kroin JS, Sendera TJ, Sobreviela T. Distribution and retrograde transport of trophic factors in the central nervous system: functional implications for the treatment of neurodegenerative diseases. Prog Neurobiol 1999; 57: 451–84

22. Schlessinger J, Lax I, Lemmon M. Regulation of growth factor activation by proteoglycans: what

is the role of the low affinity receptors? Cell 1995; 83: 357–60

23. D'Amore PA. Heparin–endothelial cell interactions. Haemostasis 1990; 20 (Suppl 1): 159–65

24. Barzu T, Lormeau JC, Petitou M, et al. Heparin-derived oligosaccharides: affinity for acidic fibroblast growth factor and effect on its growth-promoting activity for human endothelial cells. J Cell Physiol 1989; 140: 538–48

25. Ornitz DM, Herr AB, Nilsson M, et al. FGF binding and FGF receptor activation by synthetic heparan-derived di- and trisaccharides. Science 1995; 268: 432–6

26. Lindahl B, Westling C, Gimenez-Gallega G, et al. Common binding sites for beta-amyloid fibrils and fibroblast growth factor-2 in heparan sulfate from human cerebral cortex. J Biol Chem 1999; 274: 30631–5

27. Meek PD, McKeithan K, Schumock GT. Economic considerations in Alzheimer's disease. Pharmacotherapy 1998; 18: 68–73; discussion 79–82

28. Iqbal K, Grundke-Iqbal I. Ubiquitination and abnormal phosphorylation of paired helical filaments in Alzheimer's disease. Mol Neurobiol 1991; 5: 399–410

29. Mayeux R, Sano M. Treatment of Alzheimer's disease. N Engl J Med 1999; 341: 1670–9

30. Snow AD, Wight TN. Proteoglycans in the pathogenesis of Alzheimer's disease and other amyloidoses. Neurobiol Aging 1989; 10: 481–97

31. Snow AD, Sekiguchi R, Nochlin D, et al. An important role of heparan sulfate proteoglycan (Perlecan) in a model system for the deposition and persistence of fibrillar A beta-amyloid in rat brain. Neuron 1994; 12: 219–34

32. Breteler MM. Risk factors for vascular disease and dementia. J Neural Trans Gen Section 1998; 105: 773–86

33. Silverman GA, Bird PI, Carrell RW, et al. The serpins are an expanding superfamily of structurally similar but functionally diverse proteins. Evolution, mechanism of inhibition, novel functions, and a revised nomenclature. J

Biol Chem 2001; 276: 33293–6

34. Kalaria RN, Golde T, Kroon SN, Perry G. Serine protease inhibitor antithrombin III and its messenger RNA in the pathogenesis of Alzheimer's disease. Am J Pathol 1993; 143: 886–93

35. Hollister RD, Kisiel W, Hyman BT. Immunohistochemical localization of tissue factor pathway inhibitor-1 (TFPI-1), a Kunitz proteinase inhibitor, in Alzheimer's disease. Brain Res 1996; 728: 13–19

36. Janciauskiene S, Sun YX, Wright HT. Interactions of A beta with endogenous anti-inflammatory agents: a basis for chronic neuroinflammation in Alzheimer's disease. Neurobiol Dis 2002; 10: 187–200

37. Carrell RW, Lomas DA. Alpha1-antitrypsin deficiency – a model for conformational diseases. N Engl J Med 2002; 346: 45–53

38. Westrick RJ, Bodary PF, Xu Z, et al. Deficiency of tissue factor pathway inhibitor promotes atherosclerosis and thrombosis in mice. Circulation 2001; 103: 3044–6

39. Lorens SA, Guschwan M, Hata N, et al. Behavioral, endocrine, and neurochemical effects of sulfomucopolysaccharide treatment in the aged Fischer 344 male rat. Semin Thromb Hemost 1991; 17: S164–73

40. Conti L, Placidi GF, Cassano GB. Ateroid in the treatment of dementia: results of a clinical trial: Ateroid in the clinical treatment of multiinfarct dementia: a general practice trial of Ateroid 200 in 8776 patients with chronic senile cerebral insufficiency. Mod Probl Pharmacopsychiatry 1989; 23: 76–84

41. Parnetti L, Ban TA, Senim U. Glycosaminoglycan polysulfate in primary degenerative dementia. Pilot study of biologic and clinical effects. Neuropsychobiology 1995; 31: 76–80

42. Walzer M, Lorens S, Hejna M, et al. Low molecular weight glycosaminoglycan blockade of beta-amyloid induced neuropathology. Eur J Pharmacol 2002; 445: 211–20

43. Dudas B, Cornelli U, Lee JM, et al. Oral and subcutaneous administration of the glycosaminoglycan C3 attenuates Abeta(25-35)-induced abnormal tau protein immunoreactivity in rat brain. Neurobiol Aging 2002; 23: 97–104

44. Mary V, Wahl F, Uzan A, Stutzmann JM. Enoxaparin in experimental stroke: neuroprotection and therapeutic window of opportunity. Stroke 2001; 32: 993–9

45. Li PA, He QP, Siddiqui MM, Shuaib A. Post-treatment with low molecular weight heparin reduces brain edema and infarct volume in rats subjected to thrombotic middle cerebral artery occlusion. Brain Res 1998; 801: 220–3

46. Kay R, Wong KS, Yu YL, et al. Low-molecular-weight heparin for the treatment of acute ischemic stroke. N Engl J Med 1995; 333: 1588–93

47. Adams HP Jr. Emergent use of anticoagulation for treatment of patients with ischemic stroke. Stroke 2002; 33: 856–61

48. Segel GB, Francis CA. Anticoagulant proteins in childhood venous and arterial thrombosis: a review. Blood Cells Mol Dis 2000; 26: 540–60.

49. Smith MA, Kalaria RN, Perry G. Alpha 1-trypsin immunoreactivity in Alzheimer disease. Biochem Biophys Res Commun 1993; 193: 579–84

50. Ciallella JR, Figueiredo H, Smith-Swintosky V, et al. Thrombin induces surface and intracellular secretion of amyloid precursor protein from human endothelial cells. Thromb Haemost 1999; 81: 630–7

51. Haas C, Aldudo J, Cazorla P, et al. Proteolysis of Alzheimer's disease beta-amyloid precursor protein by factor Xa. Biochim Biophys Acta 1997; 1343: 85–94

52. Saporito-Irwin SM, Van Nostrand WE. Coagulation factor XIa cleaves the RHDS sequence and abolishes the cell adhesive properties of the amyloid beta-protein. J Biol Chem 1995; 270: 26265–9

53. Yasuhara O, Walker DG, McGeer PL. Hageman factor and its binding sites are present in senile plaques of Alzheimer's disease. Brain Res 1994; 654: 234–40

54. Shimizu-Okabe C, Yousef GM, Diamandis EP, et al. Expression of the kallikrein gene family in normal and Alzheimer's disease brain. Neuroreport 2001; 12: 2747–51

55. Ledesma MD, Da Silva JS, Crassaerts K, et al. Brain plasmin enhances APP alpha-cleavage and Abeta degradation and is reduced in Alzheimer's disease brains. EMBO Rep 2000; 1: 530–5

56. Rebeck GW, Harr SD, Strickland DK, Hyman BT. Multiple, diverse senile plaque-associated proteins are ligands of an apolipoprotein E receptor, the alpha 2-macroglobulin receptor/low-density-lipoprotein receptor-related protein. Ann Neurol 1995; 37: 211–17

57. Akiyama H, Barger S, Barnum S, et al. Inflammation and Alzheimer's disease. Neurobiol Aging 2000; 21: 383–421

58. Abraham CR, Selkoe DJ, Potter H. Immunochemical identification of the serine protease inhibitor alpha 1-antichymotrypsin in the brain amyloid deposits of Alzheimer's disease. Cell 1988; 52: 487–501

59. Gollin PA, Kalaria RN, Eikelenboom P, et al. Alpha 1-antitrypsin and alpha 1-antichymotrypsin are in the lesions of Alzheimer's disease. Neuroreport 1992; 3: 201–3

60. Akiyama H, Ikeda K, Kondo H, et al. Microglia express the type 2 plasminogen activator inhibitor in the brain of control subjects and patients with Alzheimer's disease. Neurosci Lett 1993; 164: 233–5

61. Turgeon VL, Houenou LJ. The role of thrombin-like (serine) proteases in the development, plasticity and pathology of the nervous system. Brain Res Brain Res Rev 1997; 25: 85–95

Chapter 29

Glycosaminoglycans and neuroprotection: effect on cholinergic neurodegeneration

B Dudas, M Rose, U Cornelli, L De Ambrosi, M Cornelli, I Hanin

ALZHEIMER'S DISEASE AND GLYCOSAMINOGLYCANS – INTRODUCTORY COMMENTS

Alzheimer's disease (AD) is a neurodegenerative disorder characterized by focal accumulation of specific proteins that have been modified by biochemical transformation of peptides normally present in the brain. Extracellularly deposited amyloid plaques are composed of fragments of a 40–42 amino acid protein, amyloid-β (Aβ),[1–4] which is formed by the abnormal cleavage of amyloid precursor protein (APP). Intracellularly developed flame-shaped tangles are made up of hyperphosphorylated and abnormal conformational forms of the naturally present tau protein.[5] Although the pathomechanism of these histological changes is not entirely known, it is believed that the deposition of these abnormal proteins leads to general neuronal loss characterized particularly by a cholinergic lesion that is responsible for the majority of the clinical symptoms of AD.

There have been several attempts to develop drugs suitable to treat AD. One major group of these compounds are inhibitors of acetylcholinesterase (AChE) that target the cholinergic damage by inhibiting the breakdown of acetylcholine. Recently, a series of studies have suggested that glycosaminoglycans (GAGs) may also be valuable adjuncts in the treatment of AD.[6–9] Ateroid®, a mixture of different GAGs including unfractionated heparin, dermatan sulfate, chondroitin sulfate and heparan sulfate, enhanced age-related cognitive deficits in rats and humans, and is currently used to improve memory functions in AD patients in several European countries.[6,7] Although the pathomechanism of the neuroprotective role of GAGs is not entirely known, it is believed that GAGs may antagonize the effect of proteoglycans (PGs), which play a pivotal role in the pathogenesis of AD. PGs were shown to increase the production of Aβ and accelerate the formation of amyloid fibrils.[10] PGs have high affinity for Aβ, and protect it from proteolysis,[11–13] leading to neurodegeneration. PGs also inhibit the clearance of amyloid by microglia,[13] induce the phosphorylation of tau protein, and stimulate the formation of paired helical filaments.[14–17]

GAGs are believed to attenuate these effects. Moreover, GAGs and other sulfated compounds inhibit the aggregation and toxicity of Aβ itself,[18–23] suggesting that GAGs play a pivotal role in the pathology of amyloid plaques. A heparin-derived low-molecular-weight oligosaccharide C3 has also been shown to increase neuronal arborization in the rat brain, possibly via influencing the release of nerve growth factor (NGF) or modulating NGF receptor expression.[24] Indeed, GAGs stimulate the effect of growth factors in cell culture[25,26] and C3 reduces the expression of cholinotoxin-stimulated growth factor receptor expression in the rat septum.[27]

Thus, based on: the neuroprotective effects of GAGs in animal models and *in vitro* cell culture studies; current experiences with these compounds in improving age-related dementia in humans; and the wide safety margin of GAGs determined in recent toxicology studies (data not shown), GAGs may be valuable drugs in the treatment of AD and other neurodegenerative disorders.

BLOOD–BRAIN ACCESSIBILITY OF GLYCOSAMINOGLYCANS

The remedial value of GAGs in neurodegenerative disorders is determined by the penetration of these compounds through the blood–brain barrier (BBB), and thus by their molecular weight. Leveugle *et al.*[28] have used *in vitro* co-culture of astrocytes and brain capillary endothelial cells as a model of the BBB and demonstrated that low-molecular-weight GAGs pass this artificial barrier and inhibit APP release. We have also shown, in rats, that the low molecular-weight GAG C3 (MW approximately 2.4 kD), can be detected in the brain tissue and cerebrospinal fluid 45 min after intravenous and subcutaneous administration[29] and 2 h after oral feeding.[30] Moreover, oral and subcutaneous administration of C3 reduced Aβ-induced abnormal tau-2 immunoreactivity,[31] and prevented AF64A-induced cholinergic lesions in the rat brain.[32] These findings, together, provide further indications that GAGs indeed penetrate

the BBB. Therefore, these compounds might be useful in the therapy of AD.

ANIMAL MODELS OF THE ALZHEIMER'S DISEASE LESION

In order to simulate the hallmarks of AD in animals, several AD models have been developed. Intracerebral injection of synthetic Aβ fragments[16,17,33–37] or senile plaque cores isolated from postmortem AD brains[15] into the rat brain induces histopathological changes characteristic of AD, including neuronal damage, amyloid deposition, and tau phosphorylation followed by its conformational change. Amyloid β neurotoxicity has also been shown in tissue culture neurons.[4] Moreover, intraventricular administration of the cholinotoxin AF64A can be used to mimic specific cholinergic damage characteristic of AD (Figure 29.1),[38,39] if it is administered in extremely low concentrations (1 nmol/2 μl per side). Using these animal models of AD, C3 has been shown to reduce Aβ-induced abnormal tau-2 immunoreactivity,[31] and to attenuate AF64A-induced cholinergic lesions in rats (Figures 29.1m–p and 29.2c).[32]

NEUROPROTECTIVE ROLE OF DIFFERENT LOW-MOLECULAR-WEIGHT GLYCOSAMINOGLYCANS

While the structural differences of low-molecular-weight GAGs are well known, the correlation between their structure and their ability to protect against neuronal damage has not yet been elucidated. Although Ateroid®, that is a mixture of GAGs, shows promising results in the treatment of age and AD-related dementia, it is not clear exactly which component of the mixture is responsible for the

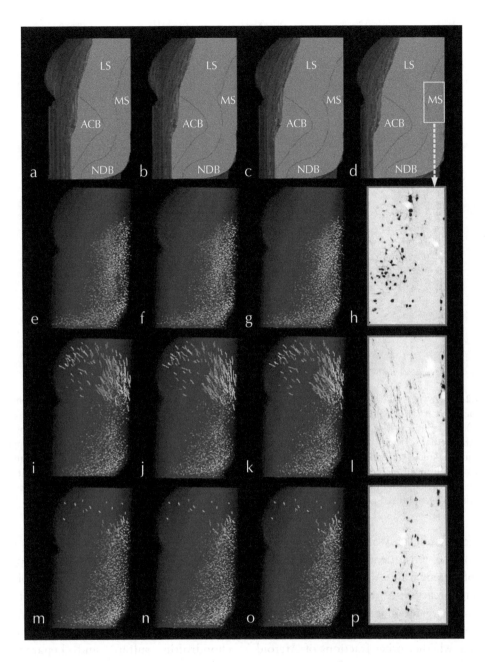

Figure 29.1 Stereoscopic images demonstrating the effect of C3 on the AF64A-induced cholinergic lesion in the septum. Images a–d show the organization of the septal region in the rat. Images i–l demonstrate the AF64A-induced choline acetyltransferase-immunoreactive (ChAT-IR) cholinergic varicosities and reduction in the number of ChAT-IR perikarya compared to the control animals (e–h). C3 attenuates this effect (m–p). LS, lateral septum; MS, medial septum; ACB, nucleus accumbens; NDB, nucleus of the diagonal band of Broca. (Stereoscopic images can be seen using parallel vision. The image is held approximately 20 in (50 cm) from the eyes. The eyes are relaxed to look into the distance until the images appear to fuse, and are then refocused by the brain.)

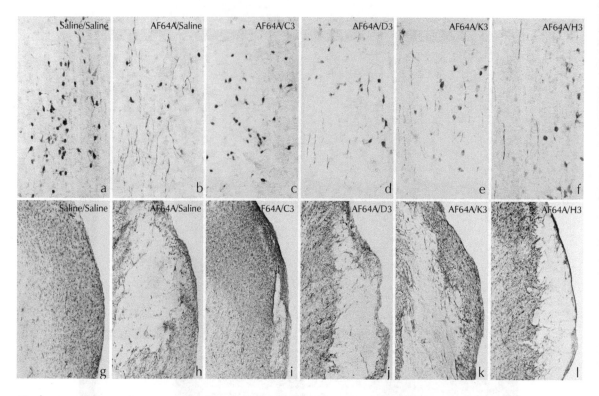

Figure 29.2 Effect of various glycosaminoglycans (GAGs) on AF64A-induced choline acetyltransferase-immunoreactive (ChAT-IR) cholinergic (a–f) and glial fibrillary acidic protein (GFAP)-IR glial (g–l) lesions in the medial (a–f) and lateral (g–l) septum. AF64A induces ChAT-IR axonal varicosities and reduces the number of ChAT-IR cells in the medial septum (b) compared to the control saline-treated animals (a). C3 attenuates the appearance of AF64A-induced axonal varicosities (c) compared to the AF64A-treated animals (b). GAGs D3, K3 and H3 have significantly smaller neuroprotective effect (d, e). AF64A treatment also reduces GFAP staining in the lateral septum (h) compared to the control rats (g). C3 attenuates this effect (i). GAGs D3, K3 and H3 have a considerably smaller impact on the AF64A-induced glial lesion (j–l)

neuroprotective effects. We have recently shown that one of the constituents of Ateroid, C3, is capable of attenuating Aβ-induced abnormal tau-2 immunoreactivity,[31] and reducing AF64A-induced cholinergic lesions in rat brains (Figures 29.1m–p and 29.2c).[32] However, these studies did not indicate whether other fractions of Ateroid might exhibit neuroprotective effects using the same animal models.

In order to examine other such compounds as potential sources for the treatment of AD and other neurodegenerative diseases, it would be crucial to determine which fraction of these

mixtures of GAGs is essential for neuroprotection. Therefore, we have recently completed a study testing the neuroprotective role of low-molecular-weight components of Ateroid, i.e. C3, D3, K3 and H3 obtained from fractionated porcine mucosal heparin, dermatan sulfate, chondroitin sulfate and heparan sulfate, respectively, by means of controlled depolymerization induced by γ-irradiation. These degraded GAGs were all oligosaccharide mixtures of 4–10 sulfated dextrose units, and were fractionated to remove high-molecular-weight fractions and to obtain a narrow-molecular-weight range of approximately 2 kDa. The relative neuroprotective effect of these compounds, if any, should therefore depend on their structural differences, e.g. electric charge of the molecules and/or the level of sulfation of these compounds.

C3, D3, K3 and H3 were tested under the same experimental conditions, using the rat model of AF64A-induced cholinergic septal lesion. The compounds were fed by oral gavage, 7 days before and 7 days after (25 mg/kg, once daily) the intraventricular. AF64A-administration (1 nmol/2 μl per side). The results of this study were in good consensus with our previous findings,[32] demonstrating that component C3 has a remarkable neuroprotective/neurorepair effect on AF64A-induced cholinergic damage in the rat septum. In addition to these data, C3 attenuated AF64A-induced glial lesions. However, the other constituents of Ateroid – D3, K3 and H3 – under the same conditions and at concentrations that we used for C3, failed to induce such neuroprotective effects. These results are illustrated in Figures 29.1 and 29.2.

Specifically, the septal cholinergic system, characterized by choline acetyltransferase (ChAT)-immunoreactive (IR) neurons in the septum, was damaged as the result of intra-ventricular AF64A treatment. Pathological changes included varicosities appearing along the neurites, axonal breakdown and reduction in cholinergic perikarya, as detected with ChAT immunohistochemistry (Figures 29.1i–l and 29.2b).[32] Moreover, AF64A administration also resulted in significant loss of glial fibrillary acidic protein (GFAP)-IR glial elements in the lateral septum (Figure 29.2h). When C3 administration was combined with AF64A injection, the cholinergic (Figures 29.1m–p and 29.2c) and glial damage (Figure 29.2i) induced by AF64A in the septum were attenuated.[32] In contrast, the other low-molecular-weight GAGs, i.e. H3, K3 and D3, had minimal protective effect on the AF64A-induced cholinergic (Figure 29.2d–f) and glial (Figure 29.2j–l) lesions, indicating that C3 is the most effective neuroprotective compound among the GAGs tested. In parallel with these findings, treatment with the GAGs alone, as controls, did not show any morphological changes in ChAT-IR or GFAP-IR elements (not shown).

DISCUSSION AND SUMMARY

The differences between the neuroprotective effects of different low-molecular-weight GAGs demonstrates the biological heterogenity of these compounds. Future studies are required to focus on determining which structural attributes of GAGs are essential for the neuroprotective effects. Such data may give us a unique opportunity in the future to develop low-molecular-weight GAG compounds with enhanced therapeutic value in the treatment of AD and other neurodegenerative disorders. In the interim, C3 has already successfully completed toxicity studies, and is in phase I testing at the time of this writing.

REFERENCES

1. Glenner GG, Wong CW, Quaranta V, Eanes ED. The amyloid deposits in Alzheimer's disease: their nature and pathogenesis. Appl Pathol 1984; 2: 357–69

2. Masters CL, Simms G, Weinman NA, et al. Amyloid plaque core protein in Alzheimer disease and Down syndrome. Proc Natl Acad Sci USA 1985; 82: 4245–9

3. Miller DL, Papayannopoulos IA, Styles J, et al. Peptide compositions of the cerebrovascular and senile plaque core amyloid deposits of Alzheimer's disease. Arch Biochem Biophys 1993; 301: 41–52

4. Roher AE, Ball MJ, Bhave SV, Wakade AR. Beta-amyloid from Alzheimer disease brains inhibits sprouting and survival of sympathetic neurons. Biochem Biophys Res Commun 1991; 174: 572–9

5. Wischik CM, Novak M, Thogersen HC, et al. Isolation of a fragment of tau derived from the core of the paired helical filament of Alzheimer disease. Proc Natl Acad Sci USA 1988; 85: 4506–10

6. Conti L, Placidi GF, Cassano GB. Ateroid in the treatment of dementia: results of a clinical trial. Mod Probl Pharmacopsychiatry 1989; 23: 76–84

7. Conti L, Re F, Lazzerini F, et al. Glycosaminoglycan polysulfate (Ateroid) in old-age dementias: effects upon depressive symptomatology in geriatric patients. Prog Neuropsychopharmacol Biol Psychiatry 1989; 13: 977–81

8. Passeri M, Cucinotta D. Ateroid in the clinical treatment of multi-infarct dementia. Mod Probl Pharmacopsychiatry 1989; 23: 85–94

9. Santini V. A general practice trial of Ateroid 200 in 8,776 patients with chronic senile cerebral insufficiency. Mod Probl Pharmacopsychiatry 1989; 23: 95–100

10. Snow AD, Sekiguchi R, Nochlin D, et al. An important role of heparan sulfate proteoglycan (Perlecan) in a model system for the deposition and persistence of fibrillar A beta-amyloid in rat brain. Neuron 1994; 12: 219–34

11. Castillo GM, Ngo C, Cummings J, et al. Perlecan binds to the beta-amyloid proteins (A beta) of Alzheimer's disease, accelerates A beta fibril formation, and maintains A beta fibril stability. J Neurochem 1997; 69: 2452–65

12. Gupta-Bansal R, Frederickson RC, Brunden KR. Proteoglycan-mediated inhibition of A beta proteolysis. A potential cause of senile plaque accumulation. J Biol Chem 1995; 270: 18666–71

13. Shaffer LM, Dority MD, Gupta-Bansal R, et al. Amyloid beta protein (A beta) removal by neuroglial cells in culture. Neurobiol Aging 1995; 16: 737–45

14. Perry G, Siedlak SL, Richey P, et al. Association of heparan sulfate proteoglycan with the neurofibrillary tangles of Alzheimer's disease. J Neurosci 1991; 11: 3679–83

15. Frautschy SA, Baird A, Cole GM. Effects of injected Alzheimer beta-amyloid cores in rat brain. Proc Natl Acad Sci USA 1991; 88: 8362–6

16. Kowall NW, McKee AC, Yankner BA, Beal MF. In vivo neurotoxicity of beta-amyloid [beta (1-40)] and the beta (25-35) fragment. Neurobiol Aging 1992; 13: 537–42

17. Sigurdsson EM, Lorens SA, Hejna MJ, et al. Local and distant histopathological effects of unilateral amyloid-beta (25-35) injections into the amygdala of young F344 rats. Neurobiol Aging 1996; 17: 893–901

18. Caughey B. Scrapie associated PrP accumulation and its prevention: insights from cell culture. Br Med Bull 1993; 49: 860–72

19. Howlett DR, Jennings KH, Lee DC, et al. Aggregation state and neurotoxic properties of

Alzheimer beta-amyloid peptide. Neurodegeneration 1995; 4: 23–32

20. Kisilevsky R, Lemieux LJ, Fraser PE, et al. Arresting amyloidosis in vivo using small-molecule anionic sulphonates or sulphates: implications for Alzheimer's disease. Nat Med 1995; 1: 143–8

21. Lorenzo A, Yankner BA. Beta-amyloid neurotoxicity requires fibril formation and is inhibited by congo red. Proc Natl Acad Sci USA 1994; 91: 12243–7

22. Podlisny MB, Ostaszewski BL, Squazzo SL, et al. Aggregation of secreted amyloid beta-protein into sodium dodecyl sulfate-stable oligomers in cell culture. J Biol Chem 1995; 270: 9564–70

23. Pollack SJ, Sadler II, Hawtin SR, et al. Sulfated glycosaminoglycans and dyes attenuate the neurotoxic effects of beta-amyloid in rat PC12 cells. Neurosci Lett 1995; 184: 113–16

24. Mervis RF, McKean J, Zats S, et al. Neurotrophic effects of the glycosaminoglycan C3 on dendritic arborization and spines in the adult rat hippocampus: a quantitative golgi study. CNS Drug Rev 2000; 6: 44–6

25. Damon DH, D'Amore PA, Wagner JA. Sulfated glycosaminoglycans modify growth factor-induced neurite outgrowth in PC12 cells. J Cell Physiol 1988; 135: 293–300

26. Lesma E, Di Giulio AM, Ferro L, et al. Glycosaminoglycans in nerve injury: 1. Low doses of glycosaminoglycans promote neurite formation. J Neurosci Res 1996; 46: 565–71

27. Dudas B, Lemes A, Cornelli U, Hanin I. Low molecular weight glycosaminoglycan C3 attenuates AF64A-stimulated, low affinity nerve growth factor (NGF) receptor-immunoreactive axonal varicosities in the rat septum. Brain Res 2004; 1033: 34–40

28. Leveugle B, Ding W, Laurence F, et al. Heparin oligosaccharides that pass the blood–brain barrier inhibit beta-amyloid precursor protein

secretion and heparin binding to beta-amyloid peptide. J Neurochem 1998; 70: 736–44

29. Ma Q, Dudas B, Hejna M, et al. The blood-brain barrier accessibility of a heparin-derived oligosaccharides C3. Thromb Res 2002; 105: 447–53

30. Cornelli U, Lorens SA, Lee JM, et al. Heparin derived oligosaccharides, Alzheimer's disease, and other age related neurological disorders. In Vossoughi J, Fareed J, Mousa SA, Karanian JW, eds. Thrombosis Research and Treatment: Bench to Bedside. Medical and Engineering Publishers, 2002

31. Dudas B, Cornelli U, Lee JM, et al. Oral and subcutaneous administration of the glycosaminoglycan C3 attenuates Abeta(25-35)-induced abnormal tau protein immunoreactivity in rat brain. Neurobiol Aging 2002; 23: 97–104

32. Rose M, Dudas B, Cornelli U, et al. Protective effect of glycosaminoglycan C3 on AF64A-induced cholinergic lesions in rats. Neurobiol Aging 2003; 24: 481–90

33. Emre M, Geula C, Ransil BJ, Mesulam MM. The acute neurotoxicity and effects upon cholinergic axons of intracerebrally injected beta-amyloid in the rat brain. Neurobiol Aging 1992; 13: 553–9

34. Giordano T, Pan JB, Monteggia LM, et al. Similarities between beta amyloid peptides (1-40) and (40-1): effects on aggregation, toxicity in vitro, and injection in young and aged rats. Exp Neurol 1994; 125: 175–82

35. Giovannelli L, Casamenti F, Scali C, et al. Differential effects of amyloid peptides beta-(1-40) and beta-(25-35) injections into the rat nucleus basalis. Neuroscience 1995; 66: 781–92

36. Rogers J, Cooper NR, Webster S, et al. Complement activation by beta-amyloid in Alzheimer disease. Proc Natl Acad Sci USA 1992; 89: 10016–20

37. Rogers J, Schultz J, Brachova L, et al. Complement activation and beta-amyloid-mediated neurotoxicity in Alzheimer's disease. Res Immunol 1992; 143: 624–30

38. Fisher A, Mantione CR, Abraham DJ, Hanin I. Long-term central cholinergic hypofunction induced in mice by ethylcholine aziridinium ion (AF64A) in vivo. J Pharmacol Exp Ther 1982; 222: 140–5

39. Fisher A, Hanin I. Potential animal models for senile dementia of Alzheimer's type, with emphasis on AF64A-induced cholinotoxicity. Annu Rev Pharmacol Toxicol 1986; 26: 161–81

Chapter 30

Orchestration of the functional subsites in the acetylcholinesterase active center – contribution to catalytic perfection and high reactivity toward specific ligands

A Shafferman, D Barak, A Ordentlich, N Ariel, C Kronman, D Kaplan, B Velan

INTRODUCTION

The enzyme acetylcholinesterase (AChE) is currently the most important molecular target for therapeutic intervention in symptomatic treatment of senile dementia of Alzheimer's type (SDAT), with four agents (tacrine, E2020, galanthamine and rivastigmine) approved for clinical use.[1] The ongoing effort to develop more therapeutically efficacious AChE inhibitors is currently driven by the remarkable progress made during the past decade in elucidating the structural and functional properties of the enzyme through X-ray crystallography[2,3] and site-directed mutagenesis.[4–8] Combination of these two powerful techniques allowed for the detailed mapping of the AChE active center, delineating the functional subsites involved in reactivity toward substrates and other non-covalent modifiers, as well as non-covalent ligands specific for the active center. These subsites include the catalytic triad (S203(200)[*], H447(440), E334(327)) as well as different combinations of the 14 aromatic amino acids which line about 40% of the human AChE (HuAChE) gorge surface e.g. the acyl pocket (F295(288) and F297(290)); the 'hydrophobic subsite' (W86(84), Y133(130), Y337(330) and F338(331)) and the cation–π interaction locus, W86(84), for charged moieties of substrates and other ligands at the active center. In addition, residues Y72(70), Y124(121), W286(279) and Y341(334), which are localized at or near the rim of the active center gorge, together with D74(72), constitute the peripheral anionic subsite (PAS) of AChE.[4,5,7]

Further examination of the functional architecture of the HuAChE active center revealed that reactivity of the enzyme toward substrates and other ligands can also be affected through perturbation of functional domains, which may include multiple subsites in the active center. Thus, enhanced conformational mobility of the catalytic histidine was recently implicated in the activity differences between human butyrylcholinesterase (HuBChE) and the hexamutant HuAChE carrying aliphatic replacements of all the active site gorge aromatic residues (Tyr72, Tyr124, Trp286, Phe295, Phe297, Tyr337) distinguishing between the two

---

[*] Residue numbers of *Torpedo californica* AChE are listed in italics with the corresponding residues of human AChE in parentheses and in plain text. Residue numbers of human AChE are listed in plain text with the corresponding numbers of *Torpedo californica* AChE in parentheses and in italics.

enzymes.[9] These include elements of the acyl pocket, the hydrophobic subsite and the PAS. Modulation of ligand interactions with the enzyme can also be affected through disruption of polar networks in the active center. One of these, the 'hydrogen bond network', includes residues Tyr133, Glu202, Glu450 as well as two strictly preserved water molecules.[10] Another one may include residues Ser229 and the catalytic triad residue Glu334 (A. Shafferman *et al.*, in preparation).

Previous investigations of HuAChE inter-actions with representative potential therapeutic agents such as edrophonium tacrine, huperzine A or the carbamates, pyridostigmine and physostigmine[8] demonstrated that an 'aromatic patch' of spatially adjacent aryl moieties of the hydrophobic subsite residues W86, Y133 and Y337 plays a dominant role in accommodation of the structurally diverse ligands.

Here we describe the role of the 'aromatic trapping' of the catalytic histidine and of the polar networks in orchestrating an optimal functional architecture of the active center for maximizing the catalytic activity of cholin-esterases (ChEs). We show the significance of this complex picture of the AChE active center to the design of new covalent or even non-covalent AChE inhibitors as potential thera-peutic agents for SDAT.

RESULTS AND DISCUSSION

Effects of butyrylization of human acetylcholinesterase

A blueprint for assessing the contributions of multiple aromatic replacements may be provided by the different amino acid compositions of the gorge linings in AChE and BChE, since the two enzymes exhibit similar reactivity toward ACh as well as toward various covalent inhibitors.[10] To investigate how this particular structural variability affects reactivity we gradually replaced all of the six aromatic residues in HuAChE by the corresponding residues in HuBChE[9] and evaluated the respective enzymes with a series of drugs used for the treatment of SDAT.

For most of the prototypical AChE inhibitors, including some of those approved for treatment of SDAT, the hexa-mutant HuAChE displayed a reactivity phenotype closely resembling that of HuBChE. These results support the accepted view that the active center architectures of AChE and BChE differ mainly by the presence of a larger void space in BChE. Nevertheless, reactivity of the hexa-mutant HuAChE toward the substrates acetyl-thiocholine (ATC) and butyrylthiocholine (BTC) as well as toward covalent inhibitors such as soman or the transition state analog TMTFA is about 45–170-fold lower than that of HuBChE. Most of this reduction in reactivity can be relat-ed to the combined replacements of the three aromatic residues at the active center: Phe295, Phe297 and Tyr337 (Figure 30.1).

The discrepancy between the capability of the hexa-mutant HuAChE to accommodate non-covalent ligands in a HuBChE-like fashion and its inferior catalytic activity toward substrates may suggest that elements of the catalytic machinery have been affected by the multiple mutations. Detailed analyses of the hexa-mutant HuAChE reactivities toward TMTFA and certain organophosphate inhibitors indicate that this enzyme, unlike BChE, is impaired in its capacity to accommo-date certain tetrahedral species in the active center, implicating the involvement of the cat-alytic His447.[9]

In order further to explore the nature of the putative array of interactions that optimize the orientation of the catalytic His447, we looked for the minimal set of replacements that would

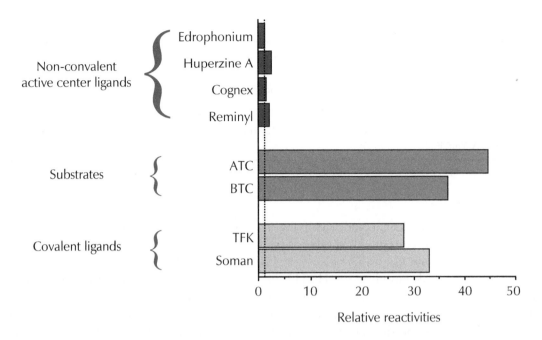

Figure 30.1 Relative reactivities of human butyrylcholinesterase and F295L/F297V/Y337A human acetylcholinesterase toward active center ligands

destabilize this residue, resulting in a decline of catalytic activity. In the process, we discovered how reactivity could also be restored through careful design of its aromatic environment.

Importance of aromatic trapping of His447 for efficient catalysis – implications for interaction with drugs for senile dementia of Alzheimer's type

According to the X-ray structure of HuAChE,[3] the catalytic His447 is within interaction distance of the aromatic residues Phe295, Phe338 and Tyr337. Nevertheless, single replacements of these aromatic residues, by alanine, had only a marginal effect on the catalytic activity of the resulting mutant enzymes.[6,11] In a further attempt to perturb the aromatic environment of His447, the double HuAChE mutants F295A/F338A and Y337A/F338A were generated.[12] For the F295A/F338A enzyme, a very dramatic decrease (680-fold) of catalytic activity toward ATC was observed. This decline in catalytic activity of the double mutant did not result from major changes in the overall architecture of the active center, since affinities of the F295A/F338A enzyme toward the active center inhibitors tacrine, BW284C51 and edrophonium were either equivalent to, or merely five-fold lower than, those of the wild-type HuAChE.[12]

The double mutant F295A/F338A HuAChE also exhibits diminished activity toward the SDAT-relevant carbamates physostigmine and exelon (Table 30.1). However, while reactivity toward physostigmine was about 50-fold lower than that of the wild-type enzyme, exelon

Table 30.1 Role of aromatic trapping in human acetylcholinesterase (HuAChE) accommodation of drugs for Alzheimer's disease

HuAChE type	Pyridostigmine K_i (10^{-4}/mol per min)	Exelon K_i (10^{-4}/mol per min)	Reminyl K_i (mol per min)	Aricept K_i (mol per min)
Wild-type	43.5	1.5	90	2
F295A/F338A	0.8	(K_i = 1200 nmol/l)	2000	400
F295A/F338A/V407F	16.5	1.0	260	1800

behaved as a non-covalent ligand, signifying a specific decline in the corresponding value of the acylation rate constant k_2.

If the enhanced mobility of His447 in F295A/F338A HuAChE and the ensuing decrease of catalytic activity are related directly to elimination of stabilizing interactions with the two aromatic residues, it seemed reasonable to assume that a compensatory interaction could be engineered through introduction of an aromatic residue in a different location adjacent to His447. Examination of the HuAChE/HuBChE sequence similarity and of molecular models of the two ChEs showed that in HuBChE an aromatic residue Phe398 appears to be vicinal to the catalytic histidine. In HuAChE the residue in an equivalent position to Phe398 is Val407, which, owing to its size, does not seem to interact with His447.

The notion that phe407 may restrict His447 mobility in the double mutant F295A/F338A was initially tested by molecular dynamic simulation of side-chain mobility within the active center of the F295A/F338A/V407F enzyme. The conformational properties of His447 in the 'theoretical' triple mutant indeed resemble those of the wild-type enzyme rather than those of the F295A/F338A HuAChE. This prediction was fully realized when the F295A/F338A/V407F HuAChE was generated and produced, since its catalytic activity was indeed 180-fold higher

than that of the F295A/F338A enzyme and only 3.5-fold lower than that of the wild-type HuAChE (Table 30.1).

Although affinity toward non-covalent inhibitors is usually not affected by the mobility of His447, the dissociation constant of the F295A/F338A HuAChE–Reminyl® complex is over 20-fold higher than that of the corresponding complex with the wild-type enzyme. Further replacement of Val407 by phenylalanine restored an almost wild-type activity toward Reminyl, indicating that in this case His447 participates in accommodation of the ligand in the active center (Table 30.1). On the other hand, the 200-fold decline in affinity of the double mutant toward Aricept® (E2020), as compared to the wild-type enzyme, cannot be compensated by substitution of phenylalanine at position 407 (the triple mutant F295A/F338A/V407F is 900-fold less reactive toward Aricept; see Table 30.1). This, in turn, suggests that the pronounced drop in the affinity of Aricept toward HuAChE with a modified acyl pocket is not a result of an enhanced His447 mobility but rather of a direct interaction of the acyl pocket[13] residues with the ligand. Such interaction is not indicated by the X-ray structure of the AChE–Aricept complex[14] and therefore this major binding characteristic of the drug, which essentially determines its selectivity toward AChE versus BChE, was missed in the comprehensive structure-based drug design study of Aricept analogs.[16]

Functional architecture of the human acetylcholinesterase active center essential for efficient interactions with covalent and non-covalent ligands is maintained by polar networks

Three acidic residues located near the bottom of the HuAChE active site gorge are a center of an intricate network of polar interactions that maintains proper orientation of key residues as well as the optimal polar environment for the catalytic process. Two of these acidic residues (Glu202, Glu450) are part of a hydrogen-bond network which also includes the hydroxyl group of Tyr133, the backbone amide nitrogens of Gly122 and Gly448, and two molecules of water.[10,11] Replacement of each of the acidic residues affects the catalytic activity of the resulting enzymes toward both charged and non-charged covalent modifiers, indicating that the effect is not due to removal of a negative charge from the vicinity of the positively charged substrate.

Substitution of residue Glu202 by the isosteric non-charged amino acid glutamine affects the affinities of the resulting enzyme toward non-covalent ligands such as the structurally diverse drugs Aricept, Reminyl,

huperzine A and Cognex®. The magnitude of the effect seems to be independent of the structural diversity, suggesting a non-specific perturbation of the binding environment rather than loss of a specific interaction (Table 30.2). These results demonstrate the importance of the polar environment of the binding site to ligand design. This element is difficult to characterize by structural analysis, which emphasizes discrete contacts with specific binding elements (Figure 30.2).

The hydrogen-bond network is connected through one of its water molecules to residue Ser229 which, in turn, is thought to maintain the functional orientation of the catalytic Glu334. Apart from the catalytic triad residues, Ser229 is the most conserved amino acid in the ChE family and its significance to the functional architecture of HuAChE is demonstrated by the finding that substitution of position 229 by alanine abolishes any observable catalytic activity.

CONCLUSIONS

Functional analysis of ligand interaction with the HuAChE, carried out through multilevel structural perturbations of its active center, is providing new information regarding the structures of enzyme–ligand complexes in solution. Such information can be converted, through molecular simulation techniques, into

Table 30.2 Efffect of the hydrogen-bond network residues on interactions with non-covalent drugs for Alzheimer's disease

HuAChE type	Relative K_i (mutant/wild type)			
	Aricept®	Reminyl®	Huperzine A	Cognex®
Wild-type	1	1	1	1
E202A	220	220	100	40

HuAChE, human acetylcholinesterase

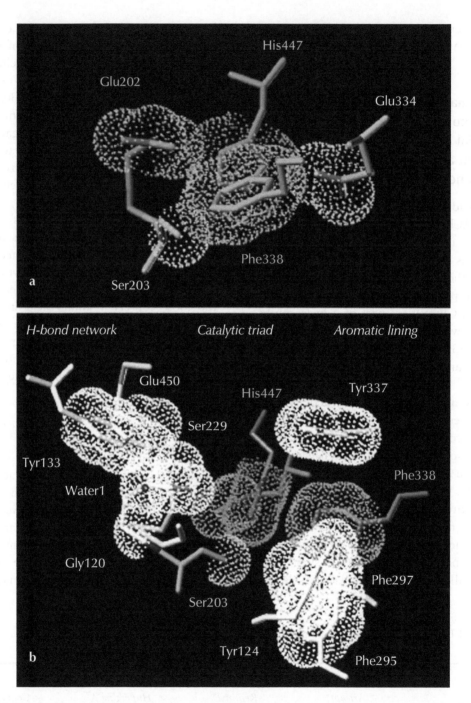

Figure 30.2 Orchestration of functional subsites in the acetylcholinesterase active center to maintain the optimal juxtaposition of residues of the catalytic triad. (a) Direct interactions of the catalytic His447 with residues Glu202 and Phe338. (b) Fine tuning of these interactions by functional domains of the active center including the H-bond network and the aromatic lining of the active center gorge

specific directions for further optimization of the inhibitor structures. Thus, combination of structural and functional analyses of HuAChE seems to be the best approach currently available for structure-based design of inhibitors as SDAT therapeutics.

ACKNOWLEDGEMENT

This work was supported in part by the US Army Medical Research and Material Command under contracts DAMD17-96-C-6088 and DAMD17-00-C-0021.

REFERENCES

1. Giacobini E. Cholinesterases and Cholinesterase Inhibitors. London: Martin Dunitz, 2000

2. Sussman JL, Harel M, Frolow F, et al. Atomic structure of acetylcholinesterase from Torpedo californica: a prototypic acetylcholine-binding protein. Science 1991; 253: 872–9

3. Kryger G, Harel M, Giles K, et al. Structures of recombinant native and E202Q mutant human acetylcholinesterase complexed with the snake-venom toxin fasciculin-II. Acta Crystallogr 2000; 56: 1385–94

4. Shafferman A, Velan B, Ordentlich A, et al. Substrate inhibition of acetylcholinesterase residues affecting signal transduction from the surface to the catalytic center. EMBO J 1992; 11: 3561–8

5. Taylor P, Radic Z. The cholinesterases. Annu Rev Pharmacol Toxicol 1994; 34: 281–320

6. Ordentlich A, Barak D, Kronman C, et al. Dissection of the human residues constituting the anionic site, the hydrophobic site, and the acyl pocket. J Biol Chem 1993; 268: 17083–95

7. Barak D, Kronman C, Ordentlich A, et al. Acetylcholinesterase peripheral anionic site degeneracy conferred by amino acid arrays sharing a common core. J Biol Chem 1994; 269: 6296–300

8. Ariel N, Ordentlich A, Barak D, et al. The 'aromatic patch' of three proximal residues in the human acetylcholinesterase active centre allows for versatile interaction modes with inhibitors. Biochem J 1998; 335: 95–102

9. Kaplan D, Orentlich A, Barak D, et al. Does 'butyrylization' of acetylcholinesterase through substitution of the six divergent aromatic amino acids in the active center gorge generate an enzyme mimic of butyrylcholinesterase? Biochemistry 2002; 41: 8245–52

10. Ordentlich A, Barak D, Kronman C, et al. Exploring the active center of human acetylcholinesterase with stereoisomers of an organophosphorus inhibitor with two chiral centers. Biochemistry 1999; 38: 3055–66

11. Ordentlich A, Kronman C, Barak D, et al. Engineering resistance to aging in phosphylated human acetylcholinesterase – role of hydrogen bond network in the active center. FEBS Lett 1993; 334: 215–20

12. Barak D, Kaplan D, Ordentlich A, et al. The 'aromatic trapping' of the catalytic histidine is essential for efficient catalysis of acetylcholinesterase. Biochemistry 2002; 41: 8245–52

13. Shafferman A, Barak D, Ordentilch A, et al. Structural and functional correlates of human acetylcholinesterase mutants for evaluating

Alzheimer's disease treatments: functional analysis of E2020 and galanthamine HuAChE complexes. In Mizuno Y, Fisher A, Hanin I, eds. Mapping the Progress of Alzheimer's and Parkinson's Disease. New York: Kluwer Academic/Plenum Publishers, 2001

14. Kryger G, Silman I, Sussman JL. Structure of acetylcholinesterase complexed with E2020 (Aricept): implications for the design of new anti-Alzheimer drugs. Structure 1999; 7: 297–307

15. Sugimoto H, Yamanishi Y, Iimura Y, Kawakami Y. Donepezil hydrochloride (E2020) and other acetylcholinesterase inhibitors. Curr Med Chem 2000; 7: 303–40

Chapter 31

Altered glycosylation of acetylcholinesterase in the Alzheimer's disease brain: involvement of α7 nicotinic acetylcholine receptors

DH Small, LR Fodero, J Sáez-Valero

INTRODUCTION

Although it is generally accepted that the accumulation of amyloid β (Aβ) in the brain is an important step in the pathogenesis of Alzheimer's disease (AD), the mechanism by which Aβ causes neuronal dysfunction is poorly understood. The cognitive loss that occurs in AD is more likely to be caused by changes in synaptic plasticity than by non-specific neurotoxicity or cell loss.[1] For this reason, there is a need to examine the effects of Aβ on biochemical mechanisms that regulate synaptic plasticity.

The entry of calcium during a dendritic action potential is a key event controlling synaptic plasticity. Calcium influx controls mechanisms of both long-term potentiation and long-term depression, both of which are important in memory storage.[2,3] L-type voltage-dependent calcium channels, α-amino-3-hydroxy-5-methyl-4-isoxazole propionic acid (AMPA) receptors, N-methyl-D-aspartate (NMDA) receptors and α7 nicotinic acetylcholine receptors (nAChRs) are all thought to play a role in calcium entry.[1]

EFFECTS OF Aβ ON α7 NICOTINIC ACETYLCHOLINE RECEPTORS

nAChRs are members of the ligand-gated ion channel superfamily.[4] The receptors consist of a pentameric arrangement of subunits around a central ion pore (Figure 31.1a), which is permeable to sodium and to a lesser extent calcium.[5] In the case of the nAChR, each subunit polypeptide contains four transmembrane domains. A number of mammalian nAChR subunits have been cloned, including nine α subunits and three β subunits.[6] Major species found in the central nervous system are the α4β2 nAChR, which contains two α4 subunits and three β2 subunits, and the α7 nAChR, which is homomeric. Because of its localization on dendritic spines and its high permeability to calcium, the α7 nAChR is thought to play a key role in synaptic plasticity.[7] For example, the level of α7 nAChRs is particularly high in the hippocampus,[8] a region of the brain that is critical for memory formation.

In 1993, we first reported that an Aβ peptide (Aβ25-35) could bind to nAChRs.[9] More recently, full-length Aβ peptides have been found

a

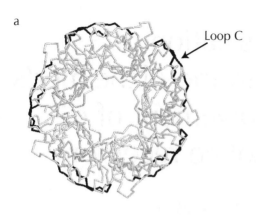

Loop C

b

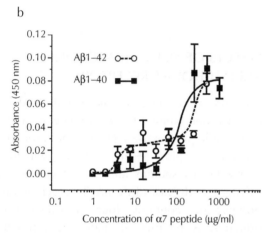

Figure 31.1 (a) Structure of the extracellular domain of the α7 nicotinic acetylcholine receptor. Part of the α-bungarotoxin binding site (loop C) is shown in black. (b) Binding of amyloid-β (Aβ) peptides to a loop C peptide. Aβ1-40 and Aβ1-42 (0.1 mg/ml in water) were coated onto a 96-well enzyme-linked immunosorbent assay plate by incubation for 1 h at ambient temperature. The plate was then incubated with a biotinyl-loop C peptide (Biotin- SGIPGKRTESFYECCKEPYPD) for 1 h. After washing, the amount of bound loop C peptide was determined using the streptavidin–peroxidase method

to bind strongly to α7 nAChRs. Wang and co-investigators[10] reported that the α7 nAChR and Aβ1-42 could be co-immunoprecipitated from human brain tissue and that neuronal cell lines overexpressing the α7 nAChR could bind Aβ1-

42. This binding was inhibited by the α7 nAChR-specific antagonist α-bungarotoxin[10].

The effect of Aβ binding on nAChR function is unclear. Aβ1-42 has been reported to inhibit[11–13] or stimulate[14,15] α7 nAChRs. Dineley and co-investigators[14] have shown that activation of α7 nAChRs by Aβ could stimulate the mitogen-activated protein kinase ERK. Stimulation of ERK and the JNK-1 pathway may, in turn, lead to increased tau phosphorylation.[16]

Although the binding site for Aβ on the α7 nAChR is unknown, it may be close to an α-bungarotoxin binding site. For example, binding of Aβ to the α7 receptor is reportedly blocked by α-bungarotoxin, which is known to bind to a region at the interface between subunits of the receptor.[10] This region contains a hairpin loop (loop C) that is stabilized by a *cys-cys* disulfide bond and is thought to be involved in binding. We have found that a peptide homologous to this loop domain could bind to Aβ1-40 and Aβ1-42 in a solid-phase binding assay (Figure 31.1).

Aβ-INDUCED CHANGES IN ACETYLCHOLINESTERASE LEVELS

Acetylcholinesterase (AChE) is the key enzyme that hydrolyzes the neurotransmitter acetylcholine.[17] Although AChE is encoded by a single gene located on chromosome 7, the enzyme exists in a variety of different molecular forms, which can be distinguished from each other by their different molecular weights and hydrodynamic properties. Splicing of AChE mRNA generates three major transcripts (R, H and T) that can be combined with non-catalytic subunits (PRiMA and ColQ) to generate a wide variety of different isoforms.[18]

Overall, the level of AChE is decreased in the AD brain. However, the levels of AChE are increased around amyloid plaques and in neurofibrillary tangle-bearing neurons in the AD brain.[19] This increase is a direct effect of Aβ on AChE expression.[20,21] When Aβ is added to neuronal cell cultures, there is an increase in the level of AChE activity in the cultures. Similarly, we have found that levels of AChE are increased in the brain of transgenic mice that express the human Aβ sequence.[22,23]

Interestingly, not all isoforms of AChE are increased by Aβ. A monomeric amphiphilic isoform of AChE encoded by the T transcript is increased when cells are incubated with Aβ.[24,25] This isoform can be distinguished from other isoforms of AChE by its unusual glycosylation pattern which lowers its affinity for the plant lectin concanavalin A.[26] As this isoform (Glyc-AChE) is increased relative to other AChE isoforms in the cerebrospinal fluid of AD patients, we have proposed that it may be a useful biomarker of AD.[27,28] Our studies suggest that the level of Glyc-AChE in the cerebrospinal fluid correlates with disease duration, suggesting that it may be useful for monitoring disease progression.[29]

The increase in Glyc-AChE is blocked by inhibitors of L-type voltage-dependent calcium channels, suggesting that calcium entry leads to increased expression of AChE.[20] The effect may be due to post-transcriptional effects, rather than to increased expression, as in myocytes, as calcium is known to increase AChE mRNA stability through activation of calcineurin.[30] Our recent studies have shown that the α7 nAChR mediates the effect of Aβ on AChE expression (L.R. Fodero et al., submitted for publication). Incubation of cortical neurons with the α7 nAChR-selective antagonists α-bungarotoxin or methyllylcaconitine (MLA) blocks the Aβ-mediated increase in AChE. Furthermore, nicotine and the α7 selective agonist choline enhance AChE expression in cortical neurons.

SUMMARY

A hypothetical scheme showing how Aβ may influence AChE expression, synaptic plasticity and tau phosphorylation is presented in Figure 31.2. We propose that membrane depolarization in the dendrite, resulting from stimulation of α7

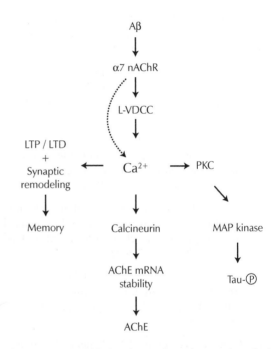

Figure 31.2 Possible biochemical mechanism by which amyloid-β (Aβ) increases acetylcholinesterase (AChE) levels and influences synaptic plasticity. The binding of Aβ to the α7 nicotinic acetylcholine receptor (nAChR) causes an influx of Na^+ and Ca^{2+} and thereby induces membrane depolarization. Entry of more Ca^{2+} occurs via L-type voltage-dependent calcium channels (VDCCs). Increased intracellular Ca^{2+} activates calcineurin, which in turn stabilizes AChE mRNA, as previously described.[30] The influx of Ca^{2+} may also stimulate tau phosphorylation via the MAP kinase pathway leading to neurofibrillary tangle formation, as suggested by Wang et al.[16] Ca^{2+} is also involved in the regulation of synaptic plasticity, long-term potentiation (LTP) and long-term depression (LDP) which are important in memory formation

nAChRs by Aβ, results in opening of voltage-dependent calcium channels. The subsequent entry of calcium could trigger increased AChE production, altered synaptic plasticity (long-term potentiation and depression) and tau phosphorylation.

REFERENCES

1. Small DH, Mok SS, Bornstein JC. Alzheimer's disease and Aβ toxicity: from top to bottom. Nat Rev Neurosci 2001; 2: 595–8

2. Magee JC, Johnston D. Synaptic activation of voltage-gated channels in the dendrites of hippocampal pyramidal neurons. Science 1997; 275: 209–13

3. Kapur A, Yeckel MF, Gray R, Johnston D. L-type calcium channels are required for one form of hippocampal mossy fiber LTP. J Neurophysiol 1998; 79: 2181–90

4. Leite JF, Cascio M. Structure of ligand-gated ion channels: critical assessment of biochemical data supports novel topology. Mol Cell Neurosci 2001; 17: 777–92

5. Cooper E, Couturier S, Ballivet M. Pentameric structure and subunit stoichiometry of a neuronal acetylcholine receptor. Nature 1991; 350: 235–8

6. Gotti C, Fornasari D, Clementi F. Human neuronal nicotinic receptors. Prog Neurobiol 1997; 53: 199–237

7. Broide RS, Leslie FM. The α7 nicotinic acetycholine receptor in neuronal plasticity. Mol Neurobiol 1999; 20: 1–16

8. Frazier CJ, Buhler AV, Weiner JL, Dunwiddie TV. Synaptic potentials mediated via α-bungarotoxin-sensitive nicotinic acetylcholine receptors in rat hippocampal interneurons. J Neurosci 1998; 18: 8228–35

9. Cheung NS, Small DH, Livett BG. An amyloid peptide, beta A4 25–35, mimics the function of substance P on modulation of nicotine-evoked secretion and desensitization in cultured bovine adrenal chromaffin cells. J Neurochem 1993; 60: 1163–6

10. Wang HY, Lee DHS, D'Andrea MR, et al. β-Amyloid$_{1-42}$ binds to α7 nicotinic acetylcholine receptor with high affinity. Implications for Alzheimer's disease pathology. J Biol Chem 2000; 275: 5626–32

11. Pettit, DL, Shao Z, Yakel JL. β-Amyloid$_{1-42}$ peptide directly modulates nicotinic receptors in the rat hippocampal slice. J Neurosci 2001; 21: RC120

12. Tozaki T, Matsumoto A, Kanno T, et al. The inhibitory and facilitatory actions of amyloid-β peptides on nicotinic ACh receptors and AMPA receptors. Biochem Biophys Res Commun 2002; 294: 42–5

13. Liu QS, Kawai H, Berg DK. β-Amyloid peptide blocks the response of α7-containing nicotinic receptors on hippocampal neurons. Proc Natl Acad Sci USA 2001; 98: 4734–9

14. Dineley KT, Westerman M, Bui D, et al. β-Amyloid activates the mitogen-activated protein kinase cascade via hippocampal α7 nicotinic acetylcholine receptors: in vitro and in vivo mechanisms related to Alzheimer's disease. J Neurosci 2001; 21: 4125–33

15. Dineley KT, Bell KA, Bui D, Sweatt JD. β-Amyloid peptide activates α7 nicotinic acetylcholine receptors expressed in Xenopus oocytes. J Biol Chem 2002; 277: 25056–61

16. Wang HY, Li W, Benedetti NJ, Lee DH. α7 nicotinic acetylcholine receptors mediate β-amyloid peptides-induced tau protein phosphorylation. J Biol Chem 2003; 278: 31547–53

17. Small DH, Michaelson S, Sberna G. Non-classical actions of cholinesterases: role in cellular differentiation, tumorigenesis and Alzheimer's disease. Neurochem Int 1996; 28: 453–83

18. Perrier AL, Massoulie J, Krejci E. PRiMA: the membrane anchor of acetylcholinesterase in the brain. Neuron 2002; 33: 275–85

19. Mesulam MM, Geula C. Shifting patterns of cortical cholinesterases in Alzheimer's disease: implications for treatment, diagnosis, and pathogenesis. Adv Neurol 1990; 51: 235–40

20. Sberna G, Sáez-Valero J, Beyreuther K, et al. The amyloid-β protein of Alzheimer's disease increases acetylcholinesterase expression by increasing intracellular calcium in embryonal carcinoma P19 cells. J Neurochem 1997; 69: 1177–84

21. Sáez-Valero J, Fodero LR, White AR, et al. Acetycholinesterase is increased in mouse neuronal and astrocyte cultures after treatment with β-amyloid peptides. Brain Res 2003; 965: 283–6

22. Sberna G, Sáez-Valero J, Li QX, et al. Acetylcholinesterase is increased in the brains of transgenic mice expressing the C-terminal fragment (CT100) of the β-amyloid protein precursor of Alzheimer's disease. J Neurochem 1998; 71: 723–31

23. Fodero LR, Sáez-Valero J, McLean CA, et al. Altered glycosylation of acetylcholinesterase in APP (SW) Tg2576 transgenic mice occurs prior to amyloid plaque deposition. J Neurochem 2002; 81: 441–8

24. Sáez-Valero J, Mok SS, Small DH. Expression of acetylcholinesterase in Alzheimer's disease: from pathogenesis to diagnosis. Acta Neurol Scand 2001; 102: 49–52

25. Sáez-Valero J, Mok SS, Marcos A, et al. Increased levels of a minor glycoform of acetylcholinesterase in Alzheimer's disease brain and cerebrospinal fluid. In Iqbal K, Sisodia SS, Winblad B, eds. Alzheimer's Disease: Advances in Etiology, Pathogenesis and Therapeutics. Chichester, UK: John Wiley & Sons, 2001: 293–301

26. Sáez-Valero J, Sberna G, McLean CA, Small DH. Molecular isoform distribution and glycosylation of acetylcholinesterase are altered in brain and cerebrospinal fluid of patients with Alzheimer's disease. J Neurochem 1999; 72: 1600–8

27. Sáez-Valero J, Sberna G, McLean CA, et al. Glycosylation of acetylcholinesterase as diagnostic marker for Alzheimer's disease. Lancet 1997; 350: 929

28. Sáez-Valero J, Barquero MS, Marcos A, et al. Altered glycosylation of acetylcholinesterase in Alzheimer lumbar cerebrospinal fluid. J Neurol Neurosurg Psychiatr 2000; 69: 664–7

29. Sáez-Valero J, Fodero LR, Sjogren M, et al. Glycosylation of acetylcholinesterase and butyrylcholinesterase changes as a function of the duration of Alzheimer's disease. J Neurosci Res 2003; 72: 520–6

30. Luo ZD, Wang Y, Werlen G, et al. Calcineurin enhances acetylcholinesterase mRNA stability during C2-C12 muscle cell differentiation. Mol Pharmacol 1999; 56: 886–94

Cholinotrophic alterations in individuals with mild cognitive impairment and Alzheimer's disease

EJ Mufson, M Fahnestock, JH Kordower, ST DeKosky

INTRODUCTION

It has been hypothesized that cholinergic basal forebrain (CBF) neurons degenerate in Alzheimer's disease (AD), owing to a loss of neurotrophic support from their cortical and hippocampal target sites that produce nerve growth factor (NGF).[1–3] Alterations in NGF receptor expression are seen within the CBF in early and late AD,[4–8] suggesting that NGF-related mechanisms required for long-term CBF survival are affected relatively early, in contrast to markers for cholinergic neurotransmission, which decline later in the disease process.[9–11] These findings suggest that therapeutic intervention with neurotrophic molecules during the early stages of the disease process might delay or prevent the degeneration of CBF neurons associated with dementia. The data presented in this chapter summarize our findings on the changes in the cholinotrophic basal forebrain projection system during the progression of AD. These observations were derived from a longitudinal clinical pathological study of aging and dementia in retired Catholic clergy studied at Rush University Medical Center in Chicago, USA.[6,9,12,13] Each participant agreed to an annual detailed clinical evaluation, brain autopsy and neuropathological analysis. The studies report-

ed in this chapter were approved by the Human Investigation Committee of Rush University Medical Center.

PHENOTYPIC DIFFERENCES IN CHOLINOTROPHIC MARKERS IN MILD COGNITIVE IMPAIRMENT

During the prodromal and earliest stages of AD, there are alterations in the phenotypic expression of CBF neurons in subjects with mild cognitive impairment (MCI) and mild AD. Stereological counts revealed that during these early stages selective changes occur in markers that are co-localized within CBF neurons (Figure 32.1a). While the number of neurons expressing choline acetyltransferase (ChAT) or the vesicular acetylcholine transporter (VAChT) were unchanged in individuals with MCI and mild AD,[9] the number of cholinergic neurons expressing p75[NTR 6] or trkA[5] were significantly reduced (Figures 32.1a and 32.2). These observations support the emerging concept that there is an absence of frank degeneration of CBF neurons in MCI. Interestingly, the reduction of p75[NTR 6] and trkA-positive[5] neurons seen in MCI occurs in the presence of normal levels of

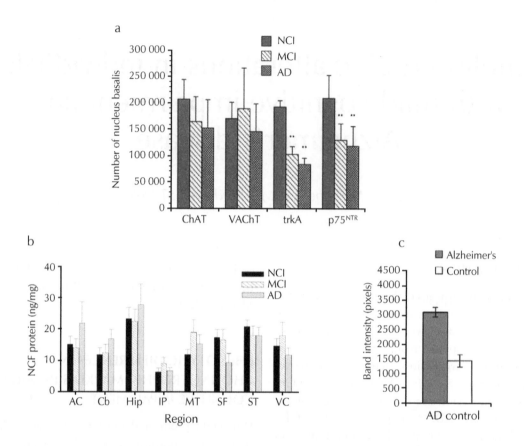

Figure 32.1 (a) Composite histogram showing the phenotypic differences in the number of choline acetyltransferase (ChAT), vesicular acetylcholine transporter (VAChT), trkA and p75[NTR]-immunoreactive nucleus basalis neurons in individuals with mild cognitive impairment (MCI) and Alzheimer's disease (AD). Note a significant reduction in nerve growth factor (NGF) receptor and not ChAT/VAChT-containing nucleus basal neurons in MCI and AD. This difference was not augmented during the transition from MCI to AD. Reproduced with the permission of Mufson *et al.*[14] (b) Histogram showing the preservation of NGF protein levels measured by enzyme linked immunosorbent assay in the anterior cingulate (AC), cerebellum (Cb), hippocampus (Hip), inferior parietal cortex (IP), middle temporal cortex (MT), superior frontal cortex (SF), superior temporal cortex (ST) and visual cortex (VC) in non-cognitive impairment (NCI), MCI and AD. Reproduced with permission of Mufson *et al.*[14] (c) Histogram showing a significant increase in intensity of proNGF measured by Western blotting in parietal cortex in end-stage AD compared to aged controls. Reproduced with permission of Fahnestock *et al.*[15]

ChAT systems,[5] suggesting that cholinergic enzyme loss is not an obligatory result of NGF receptor down-regulation at these early disease stages. Conversely, stable CBF neuronal numbers[9] and cortical ChAT activity[10,11] in MCI (Figures 32.1a and 32.3), suggest that compensa-tory repair mechanisms support the viability of these cells.[11] However, the possibility remains that the chronic reduction in both p75[NTR] and trkA is a factor underlying cholinergic dysfunc-tion, and the subsequent extensive cholinergic deficit seen in end-stage AD.[8]

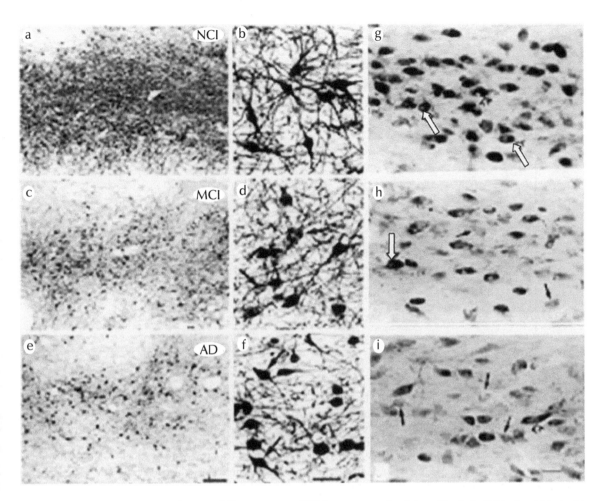

Figure 32.2 Photomicrographs showing differences in p75^NTR-immunoreactive (ir) profiles in individuals within (a, b) non-cognitive impairment (NCI), (c, d) mild cognitive impairment (MCI) and (e, f) Alzheimer's disease (AD). Note the striking reduction in p75^NTR-ir profiles in both MCI (c, d) and AD (e, f) as compared to NCI (a, b). Scale bar in a, c and e = 50 μm and in b, d and f = 100 μm. (g–i) Photomicrographs of trkA mRNA labeling in individuals categorized as NCI (g), MCI (h) and mild AD (i). Open arrows in g, h represent intense staining of trkA mRNA-expressing neurons while the closed arrows represent lightly stained (h, i) trkA mRNA-containing neurons. Note the consistently high expression of trkA mRNA within the NCI case but diminished reaction product for the gene expression in a subset of neurons from the MCI and AD cases

It remains to be determined whether the reduction of p75^NTR and trkA receptor-positive CBF neurons seen in MCI (Figures 32.1a and 32.2) is due to a down-regulation of mRNA or its translation to protein. The message for p75^NTR has been described as reduced, stable or increased in late-stage AD.[16] TrkA protein[5] and mRNA[7] are decreased within nucleus basalis neurons in MCI and mild AD (Figure 32.2), suggesting that decreased responsiveness to neurotrophins may be an early biomarker for the onset of AD. Alterations in the cellular

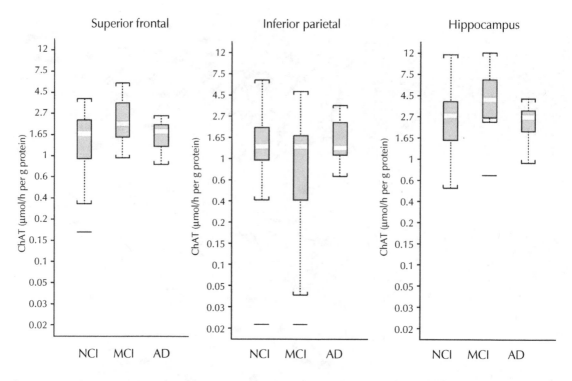

Figure 32.3 Choline acetyltransferase (ChAT) activity plotted by diagnostic group non-cognitive impairment (NCI), mild cognitive impairment (MCI) and Alzheimer's disease (AD)) in two cortical regions and the hippocampus. For each brain region, ChAT values are shown as three box-and-whisker plots for each clinical group. Black horizontal lines indicate outliers. Statistically significant differences among the three clinical groups were found only in the hippocampus ($p = 0.0026$) and frontal cortex ($p = 0.034$). Hippocampal ChAT activity was higher in the MCI group compared to both NCI and AD ($p < 0.05$). In the frontal cortex, MCI subjects had higher ChAT activity compared to NCI ($p < 0.05$), but not compared to the AD group

production of the p75[NTR] and trkA receptor, and their subsequent anterograde transport to CBF projection sites, may alter the ratio between the high- and low-affinity NGF receptors.[17] Such an imbalance may result in defective retrograde transport of NGF to CBF neurons, or alter the ability of NGF to bind to trkA, which is crucial for nuclear transcription of genes mediating signal transduction.[16] Interestingly, a loss of trkA receptor without a corresponding decrease in p75[NTR] may promote atrophy or apoptotic death of CBF neurons, since binding of NGF to p75[NTR] in the absence of trkA can trigger apoptosis.[18]

NERVE GROWTH FACTOR (NGF) AND proNGF LEVELS IN MILD COGNITIVE IMPAIRMENT AND ALZHEIMER'S DISEASE

The mature form of NGF is processed from a larger secreted precursor molecule known as proNGF.[19–21] Fahnestock and co-investigators[15,21] have demonstrated that NGF exists primarily as 32-kDa proNGF in the brain. No mature NGF is detectable in the human brain by Western blotting, suggesting that the NGF detected by enzyme-linked immunosorbent assay (ELISA) is actually proNGF, and that proNGF may be the active form of the molecule.

Although there is a reduction in trkA and p75[NTR] labeling of CBF neurons in prodromal AD,[6,7,16,22] the status of NGF synthesis in the cortex and hippocampus remains controversial. NGF mRNA expression is similar between AD and controls.[23,24] Decreased NGF immunoreactivity in the basal forebrain of AD[4] patients and increased NGF protein in the cerebral cortex and hippocampus[20,25] have generally been assumed to be due to accumulation of NGF in CBF target tissues resulting from decreased retrograde NGF transport from the cortex to the CBF.[4] Others have reported increased NGF protein levels in cortex and hippocampus in end-stage AD.[26]

Recently, we have found that NGF levels as measured by ELISA are preserved during the prodromal stages of dementia as well as in more advanced AD (Figure 32.1b),[14] despite the fact that CBF neurons exhibit reduced amounts of retrogradely transported NGF[4] and undergo extensive atrophy and degeneration in the later stages of AD.[8,12] We also found that a high-molecular-weight NGF-immunoreactive species, possibly a glycosylated intracellular form of proNGF, remains unchanged in these same subjects. In contrast, however, we recently found that 32-kDa proNGF levels measured by Western blotting were significantly increased in the cortex of individuals with MCI and mild AD[14] and severe AD (Figure 32.1c),[15] and that the accumulation of proNGF correlated with cognitive impairment.[14] Interestingly, there is up-regulation of ChAT activity in the hippocampus and superior frontal cortex of individuals with MCI (Figure 32.3),[10,11] suggesting that the CBF system undergoes a plasticity response. Perhaps this is associated with the accumulation of proNGF during the prodromal stages of AD.[21]

The role of proNGF in both the normal and the AD brain is also controversial. P75[NTR] binds a mutated, cleavage-resistant proNGF with high affinity and induces p75[NTR]-dependent apop-tosis in cultured neurons with minimal trkA activation.[19] By contrast, both native and cleavage-resistant 32-kDa proNGFs promote neurite outgrowth, survival activity and trkA activation.[21] Whether the severe reduction in NGF receptor-containing neurons seen in MCI, as well as in early and advanced AD, is related to the accumulation of proNGF in cortical and hippocampal projection sites of CBF neurons remains to be determined.

SUMMARY

The final figure of this chapter summarizes our findings at the time of writing dealing with alterations in the human cholinotrophic basal forebrain system during the progression of AD (Figure 32.4). The preservation of ChAT/VAChT-containing neurons (in the face of a reduction of trkA and p75[NTR]-expressing neurons) within the nucleus basalis in MCI and mild AD individuals indicates that there is not a frank loss of perikarya, *per se*, but a phenotypic down-regulation of NGF receptor proteins in these neurons. The preservation of ChAT-positive nucleus basalis perikarya in MCI is supported by the observation that ChAT activity within the cerebral cortex is within normal limits.[10,11] Interestingly, the presumed high molecular weight form of NGF is not altered in the disease process. Instead, the precursor molecule for NGF, proNGF, is increased in MCI and AD. Studies are currently underway to define the mechanisms underlying the alterations in trkA expression within neurons of the nucleus basalis, whether cortical areas manifest a decrease in this protein as well as p75[NTR] in individuals with MCI and early AD, and whether proNGF is transported in a retrograde manner by CBF neurons.

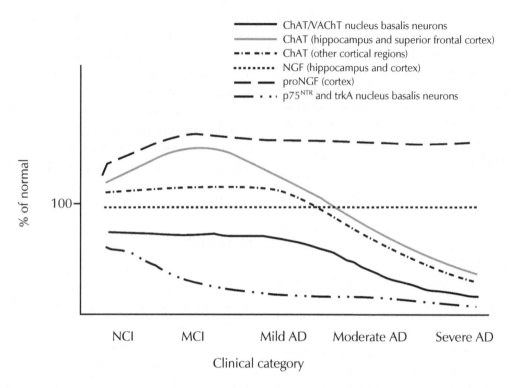

Legend:
— ChAT/VAChT nucleus basalis neurons
— ChAT (hippocampus and superior frontal cortex)
–·– ·–· ChAT (other cortical regions)
········· NGF (hippocampus and cortex)
– – proNGF (cortex)
— ·· p75NTR and trkA nucleus basalis neurons

Figure 32.4 Diagram showing alterations in the cholinotrophic basocortical projection system in individuals with mild cognitive impairment (MCI) and Alzheimer's disease (AD). Note that the cholinergic activity in the cortex and hippocampus is stable or increased in MCI and early AD. Cortical and hippocampal nerve growth factor (NGF) levels remain stable while pro nerve growth factor (NGF) increases. Note also that the number of nucleus basalis neurons containing choline acetyltransferase (ChAT)/vesicular acetylcholine transporter (VAChT) is preserved while trkA and low p75NTR receptor-containing nucleus basalis neurons are reduced in MCI and early AD. The data used to generate each line are discussed and referenced in the text. Each line is not meant to represent actual numerical values but the general trend for each variable depicted. NCI, non-cognitive impairment

ACKNOWLEDGEMENTS

This work was supported by grants AG14449, AG10688, AG09466 (E.J.M.), AG05133 (S.T.D.), CIHR and the Scottish Rite Charitable Foundation of Canada (M.F.). We acknowledge gratefully the altruism and support of the Nuns, Priests and Brothers in the Religious Orders Study of the Rush NIA Alzheimer's Disease Center (AG10161).

REFERENCES

1. Appel SH. A unifying hypothesis for the cause of amyotropic lateral sclerosis, parkinsonism, and Alzheimer disease. Ann Neurol 1981; 10: 499–505

2. Hefti F, Hartikka J, Knusel B. Function of neurotrophic factors in the adult and aging brain and their possible use in the treatment of neurodegenerative diseases. Neurobiol Aging 1989; 10: 515–33

3. Kordower JH, Mufson EJ. NGF and Alzheimer's disease: unfulfilled promise and untapped potential. Neurobiol Aging 1989; 10: 543–5

4. Mufson EJ, Conner JM, Kordower JH. Nerve growth factor in Alzheimer's disease: defective retrograde transport to nucleus basalis. Neuroreport 1995; 6: 1063–6

5. Mufson EJ, Ma SY, Cochran EJ, et al. Loss of nucleus basalis neurons containing trkA immunoreactivity in individuals with mild cognitive impairment and early Alzheimer's disease. J Comp Neurol 2000; 427: 19–30

6. Mufson EJ, Ma SY, Dills J, et al. Loss of basal forebrain P75(NTR) immunoreactivity in subjects with mild cognitive impairment and Alzheimer's disease. J Comp Neurol 2002; 443: 136–53

7. Mufson EJ, Counts SE, Ginsberg SD. Gene expression profiles of cholinergic nucleus basalis neurons in Alzheimer's disease. Neurochem Res 2002; 27: 1035–48

8. Mufson EJ, Bothwell M, Kordower JH. Loss of nerve growth factor receptor-containing neurons in Alzheimer's disease: a quantitative analysis across subregions of the basal forebrain. Exp Neurol 1989; 105: 221–32

9. Gilmor ML, Erickson JD, Varoqui H, et al. Preservation of nucleus basalis neurons containing choline acetyltransferase and the vesicular acetylcholine transporter in the elderly with mild cognitive impairment and early Alzheimer's disease. J Comp Neurol 1999; 411: 693–704

10. Davies P. Challenging the cholinergic hypothesis in Alzheimer disease. J Am Med Assoc 1999; 281: 1433–4

11. DeKosky ST, Ikonomovic MD, Styren SD, et al. Upregulation of choline acetyltransferase activity in hippocampus and frontal cortex of elderly subjects with mild cognitive impairment. Ann Neurol 2002; 51: 145–55

12. Mufson EJ, Lavine N, Jaffar S, et al. Reduction in p140-TrkA receptor protein within the nucleus basalis and cortex in Alzheimer's disease. Exp Neurol 1997; 146: 91–103

13. Bennett DA, Wilson RS, Schneider JA, et al. Natural history of mild cognitive impairment in older persons. Neurology 2002; 59: 198–205

14. Mufson E, Ikonomovic MD, Styren SD, et al. Preservation of brain nerve growth factor in mild cognitive impairment and Alzheimer's disease. Arch Neurol 2003; 60: 1143–8

15. Fahnestock M, Michalski B, Xu B, Coughlin MD. The precursor pro-nerve growth factor is the predominant form of nerve growth factor in brain and is increased in Alzheimer's disease. Mol Cell Neurosci 2001; 18: 210–20

16. Lad SP, Neet KE, Mufson E. Nerve growth factor: structure, function and therapeutic implications for Alzheimer's disease. Curr Drug Target CNS Neurol Discord 2003; 2: 315–34

17. Connor B, Young D, Lawlor P, et al. Trk receptor alterations in Alzheimer's disease. Brain Res Mol Brain Res 1996; 42: 1–17

18. Barrett GL. The p75 neurotrophin receptor and neuronal apoptosis. Prog Neurobiol 2000; 61: 205–29

19. Lee R, Kermani P, Teng KK, Hempstead BL. Regulation of cell survival by secreted pro-neurotrophins. Science 2001; 294: 1945–8

20. Fahnestock M, Scott SA, Jette N, et al. Nerve growth factor mRNA and protein levels measured in the same tissue from normal and Alzheimer's disease parietal cortex. Brain Res Mol Brain Res 1996; 42: 175–8

21. Fahnestock M, Yu G, Coughlin MD. ProNGF: a neurotrophic or an apoptotic molecule? Brain Res 2004; 146: 107–10

22. Chu Y, Cochran EJ, Bennett DA, et al. Down-regulation of trkA mRNA within nucleus basalis neurons in individuals with mild cognitive impairment and Alzheimer's disease. J Comp Neurol 2001; 437: 296–307

23. Goedert M, Fine A, Hunt SP, Ullrich A. Nerve growth factor mRNA in peripheral and central rat tissues and in the human central nervous system: lesion effects in the rat brain and levels in Alzheimer's disease. Brain Res 1986; 387: 85–92

24. Jette N, Cole MS, Fahnestock M. NGF mRNA is not decreased in frontal cortex from Alzheimer's disease patients. Brain Res Mol Brain Res 1994; 25: 242–50

25. Scott SA, Mufson EJ, Weingartner JA, et al. Nerve growth factor in Alzheimer's disease: increased levels throughout the brain coupled with declines in nucleus basalis. J Neurosci 1995; 15: 6213–21

26. Peng S, Wuu J, Mufson E, Fahnestock M. Increased proNGF levels in subjects with mild cognitive impairment and mild Alzheimer's disease. J Neuropath Exp Neurol 2004; 63: 641–9

Chapter 33

Pharmacological properties of TV3326, a cholinesterase and brain selective monoamine oxidase inhibitor for the treatment of dementia co-morbid with depression

M Weinstock, MBH Youdim

INTRODUCTION

Acetylcholinesterase (AChE) inhibitors, done-pezil, rivastigmine and galantamine have all been shown to improve cognitive function in 30–40% of patients with Alzheimer's disease (AD)[1] and may be equally effective against dementia with Lewy bodies.[2] In addition to their effect on cognitive function, AChE inhibitors reduce psychotic symptoms, such as hallucinations and delusions,[3] but they do not ameliorate depression, which is common in demented patients.[4] We have previously described the preparation and pharmacological properties of a novel drug TV3326[5] (Figure 33.1) designed to inhibit both AChE and monoamine oxidase (MAO) and to provide the neuroprotective activity reported for MAO-B inhibitors.[6]

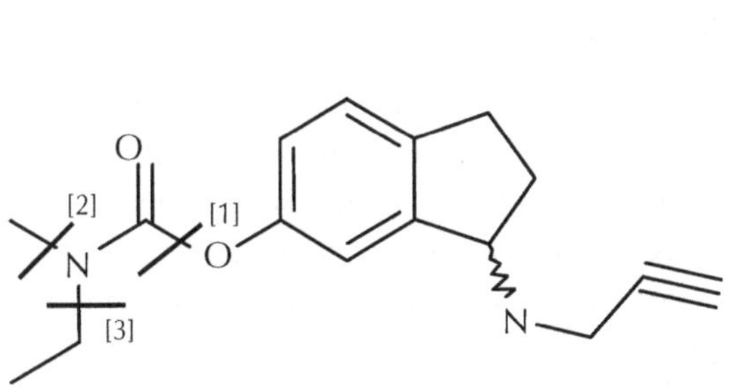

Figure 33.1 The drug TV3326. [1] Hydrolysis of carbamate group; [2] de-methylation; [3] de-ethylation

Although, like rivastigmine, TV3326 has an N-methyl, N-ethyl carbamate group, it is a much weaker inhibitor *in vitro* of both human erythrocyte AChE and rat brain MAO-B than rivastigmine and rasagiline, respectively. However, TV3326 is at least as potent as rivastigmine in inhibiting butyrylcholinesterase (BuChE) (Table 33.1). This is a potential advantage over selective AChE inhibitors, donepezil and galant-amine, since BuChE inhibition can contribute to the maintenance of acetylcholine in the AD brain after much of the AChE is lost as a result of neurodegeneration[7,8] and could explain the ability of rivastigmine to improve cognitive function in a significant proportion of patients who no longer responded to donepezil.[9]

MECHANISM OF BRAIN-SELECTIVE MONOAMINE OXIDASE INHIBITION

TV3326 showed considerably higher MAO and AChE inhibition in the brain of rats after oral administration than would have been predicted from its *in vitro* activity. This suggested that the enzyme inhibition could result from the formation of more active metabolites. Thus, when administered orally, once daily for 2 weeks

Table 33.1 Comparison between the novel drug TV3326 and rivastigmine and rasagiline[17]

Compound	Location of cleavage	IC_{50} (μmol/l)			
		AChE	BuChE	MAO-A	MAO-B
Rivastigmine		0.72	0.84	> 1000	> 1000
Rasagiline		> 1000	> 1000	0.4	0.004
TV3326		32	0.48	300	> 1000
Metabolites of TV3326					
TV3294	[1]	> 1000	> 1000	0.3	0.23
TV3724	[2]	16	0.2	40	62
TV3723	[3]	1	0.85	37	42

AChE, acetylcholinesterase; BuChE, butyrylcholinesterase; MAO, monoamine oxidase

to rats, TV3326 (26 mg/kg, 75 μmol/kg) produced more than 60% inhibition of both MAO-A and -B in the brain. Moreover, in contrast to all other irreversible MAO-A inhibitors, TV3326 did not cause any significant inhibition of this enzyme in the intestine.[5] Although TV3326 had less than one-40th of the AChE inhibitory activity of rivastigmine *in vitro*, it showed only one-seventh of the inhibitory activity of rivastigmine on rat brain AChE after oral administration.[10] The rate of onset of brain AChE inhibition by TV3326 was significantly slower than that of rivastigmine, and of longer duration.[10] This should result in a lower incidence of nausea and vomiting than is encountered with rivastigmine and may obviate the necessity for twice daily dosing.

Studies in rats and monkeys confirmed the formation of at least four active metabolites of TV3326 after oral administration. Three of them are more potent, both as AChE and MAO inhibitors, than the parent drug (Figure 33.1, Table 33.1) and are found in higher concentrations in blood within 15 min. All the active metabolites have also been detected in the brain, and both TV3723 and TV3724 inhibit brain AChE at considerably lower doses than TV3326

after parenteral administration to rats. The brain-selective inhibition of MAO after chronic oral administration of TV3326 was also obtained at much lower doses than would have been predicted from its *in vitro* activity. This could be explained by the formation in the brain, but not in the intestine, of TV3294 through hydrolysis by AChE. TV3294 is an irreversible inhibitor of MAO and at least 3000 times more potent than TV3326. Thus, daily administration of TV3326 (26 mg/kg) results in ever-increasing brain MAO inhibition until it reaches more than 80% after 2 months.[5]

ANTIDEPRESSANT-LIKE ACTIVITY OF TV3326

Although the relationship between production of immobile behavior in rats confined to a narrow cylinder of water is difficult to relate directly to depression, nevertheless the forced swim, or 'Porsolt test' has proved to be a reliable predictor of potential antidepressant drugs, including MAO-A inhibitors, tricyclics, serotonin uptake inhibitors and electro-convulsive shock.[11,12] Daily oral administration of TV3326, (26 mg/kg per day) for 2 weeks reduced the duration of immobility of rats in this test by a similar amount (about 40%) to that seen after amitriptyline (10 mg/kg per day) and the reversible MAO-A inhibitor, moclobemide (20 mg/kg per day).[13]

Irreversible MAO inhibitors are rarely given to treat depression, because of their propensity to induce potentially dangerous increases in blood pressure when tyramine-containing foods and beverages are ingested.[14] It was therefore important to determine whether the brain-selective MAO inhibition induced by TV3326 did indeed result in much less potentiation than other irreversible MAO inhibitors of the blood pressure-raising effect of tyramine. This was accomplished in conscious rabbits with in-dwelling nasopharyngeal catheters. These enabled us to administer the MAO-A inhibitors and tyramine without elevating the rabbits' blood pressure as a result of handling for oral gavage. Rabbits proved to be more sensitive than rats to the MAO-inhibiting effect of the TV3326 (26 mg/kg). After 2 weeks of daily admini-stration, brain MAO-A and -B were inhibited by more than 90%, but again there was no signifi-cant inhibition of MAO-A, the major form in the intestine. The effect of TV3326 was compared to those of moclobemide (a reversible MAO-A inhibitor), clorgyline (an irreversible MAO-A inhibitor) and tranylcypromine (a non-selective MAO-A and -B inhibitor given in doses that also caused about 90% inhibition of brain MAO-A). Clorgyline and tranylcypromine also inhibited MAO-A in the intestine by more than 90%. Compared to untreated rabbits the dose of tyramine needed to increase blood pressure by 30 mmHg was halved in those given TV3326 or moclobemide, to about 35 mg/kg, but reduced to one-sixth and one-20th in rabbits given clorgyline and tranylcypromine, respectively.[15]

CONCLUSIONS

The unique multiple actions of TV3326 combining inhibition of AChE, BuChE, MAO-A and -B make it a potentially useful drug for the treatment of dementia with depression. In addition, TV3326 has neuroprotective activity against oxidative stress in cultured neuronal cells[6] and can stimulate the processing of amyloid precursor protein (APP) to the neuroprotective soluble APPα, thereby reducing the likelihood of the formation of toxic amyloid-β (Aβ).[16] These additional properties should enable the drug to slow the progression of dementia in addition to reducing the behavioral abnormalities and cognitive deficits of AD.

REFERENCES

1. Tariot PN. Maintaining cognitive function in Alzheimer disease: how effective are current treatments? Alzheimer Dis Assoc Disord 2001; (Suppl 1): S26–33

2. Aarsland D, Ballard C, McKeith I, et al. Dementia with Lewy bodies treated with rivastigmine: effects on cognition, neuro-psychiatric symptoms, and sleep. J Neuro-psychiatry Clin Neurosci 2001; 13: 374–9

3. Mega MS, Masterman DM, O'Connor SM, et al. The spectrum of behavioral responses to cholinesterase inhibitor therapy in Alzheimer disease. Arch Neurol 1999; 56: 1388–93

4. Newman SC. The prevalence of depression in Alzheimer's disease and vascular dementia in a population sample. J Affect Disord 1999; 52: 169–76

5. Weinstock M, Goren T, Youdim MBH. Development of a novel neuroprotective drug (TV3326) for the treatment of Alzheimer's disease, with cholinesterase and monoamine oxidase inhibitory activities. Drug Dev Res 2000; 50: 216–22

6. Youdim MBH, Weinstock M. Molecular basis of neuroprotective activities of rasagiline and the anti-Alzheimer drug, TV3326, [(n-propargyl-(3r)aminoindan-5-yl)-ethyl methyl carbamate]. Cell Mol Biol 2001; 21: 555–73

7. Weinstock M. Selectivity of cholinesterase inhibition: clinical implications for the treatment of Alzheimer's disease. CNS Drugs 1999; 12: 307–23

8. Giacobini E. Selective inhibitors of butyryl-cholinesterase: a valid alternative for therapy of Alzheimer's disease? Drugs Aging 2001; 18: 891–8

9. Auriacombe S, Pere JJ, Loria-Kanza Y, Vellas B. Efficacy and safety of rivastigmine in patients with Alzheimer's disease who failed to benefit from treatment with donepezil. Curr Med Res 2002; 18: 129–38

10. Weinstock M, Gorodetsky E, Poltyrev T, et al. A novel cholinesterase and brain-selective monoamine oxidase inhibitor for the treatment of dementia co-morbid with depression and Parkinson's disease. Prog Neuropsycho-pharmacol Biol Psychiatry 2003; 27: 555–61

11. Porsolt RD, Bertin A, Blavet N, et al. Immobility induced by forced swimming in rats: effects of agents which modify central catecholamine and serotonin activity. Eur J Pharmacol 1979; 57: 201–10

12. Borsini F, Meli A. Is the forced swimming test a suitable model for revealing antidepressant activity? Psychopharmacology 1988; 94: 147–60

13. Weinstock M, Poltyrev T, Bejar C, Youdim MBH. Effect of TV3326, a novel monoamine-oxidase-cholinesterase inhibitor, in rat models of anxiety and depression. Psychopharmacol 2002; 160: 318–24

14. Blackwell B, Marley E. Interactions with cheese and its constituents with monoamine oxidase inhibitors. Br J Pharmacol Chemother 1966; 26: 120–41

15. Weinstock M, Gorodetsky E, Wang RH, et al. Limited potentiation of blood pressure response to oral tyramine by brain-selective monoamine oxidase A-B inhibitor, TV-3326 in conscious rabbits. Neuropharmacology 2002; 43: 999–1005

16. Yogev-Falach M, Amit T, Bar-Am O, et al. The involvement of mitogen-activated protein (MAP) kinase in the regulation of amyloid precursor protein processing by novel cholinesterase inhibitors derived from rasagiline. FASEB J 2002; 16: 1674–6

17. Youdim MBH, Gross A, Finberg JPM. Rasagiline [N-propargyl-1R(+)-aminoindan], a selective and potent inhibitor of mitochondrial monoamine oxidase B. Br J Pharmacol 2001; 132: 500–6

Chapter 34

Physostigmine and its analog phenserine have different effects on Alzheimer amyloid-β precursor protein

DK Lahiri, GM Alley, MR Farlow, JT Rogers, NH Greig

INTRODUCTION

One of the most prominent neuropathologic features of Alzheimer's disease is widespread cerebral deposition of a 39–43-amino acid peptide called the amyloid-β peptide (Aβ) in the form of amyloid fibrils.[1] It is generally believed that Aβ plays a central role in the progressive neurodegeneration observed in Alzheimer's disease (AD). Aβ is generated from a larger protein called the Aβ precursor protein (APP) by a group of enzymes collectively identified as secretases. Specifically, APP is proteolytically cleaved at specific amino acids by three enzymes, α-, β- and γ-secretase, to different protein fragments, including the toxic Aβ and other C-terminal fragments that are implicated in the pathogenesis of AD.[1,2] Our laboratories are engaged in studying various classes of agents that can reduce APP expression, as this is the precursor to all the Aβ toxic fragments. Over the years we have tested the effects of several clinically useful drugs/compounds on the APP metabolic pathways.[2]

Greig and colleagues have recently synthesized a family of novel cholinesterase inhibitors, phenserine and analogs, based on a common phenylcarbamate structure.[3] In rodents, phenserine was shown to improve cognitive performance, and in rats with forebrain cholinergic lesions, known to increase APP in cholinergic projection areas, phenserine prevented this rise and, additionally, reduced APP production in naive animals.[4,5] The compound is currently being assessed in phase III human clinical trials for the treatment of mild to moderate AD. Herein we report that phenserine, a structural analog of physostigmine, reduced levels of APP and Aβ while physostigmine failed to do so in neuroblastoma culture cells. The differential effects of these two closely related drugs on APP pathways contrasts with their similar potency in inhibiting acetylcholinesterase (AChE). This provides an interesting mechanism that is worthy of exploration: one that potentially lowers APP and hence Aβ deposition *in vivo*, thereby altering the neurodegenerative course of AD.

EXPERIMENTAL PROCEDURES

The human neuroblastoma (SK-N-SH) cell line was cultured in minimal essential medium (MEM) containing 10% fetal bovine serum

(FBS) to 70% confluence, as described previously.[6] For drug treatment, cells were fed with fresh media with low FBS (0.5%) and treated separately with vehicle, 10 µmol/l phenserine or physostigmine. Lactate dehydrogenase (LDH) and MTT (3-(4,5-dimethyl-thiazol-2-yl)-2,5-diphenyltetrazolium bromide)-based methods were measured as described previously.[6] Secretory APP was assayed in the conditioned medium by Western immunoblotting using 22C11 antibody, as described previously.[6] Total Aβ peptide levels were assayed in the conditioned medium samples using a sandwich enzyme-linked immunosorbent assay (ELISA) method after the modification of IBL reagents. The inhibition of human AChE and butyryl-cholinesterase by phenserine and physostigmine was measured between the concentrations of 1 µmol/l and 10 µmol/l, as described previously.[7]

RESULTS

We treated the human neuroblastoma cells with vehicle, phenserine or physostigmine, at a concentration of 10 µmol/l in the cell culture media. Cells were monitored morphologically and conditioned medium samples were collected, and subjected to various biochemical assays. First, cell membrane damage and integrity were assessed by measuring the release of the enzyme LDH. The LDH assay was sensitive and quantitative, and was carried out within a linear range. An increased activity in drug-treated cells as compared to the control indicates damage in the cell membrane and hence toxicity of the drug. As shown in Table 34.1, there was no significant increase in LDH value, as determined from optical density measurements at 490 nm wavelength, between phenserine treatment and control (0.14 vs. 0.13). Similarly, no significant increase in LDH value was observed between physostigmine treatment and control (0.08 vs. 0.13). In parallel to this toxicity assessment, cell viability was additionally determined by MTT assay. This assay measures mitochondrial function, metabolic activity and hence the cellular viability of cells. The MTT assay is sufficiently sensitive and quantitative, to suggest that an increased MTT value as compared to the control indicates increased cellular metabolic activity, and hence greater viability of the cell under the condition of assessment. Our MTT results suggest that there was no significant change in cell viability with these drug treatments. These results corroborate the LDH data, which suggest that these drugs are non-toxic to the cells under the doses and conditions used herein.

To examine the effects of these drugs on APP processing we measured levels of total secretory APP (sAPP) in the same conditioned medium

Table 34.1 Effects of phenserine and physostigmine on cellular toxicity and viability, and on levels of total secreted derivatives of amyloid-β (Aβ) precursor protein (sAPP), and Aβ, in human neuroblastoma (SK-N-SH) cells ($n = 3$)

Treatment	Dose (µg/ml)	LDH (A490 nm)	MTT (A490 nm)	sAPP (relative band density) (%)	Aβ-40 (%)
Control	—	0.13±0.02	0.34±0.03	100	100
Phenserine	5	0.14±0.02	0.44±0.03	54	64
Physostigmine	5	0.08±0.01	0.31±0.03	106	109

LDH, lactate dehydrogenase; MTT, 3-(4,5-dimethyl-thiazol-2-yl)-2,5-diphenyltetrazolium bromide

samples. We employed Western immuno-blotting, using an antibody whose epitope maps at the N-terminal part of the APP holoprotein. Phenserine treatment reduced levels of sAPP by 46% from the control. Under the same condition, physostigmine treatment did not change the level of sAPP (Table 34.1). To determine the effects of these drugs on the Aβ, we measured levels of Aβ in the same conditioned media samples by a sensitive ELISA. As shown in Table 34.1, phenserine treatment reduced levels of Aβ by 36% from the control, while physostigmine treatment marginally increased (9%) the Aβ level.

In separate experiments we determined cholinesterase inhibition associated with both drugs in human erythrocytes and plasma samples. Both phenserine and physostigmine potently inhibited AChE 1 nmol/l and 10 μmol/l. Hence, under the conditions of the cell culture study described above, cholinesterase activity can be considered to be substantially inhibited.

DISCUSSION

Our aim in these studies was to compare the effects of phenserine and physostigmine on secreted levels of APP and Aβ in cell cultures.

The reason we selected these drugs was because of their clinical utility as anticholinesterase agents, and their structural similarity; both are carbamate cholinesterase inhibitors and share the same hexahydropyrroloindole backbone[2,3] (Figure 34.1). Our hypothesis is that, in the event that the two compounds exert a similar effect on the APP pathway, there is a likelihood of convergence in the structure–activity relationship between the anticholinesterase and APP-lowering properties of the agents, suggesting a functional involvement between the two and shared mechanisms. On the other hand, their divergent influence on the APP pathway could be interpreted as independence between the anticholinesterase and APP functions, probably involving disparate mechanisms. Our results on APP and Aβ, as shown in Table 34.1, favored the second scenario.

The present results dealing with phenserine's effect on APP and Aβ are consistent with earlier observations.[8,9] Our previous cell-culture studies with human neuroblastoma cell lines, glial cell lines and PC12 cells have shown that phenserine can reduce both cellular and secreted APP levels. Subsequent detailed studies in human neuro-blastoma cells confirmed that the reduction was both time- and concentration-dependent, and occurred without a loss in cell viability (as

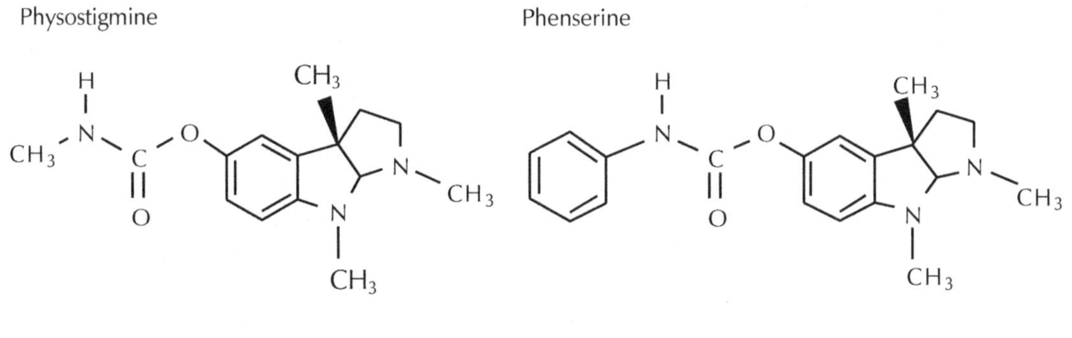

Figure 34.1 Chemical structures of physostigmine and phenserine

measured by quantifying LDH release into the conditioned media) versus untreated controls.[8] Reductions in both cellular and secreted APP resulted in a significantly lowered secretion of Aβ peptide as measured by sandwich ELISA. Here our comparative studies suggest that the effect of phenserine was not shared by its close analog, physostigmine, on Alzheimer's APP and Aβ peptide.

Such studies provide insight into the mechanism(s) underlying the phenserine-induced reductions in cellular and secreted APP in both cell culture, herein, and in prior animal studies, specifically: a lack of action of physostigmine on APP/Aβ, a close structural analog of phenserine, under similar conditions; and the divergent action of other anticholinesterases on APP in rats, indicating a non-cholinergic-mediated system. Although phenserine and physostigmine potently and similarly inhibited AChE, which, by blocking its catabolism would augment acetylcholine levels and potentially trigger muscarinic and nicotinic pathways, the sole action of phenserine on APP suggests that these pathways, which can alter APP processing,[10,11] are not primary in phenserine's APP actions.

Phenserine, which is a phenylcarbamate of (−)-eseroline, as opposed to physostigmine, which is a methylcarbamate, is a new potent and highly selective AChE inhibitor, with a >70-fold activity versus butyrylcholinesterase, and is currently in clinical trials for the treatment of AD by Axonyx, Inc. (New York, NY). The specific mechanism underpinning the differential effect of phenserine and physostigmine on APP is still unclear and is a focus of our current research. However, in accord with results from our recent studies, we are tempted to speculate on the involvement of several possible mechanisms. Although the structures of phenserine and physostigmine are very similar, they differ both solely and significantly in their carbamate groups[3,12] (Figure 34.1). Consequently, phenserine's phenylcarbamate moiety is more lipophilic, allowing greater brain delivery, and this bulky aromatic residue additionally allows both hydrophobic and π electron interactions with peptide and protein targets, due to potential π–π stacking of the phenyl group of the carbamate between closely flanking phenylalanines,[13] which are not compatible with the methyl group present in physostigmine. Whether or not the presence of this aromatic group hinders some components of APP processing machinery to operate, such as the secretase enzymes, and leads to decreased APP/Aβ formation, remains an attractive possibility that is worthy of future research. Similarly, a potential interaction with such an aromatic group could possibly interfere with the binding of APP to some important protein, such as the iron-regulatory protein (IRP).[14] Interestingly, the IRP has been shown to interact with the 5′-untranslated region (UTR) of APP mRNA and to result in translational enhancement of APP.[15] Phenserine might likewise interfere with APP translation as a result of its direct or indirect interaction at the 5′-UTR. Notably, there are several other factors that regulate APP translation through the 5′-UTR of APP mRNA.[15,16] Thus, this 5′-UTR, as a whole or in part, could be the site of phenserine's direct or indirect action that regulates APP translation.

At least a role for the hexahydropyrroloindole structure on APP reduction can be ruled out, as both phenserine and physostigmine share this backbone. This is consistent with our previous work with tacrine (9-amino-1,2,3,4-tetrahydroacridine hydrochloride) which, similar to phenserine, reduced APP/Aβ levels without having the phenylcarbamoylseroline structure.[6] These observations warrant the investigation of the effects of further analogs of phenserine on APP pathways, to determine and optimize the precise structure–activity relations and three-dimensional steric conformation requirements that are needed in a cholinesterase-inhibitor drug to provide clinically useful APP/Aβ reductions. Such research will accelerate the discovery of potential drug candidates for AD.

ACKNOWLEDGEMENTS

We acknowledge with appreciation grant support from the Alzheimer's Association, Axonyx Inc., and the National Institutes of Health (D.K.L.).

REFERENCES

1. Hardy J, Selkoe DJ. The amyloid hypothesis of Alzheimer's disease: progress and problems on the road to therapeutics. Science 2002; 297: 353–6

2. Lahiri DK, Farlow MR, Greig NH, et al. A critical analysis of new molecular targets and strategies for drug developments in Alzheimer's disease. Curr Drug Targets 2003; 4: 97–112

3. Greig NH, Pei XF, Soncrant TT, et al. Phenserine and ring C hetero-analogs: drug candidates for the treatment of Alzheimer's disease. Med Res Rev 1995; 15: 3–31

4. Patel N, Spangler E, Greig NH, et al. Phenserine, a novel acetylcholinesterase inhibitor, attenuates impaired learning of rats in a 14-unit T-maze induced by blockade of the NMDA receptor. Neuroreport 1998; 9: 171–6

5. Haroutunian V, Greig NH, Utsuki T, et al. Pharmacological modulation of Alzheimer's beta-amyloid precursor protein levels in the CSF of rats with forebrain cholinergic system lesions. Mol Brain Res 1997; 46: 161–8

6. Lahiri DK, Farlow MR, Sambamurti K. The secretion of amyloid beta-peptide is inhibited in tacrine-treated human neuroblastoma cells. Mol Brain Res 1998; 62: 131–40

7. Yu QS, Zhu X, Holloway HW, et al. Anticholinesterase activity of compounds related to geneserine tautomers – N-oxides and 1,2-oxazines. J Med Chem 2002; 45: 3684–91

8. Shaw KT, Utsuki T, Rogers J, et al. Phenserine regulates translation of beta-amyloid precursor protein mRNA by a putative interleukin-1 responsive element, a target for drug development. Proc Natl Acad Sci USA 2001; 98: 7605–10

9. Lahiri DK, Farlow MR, Hintz N, et al. Cholinesterase inhibitors, β-amyloid precursor protein, and amyloid β-peptides in Alzheimer's disease. Acta Neurol Scand 2000; 176: 60–7

10. Sambamurti K, Greig NH, Lahiri DK. Advances in the cellular and molecular biology of the beta-amyloid protein in Alzheimer's disease. Neuromolecular Med 2002; 1: 1–31

11. Lahiri DK, Farlow MR, Greig NH, Sambamurti K. Current drug targets for Alzheimer's disease treatment. Drug Dev Res 2002; 56: 267–81

12. Greig NH, De Micheli E, Holloway HW, et al. The experimental Alzheimer drug phenserine: pharmacokinetics and pharmacodynamics in the rat. Acta Neurol Scand 2000; 176: 74–84

13. Yu QS, Holloway HW, Flippen-Anderson F, et al. Methyl analogues of the experimental Alzheimer drug, phenserine: synthesis and structure/activity relationships for acetyl- and butyrylcholinesterase inhibitory action. J Med Chem 2001; 44: 4062–71

14. Rogers JT, Leiter LM, McPhee J, et al. Translation of the Alzheimer amyloid precursor protein mRNA is up-regulated by interleukin-1 through 5′-untranslated region sequences. J Biol Chem 1999; 274: 6421–31

15. Rogers JT, Cahill CM, Eder PS, et al. An iron-responsive element type II in the 5′ untranslated region of the Alzheimer's amyloid precursor protein transcript. J Biol Chem 2002; 277: 45518–28

16. Lahiri D, Chen D, Vivien D, et al. The role of cytokines in the gene expression of amyloid β-protein precursor: identification of a 5′UTR binding nuclear factor and its implications for Alzheimer's disease. J Alzheimer Dis 2003; 5: 81–90

Translation and processing of amyloid precursor protein (APP) by an M1 muscarinic agonist and an acetylcholinesterase inhibitor: the role of APP mRNA 5'-untranslated region sequences

JT Rogers, NH Greig, DK Lahiri, A Fisher

THE ALZHEIMER'S AMYLOID PRECURSOR PROTEIN

The β-amyloid precursor protein (APP) is cleaved selectively by γ-secretase and β-site APP cleaving enzyme (BACE) to produce Aβ peptide, which forms the fibrils that constitute the characteristic amyloid plaque in the brains of Alzheimer's disease (AD) patients.[1] Production and clearance of this 40–42 amino acid Aβ peptide remains an underpinning strategy to slow down the development of AD.[2] APP is encoded by the key chromosome 21 gene that remains one of the few known genetic markers linked to the pathogenesis of AD (*FAD*).[3] Our laboratory established that both iron levels and interleukin (IL)-1 regulate translation of APP through the 5'-untranslated region (APP 5'-UTR) of the precursor transcript.[4,5] In addition to the binding of the iron regulatory protein (IRP) to the APP 5'-UTR transcript,[5] a nuclear factor was also shown to bind selectively to DNA sequences encoding the APP 5'-UTR.[6] Evidently translational and transcriptional control of the APP holoprotein as mediated by APP 5'-UTR sequences is a crucial control point for the production of intracellular APP. Since the APP 5'-UTR encodes both IL-1 and iron regulatory elements, we proposed that APP is intimately involved in iron metabolism in health.[5] We also developed an RNA-based screening protocol for the selection of drugs that interact with the APP 5'-UTR to control APP holoprotein levels and hence Aβ output.[2,7] Here we discuss how the acetylcholinesterase inhibitor (AChEI) phenserine, and the M1 muscarinic agonist AF102B, influence APP gene expression through iron- and IL-1-specific pathways.

IRON, INFLAMMATION AND AMYLOID PRECURSOR PROTEIN GENE EXPRESSION (mRNA TRANSLATION)

Cytokines are physiologically relevant to the course of AD,[8,9] and influence APP gene expression at many levels, depending on the cell or tissue type in question. APP gene expression is transcriptionally controlled by IL-1 in endothelial cells and PC12 cells.[10,11] In peripheral blood lymphocytes and endothelial cells, two *cis*-acting elements in the APP 3'-UTR were shown to regulate the stability of the precursor transcript wherein addition of serum growth factors overrides the action of a 29-base sequence (2285–2313) in the APP 3'-UTR that normally destabilizes APP mRNA.[12] Transforming growth factor (TGF)β also induced a 68-kDa protein to bind to an upstream 81 nucleotide 3'-UTR motif, and thus stabilize the APP mRNA.[13]

Mbella et al.[14] observed that APP 3'-UTR sequences in between the two poly(A) selection sites enhanced APP mRNA translation in mammalian (Chinese hamster ovary) cells, and more closely mapped two guanosine residues that are crucial for this action. These authors used RNA-electrophoretic mobility shift assays (REMSA) to determine that a translational repressor protein interacts with the shorter transcript. However, the presence of the 258 nucleotide poly(A) regulatory region (PAR) (nt +3042 to +3300) removed binding of this APP mRNA repressor and facilitated longer APP mRNA translation.[14]

We found that the APP gene is upregulated by IL-1 at the translational level in astrocytes, through the action of 5'-UTR sequences by a pattern of gene expression similar to that for the universal iron storage protein, ferritin.[4,15] Interestingly, Lesne et al.[16] showed that the APP 5'-UTR (+54 to +74) is a TGFβ transcription site response site in astrocytes. These data confirmed that the APP 5'-UTR sequences (+1 to +146) is a target site for both transcriptional (nucleus) and translational control (cytoplasm), depending on the cell type and on the inducer.

As occurs during the hepatic acute-phase response (i.e. SAA in response to IL-1,[17–19]) the pathology of AD is characterized by an acute phase of astrocytic gene expression at the transcriptional level in response to IL-1. Steady-state levels of the mRNA for the amyloid-associated protein α_1-antichymotrypsin (ACT), were increased 2000-fold in IL-1-stimulated astrocytes.[20] This brain-specific genetic

induction generated an adaptive response to enhance ACT secretion (and protease inhibition) from active astrocytes during injury,[21] whereas prolonged ACT overexpression promoted amyloid plaque formation in transgenic mouse models for AD.[22,23] Using astrocytic cells we showed that APP gene expression was largely controlled at the level of message translation in response to IL-1 rather than by transcriptional mechanisms.[4] Astrocytic and endothelial cells are also known to respond to acute-phase microglial cytokines (and Aβ) during the development of amyloid plaques, wherein astrocytes can be observed to form a rim surrounding a developing plaque.[24–26] Our model predicts that IL-1 activates APP mRNA translation via the 5'-UTR element at the same time as co-activating α-secretase (Table 35.1). The release of microglial IL-1 generated the production and secretion of the neuroprotective APP ectodomain (secretory APP; sAPP) from astrocytes in response to stress.[27]

We demonstrated that the IRPs, which control intracellular iron homeostasis, selectively and specifically interacted with the APP 5'-UTR.[5] The inclusion of APP mRNA in the family of transcripts that interact with IRP-1 and IRP-2 suggests a role for APP in iron uptake and storage during health (i.e. transferrin receptor for iron uptake,[28] IRP-1 for duodenal iron efflux,[29] divalent metal ion transporter (DMT)-1 for duodenal iron uptake,[30] erythroid 5-aminolevulinate synthase (eALAS) for heme biosynthesis[31] and ferritin for iron storage.[32,33]

THE AMYLOID PRECURSOR PROTEIN 5'-UNTRANSLATED REGION IS IRON- AND INTERLEUKIN-1 RESPONSIVE

Our computer-assisted sequence alignment programs verified that APP mRNA 5'-UTR sequences (+51 to +94 in APP mRNA) show

Table 35.1 Comparative modes of action for four agents (interleukin (IL)-1, desferrioxamine, AF 102B and phenserine) in regulating amyloid precursor protein (APP) expression through the APP 5′-untranslated region (5′-UTR)

Agent	APP	sAPP	Aβ peptide	α-Secretase
Phenserine	reduced	reduced	reduced	not activated
AF102B	increased	increased	reduced	activated
Desferrioxamine	reduced	reduced	reduced	not activated
IL-1 (short term)	increased	increased	reduced	activated

sAPP, secretory APP; Aβ, amyloid-β
Phenserine and desferrioxamine lowered Aβ peptide output by suppressing APP holoprotein translation through an iron-regulator element-type II in the APP 5′-UTR (+50 to +101 nucleotide from the APP 5′ cap site). Both desferrioxamine and phenserine reduced APP holoprotein levels, leaving less of the precursor template to be cleaved by β- and γ-secretases to generate Aβ peptide. IL-1 and AF102B both stimulated APP translation and increased APP holoprotein levels. Both IL-1 and AF102B also co-activated α-secretase to increase APPs output and to lower Aβ levels, consistent with their therapeutic action

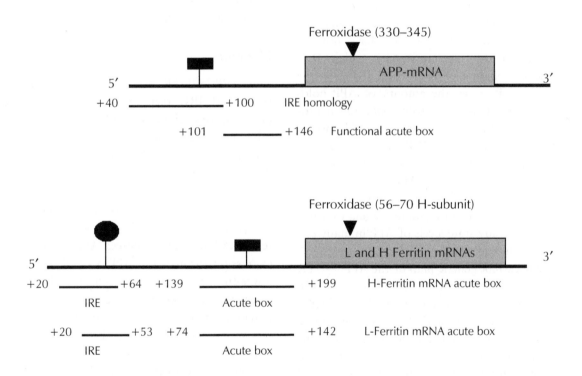

Figure 35.1 A map of the amyloid precursor protein (APP) transcript (3.2 kb) including the 146 nucleotide 5′-untranslated region (5′-UTR). Location of the interleukin (IL)-1 responsive and iron responsive elements that control the rate of APP translation. The APP 5′-UTR is an important regulatory sequence which was found to be a crossroad for the induction or suppression of cellular APP levels by iron,[2] IL-1[4] and transforming growth factor (TGF) β.[58] Structural similarity in the placement of translational regulatory elements in the 146 nucleotide APP-mRNA 5′-UTR and the L- and H-ferritin mRNA 5′-UTRs. An overlapping iron responsive element (IRE)-like sequence is present upstream of IL-1-responsive acute box translational enhancers in APP mRNA

significant identity to the known iron responsive elements (IREs), which are also encoded by the first 60 nucleotides of the mRNAs encoding the L- and H-subunits of ferritin, the universal iron storage protein (Figure 35.1). An 11 nucleotide stretch in the loop region of the predicted APP 5'-UTR stem-loop (+83 to +93) is 75% identical to the well-described canonical IREs that regulate iron-dependent translation in the 5'-UTRs of both L- and H-ferritin mRNAs.[5]

In addition to the presence of an active IRE, we previously reported the presence of a potent IL-1-responsive acute box domain in the 5'-UTR of the APP transcript (+101 to +146 in the APP 5'-UTR)[4] (Figure 35.1). The APP 5'-UTR is a crucial control point that sets the amount of APP being made by physiological signals in addition to inflammation. We have not yet established the mechanism by which IL-1 influences binding of IRP-1 and IRP-2 to the APP 5'-UTR to set the amount of APP holo-protein production in astrocytoma and neuro-blastoma cells. Any mechanism would have to account for the fact that IRP-1 is a cis-aconitase in addition to being a well-known IRE-binding protein[33,34] (and now an APP 5'-UTR-binding protein).[5] Certainly, the intracellular iron level can be seen as a major regulatory agent to determine the steady-state levels of APP in many cell types, including neurons.[5,35]

Our current genetic map of the APP 5'-UTR reflects the link between iron IL-1 and APP expression relevant to the onset of AD (Figure 35.1). Mutations in the IL-1α gene,[36] and more recently mutations in the hemochromatosis gene (Hfe),[37] were observed to accelerate the onset of AD in elderly Italian pedigrees (Hfe is involved in iron transport across the gut mucosal membrane). At the same time trisomy of the APP gene has long been associated with amyloid plaque build-up seen in Down's syndrome patients over 40 years of age.[38] Many groups have shown that APP and Ps gene mutations

independently enhance cleavage of the precursor into the Aβ peptide (Aβ1-40 and Aβ1-42) that accumulates in the brain as amyloid plaques during the onset of AD.[39] Consistent with all of these observations, both IL-1 and the acute phase protein ACT were found to be elevated in the amyloid plaques of AD patients.[8,40] Immunohistochemistry also demonstrated that the iron storage protein ferritin was present at higher amounts in the neuritic plaques of AD patients.[41,42]

DRUG TARGETING THROUGH THE AMYLOID PRECURSOR PROTEIN 5'-UNTRANSLATED REGION

Chelators

The APP 5'-UTR sequence element has a functional IRE (type II).[5] Relevant to the potential for chelation therapy for AD,[43,44] APP mRNA translation was decreased under conditions of intracellular iron chelation with desferrioxamine through APP 5'-UTR sequences[5] (Table 35.1). We predict that metal chelators, such as desferrioxamine and clioquinol (iron and copper chelators, respectively), might suppress APP holoprotein expression through the APP 5'-UTR and thus lower the amount of Aβ produced. Clioquinol (copper–zinc chelator) was reported to dissolve amyloid plaque formation in an APP transgenic mouse model.[43] Recently, clioquinol showed efficacy in a human clinical trial conducted in Melbourne, Australia.[44] The highly selective iron chelator desferrioxamine was previously shown to slow down the progression of AD in a clinical study in Toronto, Canada.[45] The therapeutic potential of metal chelators is consistent with the finding that APP is a metalloprotein.[46,47]

Amyloid precursor protein 5′-untranslated region screened

As an approach to RNA-based therapeutics beyond metal chelators for a therapeutic treatment of AD, our laboratory screened a unique library of 800 Food and Drug Administration (FDA) pre-approved drugs to identify pharmacological activity that would suppress APP 5′-UTR-directed translation of a luciferase reporter gene.[2] The library of FDA pre-approved drugs was arranged into 96-well format so that the screen could detect drugs capable of suppressing transfected reporter gene translation using an APP 5′-UTR-luciferase construct (pGAL).[2,7] Six of the original 17 drug hits were validated for their capacity to suppress reporter gene expression in stable neuro-blastoma transfectants expressing the dicistronic reporter construct.[7] Of these, paroxetine (serotonin reuptake blocker) and dimercapto-propanol (mercury chelator) exerted significant effects on APP expression (steady-state levels of APP), whereas azithromycin altered APP processing. None of these three compounds altered APLP-1 expression. Of particular interest, the APP 5′-UTR-directed drug that most actively reduced APP holoprotein expression was the metal chelator dimercapto-propanol. This finding was consistent with the presence of an IRE-type II element in the 5′-UTR of the APP transcript, which we predicted to be a site through which metal chelators suppress APP translation (and Aβ levels).[5]

CHOLINERGIC NEUROTRANSMISSION (ANTICHOLINESTERASES AND M1 MUSCARINIC AGONISTS)

In AD, acetylcholine (ACh)-mediated neuronal transmission is lowered.[48,49] Therefore, agents that restore cognitive enhancement via the ACh pathway have been extensively tested for their potential therapeutic benefit for AD.[49] We have been interested to discover the impact of both an anticholinesterase (phenserine) and an M1 muscarinic agonist (AF102B) on modulation of APP gene expression through APP 5′-UTR sequences.

Phenserine

Phenserine is a potent acetylcholinesterase inhibitor

The reduction in the levels of ACh in the AD brain can be largely offset by inhibiting its breakdown by the cholinesterase enzymes.[49] Phenserine is a new drug with reversible AChE inhibitory action[48] to have favorable pharmaco-kinetics and pharmacodynamics for use in the elderly population. Extensive medicinal chemistry, based loosely on the backbone of the classic anticholinesterase physostigmine, identi-fied the structural requirements for: selective acetyl- (AChE) vs. butyrylcholinesterase (BChE) inhibitory action; a long vs. short duration of pharmacodynamic (anticholinesterase) action; a rapid vs. slow metabolism; and a high vs. low brain delivery.[48,49] In animal cognition studies, the compound demonstrated an unusually wide therapeutic window that was coupled with a favorable toxicological profile. Multiple dose studies in older human volunteers demonstrated that phenserine tartrate was well tolerated at doses of 5 mg or 10 mg administered orally either once or twice daily for a total of 6 consecutive days. Thereafter, a 12-week phase 2 efficacy trial in subjects with mild to moderate Alzheimer's disease (10 mg b.i.d.) provided sufficient improvement in a standard battery of cognitive measures, coupled with minor adverse effects to support multiple ongoing multicenter randomized placebo-controlled double-blind trials in mild to moderate AD patients.

Phenserine suppresses the production of amyloid precursor holoprotein and reduces amyloid-β levels

Since IL-1 was reported to elevate APP levels via the 5'-UTR of the APP mRNA[4] and, thereby, to confer translational control of APP protein synthesis on neural cells, a similar mechanism was hypothesized to account for phenserine's actions to lower APP.[50] Phenserine was shown to inhibit APP 5'-UTR conferred translation independently of microtubule-associated protein (MAP) kinase and PI3 kinase pathways.[50] In vitro studies with human neuroblastoma cell lines (SK-N-SH and SH-SY-5Y) as well as glial cell lines (U373) and PC12 cells demonstrated that phenserine reduced both cellular and secreted APP levels.[50] More detailed studies in SK-N-SH human neuroblastoma cells confirmed that the reduction was both time- and concentration-dependent, and occurred without a loss in cell viability (as assessed by measuring lactate dehydrogenase release into the conditioned media versus release by untreated controls).[50] These reductions in both cellular and secreted APP resulted in a significantly lowered secretion of Aβ peptide (as assessed by sandwich enzyme-linked immunosorbent assay (ELISA)) by some 30%,[50] and occurred with no decrease in APP mRNA levels.

Phenserine and desferrioxamine appear to suppress APP translation cooperatively, partially via the APP 5'-UTR. These preliminary data suggest that the mechanism for the action of the AChEI may be to suppress APP 5'-UTR-conferred regulation of APP expression by a pathway that depends on threshold intracellular iron levels.[5] The most compelling and testable model is that phenserine operates through the conserved IRE element (+51 to +94) in the APP 5'-UTR. We have also found that APP 3'-UTR co-operates with the APP 5'-UTR element to account for the full translational response to DFO and phenserine (see reference 51 for a report accounting for the action of 5'-UTR and 3'-UTR sequences). The known enzyme inhibitory action of phenserine toward the active site cleft of AChEs may also be directed to the active site cleft of IRP-1. This IRP-1 cleft region regulates translational control of ferritin and APP mRNAs, and the RNA binding activity of IRP-1 is an interconvertible event in response to iron levels (see Thomson et al.[33] for a review and reference 5). Therefore, we will test whether phenserine can alter the cis-aconitase activity of IRP-1 leading to reduced translation of APP mRNA with beneficial therapeutic consequences.

Transgenic mouse studies showed that (-)-phenserine reduced human APP and Aβ in an in vivo mouse model of AD (N. Greig, personal communications). In this regard, a double transgene encompassing the human APP Swedish mutation and mutant PS1 was used (courtesy of the Department of Pathology, Johns Hopkins University School of Medicine, Baltimore, MD). Such mice produce large amounts of amyloid plaques as early as 5 months. (−)-Phenserine (2.5 mg/kg, i.p., daily for 3 weeks), administered to 6-month-old male mice, significantly reduced sAPP levels in cerebrospinal fluid (CSF) and APP levels in the brain. More importantly, it virtually halved brain levels of Aβ (1-40 and 1-42 aminoacids) in a manner similar to the Aβ vaccine. These studies suggested that sequences additional to the APP 5'-UTR, and also processing events, are targeted by phenserine.

AF102B

AF102B is a relatively selective M1 muscarinic agonist. Fisher[52] suggested that M1 muscarinic agonists may be used as therapeutic agents for the treatment of AD when AChEI no longer work. This is based on the assumption that M1 agonists that activate the post-synaptic M1 muscarinic ACh receptor (mAChR) do not require the production of ACh from presynaptic terminals.[52] While ACh, itself, is a highly flexible molecule capable of attaining several conformations, the AF series of drugs are rigid analogs of this neurotransmitter[53] (Figure 35.2). AF102B is currently in use clinically for the treatment of dry mouth in Sjörgren's syndrome. Additionally, AF102B has been clinically tested in AD patients and has been shown to lower amyloid in the CSF.[53,54] AF102B is a member of a new family of candidate therapeutic agents for AD which, in addition to restoration of cognitive impairment in several animal models for AD, has a potential disease-modifying property.[53]

AF102B and amyloid precursor protein processing

In terms of disease development, Aβ peptide impairs the coupling of M1 mAChR with G-proteins. This leads to decreased signal transduction and diminished secretion of the non-amyloidogenic and neuroprotective α-secretase cleavage product of APP, sAPP.[53] Studies *in vivo* support the relation between the cholinergic system and Aβ metabolism.[52] In animal models, IgG-saporin-lesioned rats exhibited lowered AChRs and decreased α-secretase activity to increase Aβ levels, an effect that was reversed by direct drug activation of mAChR signaling.[55] Activation of M1 mAChR leads also to an mAChR-mediated inhibition of

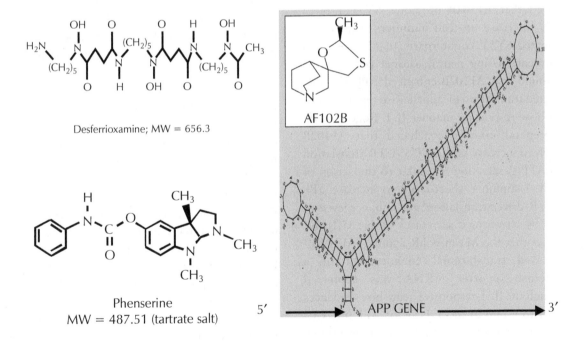

Desferrioxamine; MW = 656.3

Phenserine
MW = 487.51 (tartrate salt)

AF102B

5′ ← APP GENE → 3′

Figure 35.2 Predicted secondary structure of the amyloid precursor protein (APP) 5′-untranslated region, the site of action for three drugs that influence APP metabolism secondary to their primary known pharmacological actions. Desferrioxamine is an iron chelator used in the treatment of sickle cell disease, and transfusion iron overload in thalassemic patients

γ-secretase (T. Hartmann and A. Fisher, unpublished results).

Nitsch et al.[54] showed that activation of the ACh receptor markedly enhanced the release of sAPP[56] and this was confirmed in several other studies (see review by Fisher[52]). An increased secretion of sAPP-α in various in vitro systems resulted in decreased synthesis of Aβ following treatment with muscarinic agonists.[56,57] Like other muscarinic agonists, AF102B would be predicted to induce α-secretase activity and elevate the levels of neuroprotective sAPP in brain-specific cell types and experimental animal models.[53] This activity would lead to diminished Aβ peptide output.

Our preliminary data showed that the AF102B (like the IL-1 stimulus) appeared to increase sAPP secretion from neuroblastoma cells. Microscopic analysis of cell viability showed that AF102B promotes SY5Y growth (30% increase in cell numbers relative to untreated SY5Y counterparts ($n = 5$) over 48-h treatment). Using neuroblastoma cells (SY5Y) we found that AF102B enhanced APP 5'-UTR-directed translation of a luciferase reporter gene in a dose-responsive manner (J.T. Rogers et al., in preparation). We concluded that AF102B action to increase both APP 5'-UTR translation and APP(s) secretion is similar to the action of the IL-1 stimulus (short-term) to increase APP 5'-UTR-driven translation[4] and enhance levels of sAPP by activating α-secretase[57] (Table 35.1). We predict that the M1 mAChR agonist (AF102B)-increased translational enhancement of a luciferase reporter mRNA was conferred through the IL-1-responsive acute box sequences (+101 to +146) in the 5'-UTR of APP mRNA.[4] Our working model is that a coupling protein may co-induce the APP 5'-UTR acute box element and α-secretase activity, providing a new link between APP translation and sAPP secretion (i.e. α-secretase activation).

Comparison of the differential effects of AF102B and phenserine on APP 5'-UTR-driven expression in neuroblastoma cells suggests that both drugs (1–100 μmol/l dose) operate in a highly selective and opposite manner to modulate APP translation through 5'-UTR sequences. As an experimental control, the parental vector pGL-3 showed no response to increasing doses of AF102B or phenserine. At the maximal 100 μmol/l dose level, phenserine reduced APP 5'-UTR-driven luciferase expression > 2-fold in pGAL-transfected SY5Y neuroblastoma (Table 35.1). The AF102B increased APP 5'-UTR-directed translation > 2-fold (J.T. Rogers et al., in preparation).

CONCLUSIONS

There are two arbitrary classes of drugs associated with the 5'-UTR translational enhancer in APP mRNA. Phenserine is inhibitory (class I), whereas AF102B is stimulatory (class II).

Class I agents are typically metal chelators that reduce APP 5'-UTR directed translation (the iron chelator desferrioxamine and copper chelators). These drugs tend to suppress APP holoprotein synthesis at the level of message translation, and probably also act at the transcriptional level during prolonged usage. Phenserine, while not a chelator, appeared to operate by a mechanism consistent with the involvement of an IRE-type II) in the APP 5'-UTR (Figure 35.1 and Table 35.1), although phenserine appears to influence Aβ production at several levels.

Class II compounds are also associated with lowered Aβ output, but operate therapeutically by activating α-secretase apparently coupled to their enhancement of APP 5'-UTR-directed translation. AF102B activated α-secretase as correlated with reduced generation of

Aβ-peptide.[52] Coupled to increased secretion of sAPP, this M1 agonist stimulated translation of APP through APP 5′-UTR sequences (Figure 35.2 and Table 35.1). IL-1 (short term) also induced α-secretase activity at the same time as signaling enhanced translation through the APP 5′-UTR acute box domain.[4]

On a practical level a subset of APP 5′-UTR activating drugs should also be co-activators of α-secretase (similar to IL-1 and AF102B as class II drugs). We therefore will screen for compounds that activate α-secretase by using the APP 5′-UTR target (a significant subset of APP 5′-UTR-activating drugs are predicted to be α-secretase activators). Any drugs that activate α-secretase can be considered therapeutic for AD, based on their intrinsic capacity to lower Aβ levels.

At the levels of basic science, we note that the APP 5′-UTR is capable of interacting with the IRP that controls ferritin translation. This is consistent with the metal-related function of APP, which is a metalloprotein.[47] We note that APP 5′-UTR-directed translational enhancement is a part of an acute-phase responsive reaction leading to increased levels of APP holoprotein and sAPP secretion. Both AF102B and IL-1 (short term) activate receptor pathways to enhance the sAPP secretion into the conditioned medium, an event associated with neuroprotection. We predict the presence of IL-1 responsive cytoplasmic signaling proteins that interact with both the APP 5′-UTR (and IRP-1 and IRP-2) and the metalloprotease α-secretase (ADAM-10).

REFERENCES

1. De Strooper B. Aph-1, Pen-2, and Nicastrin with Presenilin generate an active gamma-secretase complex. Neuron 2003; 38: 9–12

2. Rogers JT, Randall J, Eder PS, et al. Alzheimer's disease drug discovery targeted to the APP mRNA 5′-untranslated region. J Mol Neurosci 2002; 19: 77–82

3. Hardy J, Selkoe DJ. The amyloid hypothesis of Alzheimer's disease: progress and problems on the road to therapeutics. Science 2002; 297: 353–6

4. Rogers JT, Leiter LM, McPhee J, et al. Translation of the Alzheimer amyloid precursor protein mRNA is up-regulated by interleukin-1 through 5′-untranslated region sequences. J Biol Chem 1999; 274: 6421–31

5. Rogers JT, Cahill CM, Eder PS, et al. An iron-responsive element type II in the 5′-untranslated region of the Alzheimer's amyloid precursor protein transcript. J Biol Chem 2002; 227: 45518–28

6. Lahiri D, Chen D, Vivien D, et al. The role of cytokines in the gene expression of amyloid β-protein precursor: identification of a 5′-UTR binding nuclear factor and its implications for Alzheimer's disease. J Alzheimer's Dis 2003; 5: 81–90

7. Payton S, Cahill C, Randall J, et al. Alzheimer's disease drug discovery targeted to the APP mRNA 5′-untranslated region; paroxetine and dimercaptopropanol are drug hits. J Mol Neurosci 2004; 20: 267–75

8. Griffin WS, Stanley LC, Ling C, et al. Brain interleukin 1 and S-100 immunoreactivity are elevated in Down syndrome and Alzheimer disease. Proc Natl Acad Sci USA 1989; 86: 7611–15

9. Blasko I, Stampfer-Kountchev M, Saurwein-Teissl M, et al. Co-stimulatory effects of interferon-gamma and interleukin-1beta or tumor necrosis factor alpha on the synthesis of Abeta1-40 and Abeta1-42 by human astrocytes. Neurobiol Dis 2000; 7: 682–9

10. Goldgaber D, Harris HW, Hla T, et al. Interleukin 1 regulates synthesis of amyloid beta-protein precursor mRNA in human endothelial cells. Proc Natl Acad Sci USA 1989; 86: 7606–10

11. Lahiri DK NC. Promoter activity of the gene encoding the beta-amyloid precursor protein is up-regulated by growth factors, phorbol ester, retinoic acid and interleukin-1. Brain Res Mol Brain Res 1995; 32: 233–40

12. Rajagopalan LE, Malter JS. Growth factor-mediated stabilization of amyloid precursor protein mRNA is mediated by a conserved 29-nucleotide sequence in the 3′-untranslated region. J Neurochem 2000; 74: 52–9

13. Amara FM, Junaid A, Clough RR, Liang B. TGF-beta(1), regulation of Alzheimer amyloid precursor protein mRNA expression in a normal human astrocyte cell line: mRNA stabilization. Brain Res Mol Brain Res 1999; 71: 42–9

14. Mbella EG, Bertrand S, Huez G, Octave JN. A GG nucleotide sequence of the 3′ untranslated region of amyloid precursor protein mRNA plays a key role in the regulation of translation and the binding of proteins. Mol Cell Biol 2000; 20: 4572–9

15. Rogers JT. Ferritin translation by interleukin-1: the role of sequences upstream of the start codons of the heavy and light subunit genes. Blood 1996; 87: 2525–37

16. Lesne S, Docagne F, Gabriel C, et al. Transforming growth factor-beta 1 potentiates amyloid-beta generation in astrocytes and in transgenic mice. J Biol Chem 2003; 278: 18408–18

17. Steel D, DeBeer M, DeBeer F, Whitehead AS. Biosynthesis of human acute-phase serum amyloid A protein (A-SAA) in vitro: the roles of mRNA accumulation, poly(A) tail shortening and translational efficiency. J Biochem 1993; 291: 701–7

18. Kindy MS, Yu J, de Beer FC. Expression of mouse acute-phase (SAA1.1) and constitutive (SAA4) serum amyloid A isotypes: influence on lipoprotein profiles. Arterioscler Thromb Vasc Biol J 2000; 20: 1543–50

19. Morrone G, Ciliberto G, Oliviero S, et al. Recombinant interleukin-6 regulates the transcriptional activation of a set of human acute phase response genes. J Biol Chem 1988; 263: 12554–8

20. Das S, Potter H. Expression of the Alzheimer amyloid-promoting factor antichymotrypsin is induced in human astrocytes by IL-1. Neuron 1995; 14: 447–56

21. Kordula T, Bugno M, Rydel RE, Travis J. Mechanism of interleukin-1- and tumor necrosis factor alpha-dependent regulation of the alpha 1-antichymotrypsin gene in human astrocytes. J Neurosci 2000; 20: 7510–16

22. Nilsson LN, Bales KR, DiCarlo G, et al. Alpha-1-antichymotrypsin promotes beta-sheet amyloid plaque deposition in a transgenic mouse model of Alzheimer's disease. J Neurosci 2001; 21: 1444–51

23. Abraham CR, McGraw WT, Slot F, Yamin R. Alpha 1-antichymotrypsin inhibits Abeta degradation in vitro and in vivo. Ann NY Acad Sci 2000; 920: 245–8

24. Itagaki S, McGeer PL, Akiyama H, et al. Relationship of microglia and astrocytes to amyloid deposits of Alzheimer's disease. J Neuroimmuno 1989; 24: 173–82

25. Giulian D, Baker TJ, Shih LN, Lachman LB. Interleukin-1 of the central nervous system is produced by ameboid microglia. J Exp Med 1986; 164: 594–604

26. Thomas T, Thomas G, Mclendon C, et al. Beta-Amyloid-mediated vasoactivity and vascular endothelial damage. Nature 1996; 380: 168–71

27. Karin M. The regulation of AP-1 activity by mitogen-activated protein kinases. J Biol Chem 1995; 270: 16483–6

28. Klausner R, Rouault TA, Harford JB. Regulating the fate of mRNA: the control of cellular iron metabolism. Cell 1993; 72: 19–28

29. McKie AT, Marciani P, Rolfs A, et al. A novel duodenal iron-regulated transporter, IREG implicated in the basolateral transfer of iron to the circulation. Mol Cell 2000; 5: 299–309

30. Gunshin H, Allerson CR, Polycarpou-Schwarz M, et al. Iron-dependent regulation of the divalent metal ion transporter. FEBS Lett 2001; 509: 309–16

31. Cox TC, Bawden MJ, Martin A, May BK. Human erythroid 5-aminolevulinate synthase: promoter analysis and identification of an iron-responsive element in the mRNA. EMBO J 1991; 10: 1891–902

32. Leedman P, Stein AR, Chin WW, Rogers JT. Thyroid hormone modulates the interaction between the iron regulatory protein and ferritin mRNA iron-responsive elements. J Biol Chem 1996; 271: 12017–23

33. Thomson AM, Rogers JT, Leedman PJ. Iron-regulatory proteins, iron-responsive elements and ferritin mRNA translation. Int J Biochem Cell Biol 1999; 31: 1139–52

34. Thomson AM, Rogers JT, Leedman PJ. Thyrotropin-releasing hormone and epidermal growth factor regulate iron- regulatory protein binding in pituitary cells via protein kinase C-dependent and -independent signaling pathways [In Process Citation]. J Biol Chem 2000; 275: 31609–15

35. Bodovitz S, Falduto MT, Frail DE, Klein WL. Iron levels modulate alpha-secretase cleavage of amyloid precursor protein. J Neurochem 1995; 64: 307–15

36. Grimaldi LM, Casadei VM, Ferri C, et al. Association of early-onset Alzheimer's disease with an interleukin-1alpha gene polymorphism [In Process Citation]. Ann Neurol 2000; 47: 361–5

37. Sampietro M, Caputo L, Casatta A, et al. The hemochromatosis gene affects the age of onset of sporadic Alzheimer's disease. Neurobiol Aging 2001; 22: 563–8

38. Wisniewski KE, Wisniewski HM, Wen G. Occurrence of neuropathological changes and dementia of Alzheimer's disease in Down's syndrome. Ann Neurol 1985; 17: 278–82

39. Levy-Lahad E, Wasco W, Poorkaj P, et al. Candidate gene for the chromosome 1 familial Alzheimer's disease locus. Science 1995; 269: 973–7

40. Abraham C, Selkoe DJ, Potter H. Immunochemical identification of the serine protease inhibitor α1-antichymotrypsin in the brain amyloid deposits of Alzheimer's disease. Cell 1988; 52: 487–501

41. Robinson S, Noone DF, Kril J, Haliday GM. Most amyloid plaques contain ferritin rich cells. Alzheimer's Res 1995; 1: 191–3

42. Connor JR, Menzies SL, St. Martin SM, Mufson EJ. A histochemical study of iron, transferrin, and ferritin in Alzheimer's diseased brains. J Neurosci Res 1992; 31: 75–83

43. Cherny R, Atwood CS, Xilinas ME, et al. Treatment with copper–zinc chelator markedly and rapidly inhibits beta-amyloid accumulation in Alzheimer's disease transgenic mice. Neuron 2001; 30: 641–2

44. Ritchie CW, Bush AI, Mackinnon A, et al. Metal-protein attenuation with iodochlorhydroxyquin (clioquinol) targeting Aβ amyloid deposition and toxicity in Alzheimer's disease: a pilot phase 2 clinical trial. Arch Neurol 2004; in press

45. Crapper McLachlan D, Dalton AJ, Kruck TPA, et al. Intramuscular desferrioxamine in patients with Alzheimer's disease. Lancet 1991; 337: 1304–8

46. Multhaup G, Schlicksupp A, Hesse L, et al. The amyloid precursor protein of Alzheimer's disease in the reduction of copper(II) to copper(I). Science 1996; 271: 1406–9

47. Bush AI. The metallobiology of Alzheimer's disease. Trends Neurosci 2003; 26: 207–14

48. Greig NH, Pei XF, Soncrant TT, et al. Phenserine and ring C hetero-analogues: drug candidates for the treatment of Alzheimer's disease. Med Res Rev 1995; 15: 3–31

49. Giacobini E. In Becker R Giacobini E, eds. Alzheimer's Disease: from Molecular Biology to Therapy. Boston: Birkhäuser, 1997: 187–204

50. Shaw KT, Utsuki T, Rogers J, et al. Phenserine regulates translation of beta-amyloid precursor protein mRNA by a putative interleukin-1 responsive element, a target for drug development. Proc Natl Acad Sci USA 2001; 98: 7605–10

51. Preiss T, Hentze MW. Dual function of the messenger RNA cap structure in poly(A)-tail-promoted translation in yeast. Nature 1998; 392: 516–20

52. Fisher A. Therapeutic strategies in Alzheimer's disease: m1 muscaric agonists. Jpn J Pharmacol 2000; 84: 101–12

53. Fisher A, Michaelson DM, Brandeis R, et al. M1 muscarinic agonists as potential disease-modifying agents in Alzheimer's disease. Rationale and perspectives. Ann NY Acad Sci 2000; 920: 315–20

54. Nitsch RM, Deng M, Tennis M, et al. The selective muscarinic M1 agonist AF102B decreases levels of total Abeta in the cerebrospinal fluid of patients with Alzheimer's disease. Ann Neurol 2000; 48: 913–18

55. Lin L, Georgievska B, Mattsson A, Isacson O. Cognitive changes and modified processing of amyloid precursor protein in the cortical and hippocampal system after cholinergic synapse loss and muscarinic receptor activation. Proc Natl Acad Sci USA 1999; 96: 12108–13

56. Nitsch RM, Slack BE, Wurtman RJ, Growdon JH. Release of Alzheimer amyloid precursor derivatives stimulated by activation of muscarinic acetylcholine receptors. Science 1992; 258: 304–7

57. Buxbaum J, Oishi M, Chen HI, et al. Cholinergic agonists and interleukin-1 regulate processing and secretion of the Alzheimer β/A4 amyloid precursor. Proc Natl Acad Sci USA 1992; 89: 10075–8

Chapter 36

Modulation of Alzheimer's amyloidosis by statins: possible mechanisms of action

S Petanceska, M Pappolla, LM Refolo

INTRODUCTION

Being the major cause of dementia in the elderly population of the world, Alzheimer's disease (AD) poses a health problem of pandemic proportions. Currently, there are 35 million people affected by AD worldwide, and it is estimated that by the year 2030 this number will be greater than 60 million. AD is extremely costly to the patients, their families and society as a whole; in 2003 an estimated $100 billion was spent in the USA alone on health-care expenses and lost wages for AD patients and their caregivers. The prediction is that, by the year 2030, $375 billion will be spent annually in the USA on AD. Faced with these harrowing statistics, scientists are hurrying to find new medicines for the prevention and treatment of AD. In the case of AD, the very difficult and costly process of drug discovery is further complicated by the fact that the exact cause(s) of the disease are still unknown and that early diagnosis of the disease is not available.

A multiplicity of genetic and environmental factors determine the degree of risk and age of onset of AD. The majority of AD cases (more than 90%) are sporadic, with an age of onset of 65 or older. The identification of factors that influence the onset or progression of the sporadic form of the disease, or both, is a key step towards understanding its mechanism(s) and for developing successful rational therapies. A small percentage of AD cases are inherited in an autosomal dominant fashion due to mutations in one of three familial AD genes: the amyloid precursor protein (*APP*), presenilin 1 (*PS1*) and presenilin 2 (*PS2*).[1]

Although the pathogenesis of AD is complex, there is compelling evidence that the neuritic dystrophy, neurofibrillary tangle formation, microglial reactivity, gliosis and other degenerative changes observed in the brains of AD patients are a result of the cerebral accumulation and deposition of amyloid β (Aβ) peptides.[2,3] Aβ peptides are generated by proteolytic processing of the amyloid precursor protein (APP), a type I, single transmembrane glycoprotein, as a result of the action of β- and γ-secretase activities. Alternatively, APP can be cleaved by α-secretase, which precludes the formation of Aβ. The relative utilization of each processing route is controlled by numerous signal transduction pathways.[4] Since cerebral accumulation and subsequent deposition of Aβ seem necessary for both disease initiation and its clinical progression, therapies that attenuate these processes might delay onset and/or retard disease progression.

CHOLESTEROL METABOLISM AS A THERAPEUTIC TARGET FOR ALZHEIMER'S DISEASE

A number of epidemiological studies point to a link between cholesterol metabolism and AD pathology (reviewed in reference 5). Several studies have identified a significant correlation between hypercholesterolemia and the risk of developing AD; other studies, however, have not observed such a correlation.[6–10] Experimental studies support the proposed link between hypercholesterolemia and AD, and point to Aβ metabolism as the mechanistic connection. Numerous *in vitro* studies with neuronal and non-neuronal cells have shown that changes in cellular cholesterol content are associated with changes in APP processing, such that an increase in cellular cholesterol content leads to elevated production of Aβ peptides, and that the decrease in cellular cholesterol results in reduced production of Aβ peptides and/or in increased secretion of secretary APPα (sAPPα), the product of non-amyloidogenic processing.[11–18]

The exact mechanism by which cholesterol regulates Aβ production at the cellular level is not known, but there is evidence that changes in membrane cholesterol content or in the ratio of membrane cholesterol to cytosolic cholesterol esters affect the activity and subcellular distribution of APP secretases and consequently Aβ production.[11,15,17,19] This is to be expected, bearing in mind that cholesterol is a key component of all eukaryotic membranes and that both APP and the secretases are transmembrane proteins. The cholesterol content of cellular membranes not only determines their physical properties, such as ordering, rigidity and fluidity, but also regulates vesicular trafficking.[20]

Moreover, since all of the secretase cleavage sites lie within, or near, the transmembrane domain of APP, as membrane cholesterol levels change so does the accessibility of the processing sites, β- and γ- in particular, to their cognate secretases.

Studies with animal models, such as rabbits, guinea pigs and Aβ-depositing transgenic mice, have provided proof-of-concept that cholesterol modulates brain Aβ accumulation and deposition. Diet-induced hypercholesterolemia has been associated with increased brain Aβ accumulation and deposition, while pharmacologically induced hypocholesterolemia attenuated brain Aβ accumulation and deposition.[21–24] Diet- or pharmacologically induced changes in plasma and brain cholesterol also have been associated with changes in APP processing, suggesting that altering brain and/or plasma cholesterol content leads to changes in Aβ production.[22,23]

APOLIPOPROTEIN E, A MECHANISTIC LINK BETWEEN CHOLESTEROL AND Aβ METABOLISM

Apolipoprotein E (apoE) is the major lipid carrier protein in the central nervous system (CNS) involved in brain development and in brain regeneration after injury.[25] In conjunction with the low-density lipoprotein (LDL) receptor family, apoE mediates the exchange of cholesterol between brain cells.[26] The human *apoE* gene has three alleles (ε2, ε3, ε4) coding for three protein isoforms: apoE2, apoE3 and apoE4. The *apoE* ε4 allele is associated with an increased risk for late-onset AD.[27] Individuals with two copies of the *apoE4* allele are also predisposed to elevated serum cholesterol levels, and are at greater risk for developing cardiovascular disease.

ApoE binds Aβ and has been shown to affect the process of Aβ fibrillogenesis *in vitro* and *in vivo* (reviewed in reference 5). Studies with transgenic mice carrying human APP transgenes and different isoforms of human apoE have revealed a role of apoE as a chaperone that facilitates the conversion of Aβ into the insoluble fibrillar form of amyloid in an isoform-specific manner.[28] Under conditions when the production of Aβ remains constant, the extent of neuritic plaque formation is proportional to the amount of apoE3 expressed in the brain, and this process is further enhanced in mice expressing human apoE4.[29,30] In support of the role of apoE in Aβ deposition is the finding that human APP-carrying mice that are apoE-deficient fail to form amyloid deposits.[31] There is also evidence that both human and mouse apoE significantly affect the age of onset, as well as the levels, structure and anatomical distribution, of brain Aβ deposits in a transgenic mouse model of Alzheimer's amyloidosis.[32]

Cholesterol regulates apoE expression *in vitro* and *in vivo*. In rats, diet-induced hypercholesterolemia resulted in an increase in apoE in both serum and liver and increased the levels of apoE mRNA in liver.[33–35] A diet high in lipids was also shown to result in elevation of apoE levels in mouse and rabbit brain.[14,36] While the mechanism for the upregulation of brain apoE by cholesterol remains unknown, this regulation may in part explain the link between cholesterol metabolism, the apoE genotype and the risk for developing AD. In support of this hypothesis are findings that the levels of apoE are higher in the brains and plasma of AD patients compared to age-matched controls, and evidence that certain polymorphisms of the apoE promoter conferring higher apoE expression are associated with increased risk for AD, independent of the risk due to the *apoE* ε4 allele.[7,9,37,38]

STATINS FOR ALZHEIMER'S DISEASE THERAPY

In support of the hypothesis that hypercholesterolemia is a risk factor for AD are the results of retrospective epidemiological studies that have reported a marked reduction in AD prevalence or risk of developing AD in patients taking statins for the treatment of coronary artery disease (CAD) compared to individuals taking non-statin therapies or not receiving treatment for this condition.[39–42] Statins are the most widely prescribed medications for the treatment of hypercholesterolemia and hyperlipidemia-related CAD. These compounds are inhibitors of 3-hydroxy 3-methylglutaryl (HMG) CoA reductase, the enzyme that catalyzes the first, rate-limiting step in the *de novo* pathway of cholesterol biosynthesis; the resulting decrease in cellular cholesterol leads to a compensatory increase in cholesterol uptake by the LDL receptors and to a concomitant decrease in total plasma cholesterol and LDL-cholesterol.[43] Although the above-mentioned epidemiological studies used a retrospective, case–control design, they offered great hope that statin therapy would be efficacious in preventing and/or treating AD. Currently, five statins are on the market in the USA: atorvastatin (Lipitor®), simvastatin (Zocor®), pravastatin (Pravacol®), fluvastatin (Lescol®) and lovastatin (Mevacor®). Perhaps the most attractive feature of a potential statin therapy for AD is that they are approved by the Food and Drug Assosciation (FDA) and well tolerated when used chronically. This is a considerable advantage over other potential Aβ-reducing therapies (e.g. secretase inhibitors and Aβ vaccine) that are currently in the AD therapeutics pipeline.

A number of experimental studies imply that a likely mechanism by which statins reduce the risk of developing AD is by modulating Aβ metabolism. Statin treatment of cultured neuronal cells increases the production of sAPPα and/or reduces the production of Aβ.[12,15,21] Chronic simvastatin treatment of guinea pigs resulted in a significant decrease in Aβ peptides in the cerebrospinal fluid (CSF).[21] The results of two recent randomized placebo-controlled clinical trials are also encouraging. A dose-dependent decrease in plasma Aβ levels was observed in hypercholesterolemic subjects treated with lovastatin for 3 months.[12] Chronic simvastatin treatment of normocholesterolemic subjects diagnosed with mild or moderate AD resulted in a significant decrease in CSF Aβ40 in a *post hoc* analysis of subjects with mild AD compared to placebo-treated patients. This decrease correlated with a decrease in 24S-hydroxycholesterol, a product of brain cholesterol metabolism. Most importantly, the patients receiving simvastatin underwent a slower cognitive decline over time compared to the placebo-treated patients.[44]

These clinical observations emphasize the need for preclinical studies in animal models of AD so that one can determine: which AD-related pathological features are being alleviated in response to statin treatment; the relative efficacy with which different statins alleviate such features; and the mechanism by which they act to attenuate these disease phenotype(s). Here, we discuss the results of a previously reported preclinical study aimed at testing the ability of atorvastatin (Lipitor) to attenuate brain Aβ accumulation in the PSAPP transgenic mouse model of Alzheimer's amyloidosis.[45–47]

ATORVASTATIN DELAYS THE ONSET OF Aβ DEPOSITION IN THE PSAPP MOUSE MODEL OF ALZHEIMER'S AMYLOIDOSIS

We tested the ability of atorvastatin (Lipitor) to delay the onset of Aβ deposition in the PSAPP transgenic mouse model using a chronic treat-ment paradigm.[23] Atorvastatin was chosen because it is the most widely prescribed statin and because it was the first statin used in a phase II therapeutic trial with patients with probable AD. Chronic (8 weeks) atorvastatin treatment, beginning at an age prior to the onset of Aβ deposition, reduced the levels of total cholesterol in the plasma without altering the levels of total cholesterol in the cortex or cerebellum (Figure 36.1).[47] This was in contrast with previous observations, where treatment with BM15.766, a cholesterol-lowering drug that inhibits 7-dehydrocholesterol-Δ-reductase, the enzyme that catalyzes the last step in the *de novo* cholesterol biosynthesis pathway, resulted in a modest but significant decrease in total brain cholesterol.[23] This difference was probably due to the fact that: atorvastatin is hydrophilic and has much lower blood–brain barrier (BBB) permeability compared to BM15.766;[48] or because inhibitors of sterol reductases, such as BM15.766, are more powerful inhibitors of total sterol biosynthesis than are HMG CoA-reductase inhibitors.[49]

The atorvastatin-induced hypocholes-terolemia was associated with a significant reduction in brain Aβ40 and brain Aβ42 levels (Figure 36.2).[47] On average, approximately 2.5-fold reduction was observed for each peptide in response to drug treatment, compared to vehicle treament. This reduction in brain Aβ levels was accompanied by a similar (more than 2-fold) reduction in amyloid load (Figure 36.3).[47] The steady-state levels of full-length APP, as well as the levels of the products of non-amyloidogenic processing (sAPPα) or amyloidogenic processing (β-C-terminal fragment (CTF)-APP) did not change significantly in response to atorvastatin as determined by semiquantitative Western blot and immunoprecipitation/Western blot analyses of the same extracts used for measuring brain Aβ levels (unpublished observation). The effects of atorvastatin on APP processing were different

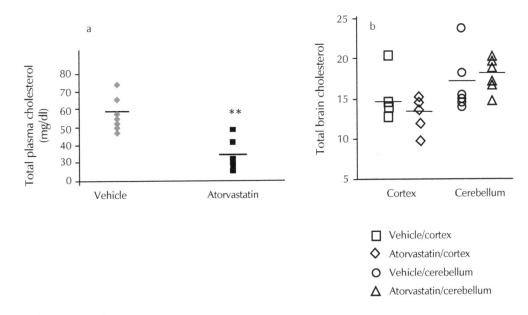

Figure 36.1 Atorvastatin treatment lowers total plasma cholesterol but does not alter central nervous system cholesterol levels. (a) Eight-week-old PSAPP mice were treated with Lipitor® (30 mg atorvastatin/kg body weight per day, p.o.) or vehicle (0.5% methylcellulose in strawberry drink) for 8 weeks. Total cholesterol levels in plasma were determined by gas chromatography. ** $p = 0.001$. (b) Cortices and cerebella were dissected out and processed for measuring total cholesterol by gas chromatography

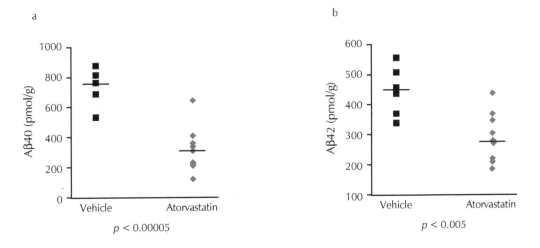

Figure 36.2 Atorvastatin treatment reduces brain amyloid β (Aβ) levels. Eight-week-old PSAPP mice were given atorvastatin ($n = 10$) or vehicle ($n = 6$), for 8 weeks. Brain hemispheres were removed and homogenized in 70% formic acid. High-speed supernatants were generated and, after being neutralized, were used for measuring Aβ40 (a) and Aβ42 (b) levels by enzyme-linked immunosorbent assays. From references 22 and 23

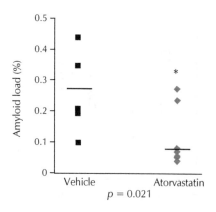

$p = 0.021$

Figure 36.3 Atorvastatin treatment reduces amyloid load. Amyloid β deposits in the brains of PSAPP mice treated with either atorvastatin ($n = 10$) or vehicle ($n = 6$) were visualized by immunostaining with the monoclonal antibody 4G8 (Signet). For each animal, two sets of three serial 5 μm-thick sections, that were 2 mm apart, were immunostained with 4G8, and the amyloid load was quantified by image analysis using a digital computerized system (Olympus Instruments)

from the effects of BM15.766; BM15.766 treatment decreased the amyloidogenic processing of APP, reflected in decreased levels of the processing intermediate β-CTF-APP, and increased the non-amyloidogenic processing of APP, reflected in increased levels of sAPPα.[23]

The observation that BM15.766 and atorvastatin both attenuated Aβ accumulation, but exhibited different effects on APP processing, implies that statins with different biophysical properties (i.e. relative hydrophilicity) might attenuate brain amyloidosis via different mechanisms. Changes in APP processing were observed in the brains of mice treated with BM15.766, a lypophilic, brain-penetrant compound that significantly reduced total brain cholesterol levels.[23] Treatment with atorvastatin, a hydrophilic compound with poor BBB permeability, had no effect on total brain cholesterol and was not associated with significant changes in brain APP processing. Based on these

observations, we propose that changes in brain cholesterol drive changes in brain APP processing. Examining changes in APP processing in the brain, in response to treatment with a statin with both high BBB permeability and an ability to lower brain cholesterol-lowering (e.g. simvastatin, or lovastatin), would test this hypothesis. The relative lipophilicity, i.e. BBB permeability of statins, could be a key determinant of the efficacy and the mechanism with which they will reduce brain amyloidosis, and consequently will affect their therapeutic value for AD.

The hypocholesterolemia induced by chronic atorvastatin treatment was also associated with reduced apoE levels in the brain, as determined by semiquantitative Western blotting of protein from the extracts used for Aβ enzyme-linked immunosorbent assays (ELISAs) (unpublished observations). This is in agreement with the strong positive correlation that we observed between total plasma cholesterol, brain apoE levels and the levels of formic-acid extractable brain Aβ in a PSAPP transgenic mouse model (Figure 36.4).[22,23,47] The strong positive correlation between the levels of cholesterol and brain apoE suggests that cholesterol, or one of its metabolites, regulates *apoE* gene expression in brain. This hypothesis is supported by the previously reported findings that cholesterol regulates hepatic apoE gene expression and that 25S-hydroxycholesterol, a metabolite formed by hydroxylation of cholesterol in the brain, is a potent regulator of apoE gene transcription.[50]

A WORKING HYPOTHESIS

The study described in this chapter provides experimental evidence that statin treatment can attenuate cerebral Aβ accumulation. Together with observations by other groups, this study supports the hypothesis that one of the ways by which statins act to decrease the prevalence or

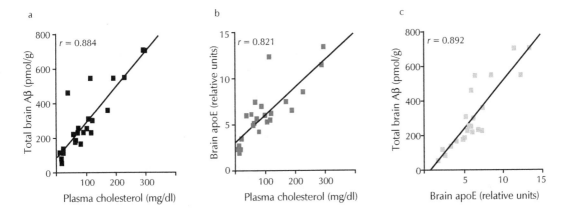

Figure 36.4 Positive correlation between total plasma cholesterol levels, brain apolipoprotein E (apoE) levels and brain amyloid β (Aβ). Data points for total plasma cholesterol, brain apoE and total brain Aβ (a–c) from a high-cholesterol experimental group, a BM15.766-treated group and a basal-diet group of PSAPP mice were used for each correlation analysis. From references 22 and 23

the risk of developing AD is by attenuating the process of brain Aβ accumulation. The mechanisms of the *in vivo* Aβ-lowering activity of statins can be multiple (Figure 36.5). The existing evidence suggests that the effects of statins on brain amyloidosis are a result of their ability to decrease the amyloidogenic processing of APP and/or a result of their apoE-reducing effect, and that both of these effects are a function of their lipid-lowering activity. However, a number of other activities of statins that are largely independent of their lipid-lowering effects might also contribute to their effect on brain Aβ accumulation, such as their anti-inflammatory, vascular and antioxidant effects.[51,52] In support of this notion are the findings of one retrospective epidemiological study showing that non-statin lipid-lowering drugs were not associated with decreased prevalence of AD.[39]

The anti-inflammatory activities of statins are of particular interest when evaluating these compounds as potential AD therapy, since chronic inflammation is one of the salient

features of AD pathology,[53] and an abundance of clinical studies have shown decreased prevalence of AD in populations taking non-steroidal anti-inflammatory drugs.[54] Moreover, studies with different transgenic mouse models of Alzheimer's amyloidosis have shown that chronic treatment with anti-inflammatory and immunomodulatory compounds significantly reduced brain amyloidosis.[55–57] Recent experimental evidence points to the peroxisome proliferator activated receptors (PPAR), as one of the likely mediators of the anti-inflammatory effects of statins in the brain. Atorvastatin can activate PPARγ in peripheral monocytes;[58] other *in vitro* studies have shown that the activation of this receptor can prevent Aβ-induced neurotoxicity mediated by microglia[59] as well as reversing the increase in Aβ production by neuronal cells in response to pro-inflammatory cytokines.[60] In light of these observations and the growing appreciation of statins as anti-inflammatory and immunomodulatory agents,[61] it is important to examine their effect on the inflammatory response in the brain and to

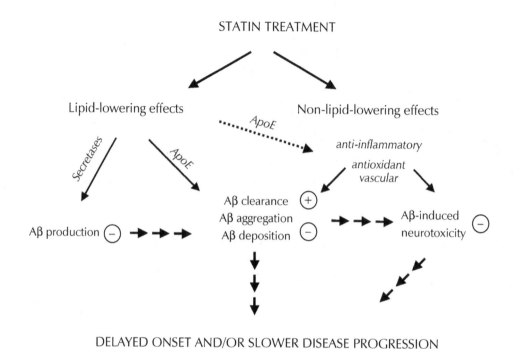

Figure 36.5 A working hypothesis of the mechanisms by which statins might attenuate brain amyloidosis

evaluate the contribution of these activities to the overall Aβ-lowering effect of statins *in vivo*.

Statins also exert multiple beneficial effects on the vasculature, independent of their lipid-lowering effect.[51,52] Recently lovastatin was shown to inhibit Aβ-induced vasoconstriction of rat aortic rings *in vitro*.[62] It would be of relevance to explore whether statins reduce brain amyloidosis, in part, by altering the Aβ equilibrium between the CNS and the plasma through their vascular effects.

Applying different statin-treatment regimens to the available transgenic mouse models of AD in conjunction with extensive biochemical and immunohistochemical analyses will help to elucidate the mechanisms by which statins attenuate brain amyloidosis. Such studies, in parallel with the assessment of behavioral outcomes of chronic statin treatment in these animals models, will be of great value for the design of future randomized clinical trials, and will facilitate the design of efficacious and safe statin-like drugs for AD treatment and/or prevention.

ACKNOWLEDGEMENTS

This work was supported by the Alzheimer's Association, the Institute for the Study of Aging, and the National Institute for Aging. The monoclonal antibodies used in the ELISA assays to detect Aβ40 and Aβ42 antibodies were generously provided by Dr Mark Mercken from Johnson and Johnson Pharmaceuticals.

REFERENCES

1. Hutton M, Perez-Tur J, Hardy J. Genetics of Alzheimer's disease Essays Biochem 1998; 33: 117

2. Naslund J, Haroutunian V, Mohs R, et al. Correlation between elevated levels of amyloid beta-peptide in the brain and cognitive decline. J Am Med Assoc 2000; 283: 1571

3. Parvathy S, Davies P, Haroutunian V, et al. Correlation between Abetax-40-, Abetax-42-, and Abetax-43-containing amyloid plaques and cognitive decline. Arch Neurol 2001; 58: 2025

4. Gandy S, Petanceska S. Regulation of Alzheimer beta-amyloid precursor trafficking and metabolism. Biochim Biophys Acta 2000; 492: 44

5. Tomiyama T, Corder EH, Mori H. Molecular pathogenesis of apolipoprotein E-mediated amyloidosis in late-onset Alzheimer's disease. Cell Mol Life Sci 1999; 56: 268

6. Jarvik GP, Austin MA, Fabsitz RR, et al. Genetic influences on age-related change in total cholesterol, low density lipoprotein-cholesterol, and triglyceride levels: longitudinal apolipoprotein E genotype effects. Genet Epidemiol 1994; 11: 375

7. Jarvik GP, Wijsman EM, Kukull WA, et al. Interactions of apolipoprotein E genotype, total cholesterol level, age, and sex in prediction of Alzheimer's disease: a case-control study. Neurology 1995; 45:1092

8. Kivipelto M, Laakso MP, Tuomolehto J, et al. Hypertension and hypercholesterolaemia as risk factors for Alzheimer's disease: potential for pharmacological intervention. CNS Drugs 2002; 16: 435

9. Notkola IL, Sulkava R, Pekkanen J, et al. Serum total cholesterol, apolipoprotein E epsilon 4 allele, and Alzheimer's disease. Neuroepidemiology 1998; 17: 14

10. Romas SN, Tang MX, Berglund L, Mayeux R. APOE genotype, plasma lipids, lipoproteins, and AD in community elderly Neurology 1999; 53: 517

11. Bodovitz S, Klein WL. Cholesterol modulates alpha-secretase cleavage of amyloid precursor protein. J Biol Chem 1996; 271: 4436

12. Buxbaum JD, Cullen EI, Friedhoff LT. Pharmacological concentrations of the HMG-CoA reductase inhibitor lovastatin decrease the formation of the Alzheimer beta-amyloid peptide in vitro and in patients. Front Biosci 2002; 7: 50

13. Frears ER, Stephens DJ, Walters CE, et al. The role of cholesterol in the biosynthesis of beta-amyloid. Neuroreport 1999; 10: 1699

14. Howland DS, Trusko SP, Savage MJ. Modulation of secreted beta-amyloid precursor protein and amyloid beta-peptide in brain by cholesterol. J Biol Chem 1998; 273: 16566

15. Kojro E, Gimpi G, Lammich S, et al. Low cholesterol stimulates the nonamyloidogenic pathway by its effect on the alpha -secretase ADAM 10 Proc Natl Acad Sci USA 2001; 98: 5815

16. Mizuno T, Haass C, Michikawa M, Yanagisawa K. Cholesterol-dependent generation of a unique amyloid beta-protein from apically missorted amyloid precursor protein in MDCK cells Biochim Biophys Acta 1998; 1373: 119

17. Puglielli L, Konopka G, Pack-Chung E, et al. Acyl-coenzyme A: cholesterol acyltransferase modulates the generation of the amyloid beta-peptide. Nat Cell Biol 2001; 3: 905

18. Simons M, Keller P, De Strooper B, et al. Cholesterol depletion inhibits the generation of beta-amyloid in hippocampal neurons. Proc Natl Acad Sci USA 1998; 95: 6460

19. Riddell DR, Christie G, Hussain I, Dingwall C. Compartmentalization of beta-secretase (Asp2) into low-buoyant density, noncaveolar lipid rafts. Curr Biol 2001; 11: 1288

20. Prinz W. Cholesterol trafficking in the secretory and endocytic systems. Cell Dev Biol 2002; 13: 197

21. Fassbender K, Simons M, Bergmann C, et al. Simvastatin strongly reduces levels of Alzheimer's disease beta-amyloid peptides

Abeta 42 and Abeta 40 in vitro and in vivo. Proc Natl Acad Sci USA 2001; 98: 5856

22. Refolo LM, Malester B, LaFrancois J, et al. Hypercholesterolemia accelerates the Alzheimer's amyloid pathology in a transgenic mouse model. Neurobiol Dis 2000; 7: 321

23. Refolo LM, Pappolla MA, LaFrancois J, et al. A cholesterol-lowering drug reduces beta-amyloid pathology in a transgenic mouse model of Alzheimer's disease. Neurobiol Dis 2001; 8: 890

24. Sparks DL. Intraneuronal beta-amyloid immunoreactivity in the CNS. Neurobiol Aging 1996; 17: 291

25. Laskowitz DT, Horburgh K, Roses AD. Apolipoprotein E and the CNS response to injury. J Cereb Blood Flow Metab 1998; 18: 465

26. Dietschy JM, Turley SD. Cholesterol metabolism in the brain. Curr Opin Lipid 2001; 12: 105

27. Roses AD, Saunders AM, Corder EH, et al. Influence of the susceptibility genes apolipoprotein E-epsilon 4 and apolipoprotein E-epsilon 2 on the rate of disease expressivity of late-onset Alzheimer's disease. Arzneimittelforschung 1995; 45: 413

28. Holtzman DM. Role of apoe/Abeta interactions in the pathogenesis of Alzheimer's disease and cerebral amyloid angiopathy. J Mol Neurosci 2001; 17: 147

29. Bales KR, Verina T, Cummins DJ, et al. Apolipoprotein E is essential for amyloid deposition in the APP(V717F) transgenic mouse model of Alzheimer's disease. Proc Natl Acad Sci USA 1999; 96: 15233

30. Fagan A, Holtzman DM. Astrocyte lipoproteins, effects of apoE on neuronal function, and role of apoE in amyloid-beta deposition in vivo. Microscopy Res Techn 2000; 49: 297

31. Holtzman DM, Fagan AM, Mackey B, et al. Apolipoprotein E facilitates neuritic and cerebrovascular plaque formation in an Alzheimer's disease model. Ann Neurol 2000; 47: 739

32. Fagan AM, Watson M, Parsadanian M, et al. Human and murine ApoE markedly alters A beta metabolism before and after plaque forma-

tion in a mouse model of Alzheimer's disease. Neurobiol Dis 2002; 9: 305

33. Santillo M, Migliaro A, Mondola P, et al. Dietary and hypothyroid hypercholesterolemia induces hepatic apolipoprotein E expression in the rat: direct role of cholesterol. FEBS Lett 1999; 463: 83

34. Srivastava R. Regulation of the apolipoprotein E by dietary lipids occurs by transcriptional and post-transcriptional mechanisms. Mol Cell Sci 1996; 155: 153

35. Wong L, Rubenstein D. The levels of apolipoprotein-E in hypercholesterolemic rat serum. J Biochem 1997; 56: 161

36. Sparks DL, Liu H, Gross DR, Scheff SW. Increased density of cortical apolipoprotein E immunoreactive neurons in rabbit brain after dietary administration of cholesterol. Neurosci Lett 1995; 187: 142

37. Bullido MJ, Valdivieso F. Apolipoprotein E gene promoter polymorphisms in Alzheimer's disease. Microscopy Res Techn 2000; 50: 261

38. Wang JC, Kwon JM, Shah P. Effect of APOE genotype and promoter polymorphism on risk of Alzheimer's disease. Neurology 2000; 55: 1644

39. Jick H, Zornberg GL, Jick SS, et al. Statins and the risk of dementia. Lancet 2000; 356: 1627

40. Rockwood K, Kirkland S, Hogan, DB, et al. Use of lipid-lowering agents, indication bias, and the risk of dementia in community-dwelling elderly people. Arch Neurol 2002; 59: 223

41. Yaffe K, Barrett-Connor E, Lin F, Grady D. Serum lipoprotein levels, statin use, and cognitive function in older women. Arch Neurol 2002; 59: 378

42. Wolozin B, Kellman W, Ruosseau P, et al. Decreased prevalence of Alzheimer disease associated with 3-hydroxy-3-methylglutaryl coenzyme A reductase inhibitors. Arch Neurol 2000; 57: 1439

43. Moghadasian M. Clinical pharmacology of 3-hydroxy-3-methylglutaryl coenzyme A reductase inhibitors. Life Sci 1999; 65: 1329

44. Simons M, Schwarzler F, Lutjohann D, et al. Treatment with simvastatin in normocholesterolemic patients with Alzheimer's disease: A 26-week randomized, placebo-controlled, double-blind trial. Ann Neurol 2002; 52: 346

45. Holcomb L, Gordon MN, McGowan E, et al. Accelerated Alzheimer-type phenotype in transgenic mice carrying both mutant amyloid precursor protein and presenilin 1 transgenes. Nat Med 1998; 4: 97

46. Petanceska SS, DeRosa S, Olm V, et al. Statin therapy for Alzheimer's disease: will it work? J Mol Neurosci 2002; 19: 155

47. Refolo L, Petanceska S, DeRosa S, et al. Cholesterol Metabolism: a Potential Target for Alzheimer's Disease Therapy Soc. Neurosci Abstr 2001; 31: 583–7

48. Hamelin BA, Turgeon T. 1998. Hydrophilicity/lipophilicity: relevance for the pharmacology and clinical effects of HMG-CoA reductase inhibitors. Trends Pharm Sci 1998; 19: 26

49. Honda A, Salen G, Nguyen LB, et al. Down-regulation of cholesterol biosynthesis in sitosterolemia: diminished activities of acetoacetyl-CoA thiolase, 3-hydroxy-3-methyl-glutaryl-CoA synthase, reductase, squalene synthase, and 7-dehydrocholesterol delta7-reductase in liver and mononuclear leukocytes. Hepatology 1998; 27: 153

50. Gueguen Y, Bertrand P, Ferrari L, et al. Control of apolipoprotein E secretion by 25-hydroxycholesterol and proinflammatory cytokines in the human astrocytoma cell line CCF-STTG1. Cell Biol Toxicol 2001; 17: 191

51. Corsini A. Fluvastatin: effects beyond cholesterol lowering. J Cardiovasc Pharmacol Ther 2000; 5: 161

52. Cucchiara B, Kasner SE. Use of statins in CNS disorders. J Neurol. Sci 2001; 187: 81

53. Neuroinflammation Working Group. Inflammation, autotoxicity and Alzheimer disease. Neurobiol Aging 2000; 21: 383

54. McGeer PL, McGeer EG. Inflammation, autotoxicity and Alzheimer disease. Neurobiol Aging 2001; 22:799

55. Frautschy SA, Hu W, Kim SA, et al. Phenolic anti-inflammatory antioxidant reversal of Abeta-induced cognitive deficits and neuropathology. Neurobiol Aging 2001; 22: 993

56. Jantzen PT, Connor KE, DiCarlo G, et al. Microglial activation and beta-amyloid deposit reduction caused by a nitric oxide-releasing nonsteroidal anti-inflammatory drug in amyloid precursor protein plus presenilin-1 transgenic mice. J Neurosci 2002; 22: 2246

57. Lim GP, Yang F, Chen P, et al. Ibuprofen suppresses plaque pathology and inflammation in a mouse model for Alzheimer's disease. J Neurosci 2001; 20: 5709

58. Grip S, Lindgren J, Lindgren S. Atorvastatin activates PPAR-gamma and attenuates the inflammatory response in human monocytes. Inflamm Res 2002; 51: 58

59. Combs CK, Johnson DE, Karlo JC, et al. Inflammatory mechanisms in Alzheimer's disease: inhibition of beta-amyloid-stimulated proinflammatory responses and neurotoxicity by PPARgamma agonists. J Neurosci 2000; 20: 558

60. Sastre M, Landreth G, Bayer TA, et al. Nonsteroidal anti-inflammatory drugs and peroxisome proliferator-activated receptor-gamma agonists modulate immunostimulated processing of amyloid precursor protein through regulation of beta-secretase. Soc Neurosci Abstr 2002; 32: 483–3

61. Kwak B, Mulhaupt F, Myit S, Mach F. Statins as a newly recognized type of immunomodulator. Nat Med 2000; 6: 1399

62. Paris D, Townsend, KP, Humphrey J, et al. Statins inhibit A beta-neurotoxicity in vitro and A beta-induced vasoconstriction and inflammation in rat aortae. Atheroscler 2002; 19: 293

Chapter 37

β-Secretase – progress and questions

M Citron

INTRODUCTION: WHY CARE ABOUT β-SECRETASE?

The unmet medical need for disease-modifying pharmacotherapy of Alzheimer's disease (AD) continues to grow. Much of AD research over the past 20 years has been focused on the amyloid cascade hypothesis, which states that amyloid-β (Aβ)42, a proteolytic derivative of the large transmembrane amyloid precursor protein (APP), plays an early and critical role in all cases of AD.[1] Consequently, blocking the production of Aβ42, by specific inhibition of the key proteases β- and γ-secretase, which cleave APP to generate Aβ and thus initiate the amyloid cascade, is a major focus of AD therapy research. The identification of β-secretase, the aspartic protease that generates the amino-terminus of Aβ, has triggered many studies to characterize this enzyme. At the same time, improved understanding of the nature of the γ-secretase complex (for a recent review see DeStrooper[2]) has led to concerns about the therapeutic feasibility of γ-secretase inhibition, making the identification of drug-like β-secretase inhibitors all the more important.

CHARACTERIZATION OF β-SECRETASE

We initially identified β-secretase using an expression cloning strategy,[3] and subsequently three other groups reported identification of the same enzyme using different approaches.[4–6] β-Secretase was identified as the transmembrane aspartic protease BACE1, which, together with its subsequently discovered homolog BACE2,[7] forms a new branch of the pepsin family. While the transmembrane domain is unprecedented in mammalian aspartic proteases, the enzyme is otherwise relatively similar to pepsin – this protease would not attract much interest, if it were not involved in AD. BACE1 is a 501-amino acid protein with an amino-terminal signal peptide of 21 amino acids, followed by a pro-protein spanning amino acids 22–45. The luminal domain of the mature protein extends from residues 46 to 460 and is followed by a transmembrane domain of 17 residues and a short cytosolic tail of 24 amino acids. BACE1 contains two active site motifs at amino acids 93–96 and 289–292 in the luminal domain, each containing the highly conserved signature motif of aspartic proteases D T/S G T/S. BACE1 is predicted to be a type 1 transmembrane protein with the active site on the luminal side of the membrane, where APP is cleaved. We have demonstrated that BACE1 exhibits all the properties of β-secretase[3] and we localized the BACE1 gene to chromosome 11q23.3,[7] but no FAD locus or AD risk factor has yet been mapped to this region. However, three intriguing recent studies have suggested that β-secretase may be up-regulated in sporadic AD brains. Whether this up-regulation has a causal role in the disease process or is a late consequence remains to be seen.[8–10] The homolog BACE2 initially attracted much attention: it is localized to the obligate Down's syndrome region of chromosome 21, and its relationship to BACE1 suggested that it may be involved in APP processing as well. However, its brain expression is low[11] and, upon overexpression, it cleaves at the α- rather than the β-secretase cleavage sites of APP,[12] so it is currently proposed to play an anti-amyloidogenic rather than an amyloidogenic role *in vivo*.[13] Several publications have addressed the cell biology and the post-translational modifications of BACE1. The six cysteine residues in the ecto-domain all form intramolecular disulfide bonds in a pattern that is not conserved in other aspartic proteases.[14] BACE1 is initially synthesized as a proprotein that is cleaved at residue E46 to form the mature enzyme. Interestingly, both the proprotein and the mature protein are proteolytically active and the prodomain does not suppress activity as in a strict zymogen, but appears to facilitate proper folding of the active enzyme.[15] The prodomain cleavage is not autocatalytic, as in some other aspartic proteases. Instead, furin, or a furin-like protease, is probably responsible for the pro-peptide cleavage.[16] After full maturation, BACE1 can be phosphorylated within its cytoplasmic domain at Ser498. The phosphorylation regulates retrieval of BACE1 from endocytosed vesicles, a mechanism reminiscent of furin trafficking.[17] Endogenous BACE1 was shown

primarily to localize to the trigerminal nucleus (TGN), from which a small portion is delivered to the plasma membrane, from which it then recycles to endocytic compartments.[18,19] It appears that the BACE1 transmembrane domain contains a TGN targeting signal.[20] Endosomal targeting of BACE1 depends on a cytoplasmic dileucine motif (residues 499 and 500).[18]

CONSIDERATIONS FOR β-SECRETASE INHIBITION

Two sets of data are most desirable to assess the feasibility of therapeutic β-secretase inhibition: analysis of the β-secretase active site crystal structure, which provides information on the opportunities and challenges of small molecule inhibitor development; and study of β-secretase knockout mice, which could highlight potential liabilities of β-secretase inhibition. The X-ray crystal structure of the recombinant BACE1 protease domain complexed to a peptidic inhibitor became available in 2000, just 1 year after publication of the enzyme structure. It was shown that six residues of the inhibitor (P4 to P2′) are bound in the active site of the enzyme. The overall structure of the enzyme is similar to that of other known aspartic proteases, but there are differences in the details of the active site, which is generally more open and less hydrophobic than in other aspartic proteases.[21] Using this information and data on the subsite specificity of BACE1 obtained with a combinatorial peptide library,[22] potent peptidic transition state inhibitors of BACE1 have been generated.[22,23] The main drug-development challenge now is to move from such large peptidic inhibitors to drug-like small molecules with the desired pharmacokinetic properties, in particular brain penetration. As a first step towards this goal, smaller peptidic molecules which achieve cell penetration have been generated.[24] However, going from such research tools to drugs that are stable, orally available and brain penetrant, and which can be manufactured at reasonable cost on a large scale, remains a major challenge.

We and others generated β-secretase knockout mice, because such mice could point to potential liabilities of chronic β-secretase inhibition. In the worst case they could show that mechanism-based toxicity of β-secretase inhibitors precludes the development of such compounds for therapeutic purposes. The finding that β-secretase knockout mice are deficient in Aβ production, independently reported by us and two other groups, was not unexpected, but it did provide ultimate *in vivo* validation of BACE1 as β-secretase and it demonstrated that in mice no compensatory mechanism for β-secretase cleavage exists.[25–27] The more exciting and unexpected aspect of the knockout studies was the absence of major problems due to β-secretase ablation. We analyzed the phenotype of young BACE1 knockout mice and found them to be healthy and fertile. A detailed analysis demonstrated that the knockout mice are normal in terms of gross morphology and anatomy, tissue histology, hematology and clinical chemistry.[25] We have recently extended these studies to include both gene expression profiling and phenotypic assessment of older BACE1 knockout mice. We did not detect global compensatory changes in neural gene expression in young BACE1

knockout mice. In particular, expression of BACE2 was not up-regulated. In BACE1 knockout mice aged to 14 months we found no structural alterations in any organ, including all central and peripheral neural tissues. Aged BACE1 knockout mice engineered to overexpress APP did not develop amyloid deposits, reinforcing the notion that mouse brain has no significant compensatory mechanism for APP cleavage that could avert the absence of BACE1 and drive plaque formation over time.[28] Initial behavioral analysis of the knockout mice generated by Roberds *et al.* showed no obvious deficits in basal neurological and physiological functions.[27] However, a recent poster at the 2002 meeting of the Society for Neuroscience reported a timid and less exploratory pattern of behavior correlating with increased 5-hydroxytryptamine turnover in the hippocampus of BACE1 knockout mice, raising the possibility that BACE1 could play a role in neurotransmitter turnover or release.[29]

Clearly, more studies on behavior of BACE1 knockout mice are needed for full understanding of the more subtle cognitive and behavioral consequences of β-secretase ablation. While one should be cautious not to overinterpret mouse data, no liabilities of β-secretase inhibition have surfaced to suggest that this target should be abandoned. Ultimately, only a clinical trial in humans will test whether β-secretase inhibition can live up to its promise, but it may take some time until drug-like inhibitors are ready.

REFERENCES

1. Hardy J, Selkoe DJ. The amyloid hypothesis of Alzheimer's disease: progress and problems on the road to therapeutics. Science 2002; 297: 353–6

2. DeStrooper B. Aph-1, Pen-2, and nicastrin with presenilin generate an active γ-secretase complex. Neuron 2003; 38: 9–12

3. Vassar R, Bennett BD, Babu-Khan S, et al. β-secretase cleavage of Alzheimer's amyloid precursor protein by the transmembrane aspartic protease BACE. Science 1999; 286: 735–41

4. Sinha S, Lieberburg I. Cellular mechanisms of β-amyloid production and secretion. Proc Natl Acad Sci USA 1999; 96: 11049–53

5. Yan R, Bienkowski MJ, Shuck ME, et al. Membrane-anchored aspartyl protease with Alzheimer's disease β-secretase specificity. Nature 1999; 402: 533–7

6. Hussain I, Powell D, Howlett DR, et al. Identification of a novel aspartic protease (Asp2) as β-secretase. Mol Cell Neurosci 1999; 14: 419–27

7. Saunders AJ, Kim T-W, Tanzi RE, et al. BACE maps to chromosome 11 and a BACE homolog, BACE2, resides in the obligate Down syndrome region of chromosome 21. Science 1999; 286: 1255a

8. Fukumoto H, Cheung BS, Hyman BT, Irizarry MC. β-secretase protein and activity are increased in the neocortex in Alzheimer disease. Arch Neurol 2002; 59: 1381–9

9. Holsinger RMD, McLean CA, Beyreuther K, et al. Increased expression of the amyloid precursor β-secretase in sporadic Alzheimer's disease. Ann Neurol 2002; 51: 783–6

10. Yang LB, Lindholm K, Yan R, et al. Elevated β-secretase expression and enzymatic activity detected in sporadic Alzheimer disease. Nat Med 2003; 9: 3–4

11. Bennett BD, Babu-Khan S, Loeloff R, et al. Expression analysis of BACE2 in brain and peripheral tissues. J Biol Chem 2000; 275: 20647–51

12. Farzan M, Schnitzler CE, Vasilieva N, et al. BACE2, a β-secretase homolog, cleaves at the β-site and within the amyloid-β region of the amyloid-β precursor protein. Proc Natl Acad Sci USA 2000; 97: 9712–17

13. Basi G, Frigon N, Barbour R, et al. Antagonistic effects of β-site amyloid precursor protein-cleaving enzymes 1 and 2 on Aβ production in cells. J Biol Chem 2003; 278: 31512–20

14. Haniu M, Denis P, Young Y, et al. Characterization of Alzheimer's β-secretase protein BACE – a pepsin family member with unusual properties. J Biol Chem 2000; 275: 21099–106

15. Shi XP, Chen E, Yin KC, et al. The pro domain of β-secretase does not confer strict zymogen-like properties but does assist proper folding of the protease domain. J Biol Chem 2001; 276: 10366–73

16. Bennett BD, Denis P, Haniu M, et al. A furin-like convertase mediates propeptide cleavage of BACE, the Alzheimer's β-secretase. J Biol Chem 2000; 275: 37712–17

17. Walter J, Fluhrer R, Hartung B, et al. Phosphorylation regulates intracellular trafficking of β-secretase. J Biol Chem 2001; 276: 14634–41

18. Huse JT, Pijak DS, Leslie GJ, et al. Maturation and endosomal targeting of β-site amyloid precursor protein-cleaving enzyme. J Biol Chem 2000; 275: 33729–37

19. Capell A, Steiner S, Willem M, et al. Maturation and pro-peptide cleavage of β-secretase. J Biol Chem 2000; 275: 30849–54

20. Yan R, Han P, Miao H, et al. The trans-membrane domain of the Alzheimer's

β-secretase (BACE1) determines its late Golgi localization and access to β-amyloid precursor protein (APP) substrate. J Biol Chem 2001; 276: 36788–96

21. Hong L, Koelsch G, Lin X, et al. Structure of the protease domain of memapsin 2 (β-secretase) complexed with inhibitor. Science 2000; 290: 150–3

22. Turner RT, Koelsch G, Hong L, et al. Subsite specificity of memapsin 2 (β-secretase): implications for inhibitor design. Biochemistry 2001; 40: 10001–6

23. Ghosh AK, Bilcer G, Harwood C, et al. Structure-based design: potent inhibitors of human brain memapsin 2 (β-secretase). J Med Chem 2001; 44: 2865–8

24. Hom RK, Fang LY, Mamo S, et al. Design and synthesis of statin-based cell-permeable peptidomimetic inhibitors of human β-secretase. J Med Chem 2003; 46: 1799–802

25. Luo Y, Bolon B, Kahn S, et al. Mice deficient in BACE1, the Alzheimer's β-secretase, have normal phenotype and abolished β-amyloid generation. Nat Neurosci 2001; 4: 231–2

26. Cai H, Wang Y, McCarthy D, et al. BACE1 is the major β-secretase for generation of Aβ peptides by neurons. Nat Neurosci 2001; 4: 233–4

27. Roberds SL, Anderson J, Basi G, et al. BACE knockout mice are healthy despite lacking the primary β-secretase activity in brain: implications for Alzheimer's disease therapeutics. Hum Mol Genet 2001; 10: 1317–24

28. Luo Y, Bolon B, Damore MA, et al. BACE1 (β-secretase) knockout mice do not acquire compensatory gene expression changes or develop neural lesions over time. Neurobiol Dis 2003; 14: 81–8

29. Harper AJ, Pugh P, Harrison S, et al. Unexpected phenotype in BACE1 mice. Poster presented at the Meeting of the Society for Neuroscience, 2002

Chapter 38

Tau phosphorylation and assembly in tauopathies

J Avila, M Pérez, A Gómez-Ramos, JJ Lucas, F Hernández

INTRODUCTION

Alzheimer's disease (AD) is characterized by the presence of two aberrant structures, senile plaques, composed of amyloid-β protein (Aβ), and neurofibrillary tangles (NFT), composed of paired helical filaments (PHF). Isolated PHF are characterized by three different methods: amino acid analysis, gel electrophoresis and immuno-electron microscopy. These have indicated the presence of a high proportion (3–4%) of phosphoserine and threonine residues in PHF protein; an abnormal electrophoretic mobility of tau protein present in PHF, which can be reversed by phosphatase treatment; and the binding of antibodies recognizing phospho-epitopes of tau protein in PHF. These three features support the pioneer observation that tau protein in PHF is in a hyperphosphorylated state.[1,2]

TAU PHOSPHORYLATION

Different kinases have been involved in tau phosphorylation[3] and different motifs for those kinases are present in the tau molecule. The motif S/TXXXS/T, which is the sequence modified by GSK3 kinase, is repeated 22 times in the tau molecule, and several of these sites have been confirmed *in vivo*.[4,5]

Furthermore, a transgenic mouse overexpressing GSK3 has been generated, resembling some pathological tau features observed in AD,[6] including behavior deficits, as determined by the Morris water maze test.[7] However, in this transgenic mouse the formation of PHF-like structures was not observed, although the presence of aggregated phosphorylated tau was not excluded.[6] This observation suggests that tau phosphorylation might be unrelated to tau filament formation; or that it could be necessary, but not sufficient, for that assembly.

TAU PHOSPHORYLATION AND ASSEMBLY

In vitro studies to promote phosphorylated tau filament formation have yielded controversial results. For tau polymerization induced by the addition of polyanions such as heparin, phosphorylated tau showed a decreased capacity to polymerize compared to unmodified tau[8] (M. Pérez, unpublished results). However, when tau polymerization was promoted by compounds such as hydroxynonenal (HNE), phosphorylated

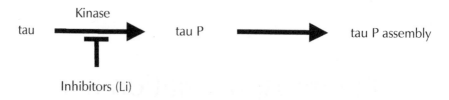

Figure 38.1 Tau phosphorylation (P) leading to tau assembly. Li, lithium

tau, but not unmodified tau, could assemble into filamentous polymers.[9] Little is known about the capacity of phosphorylated tau to polymerize in the presence of fatty acids such as arachidonic acid.[10,11]

On the other hand, in other tauopathy-like frontotemporal dementias associated with chromosome 17 (FTDP-17), tau can assemble into filamentous polymers[12] in a hyperphosphorylated form. This suggests a possible correlation between tau phosphorylation and tau assembly. Tau phosphorylation may take place because mutations in the tau molecule, characteristic of FTDP-17, might prevent the binding of phosphatase PP2A to phosphorylated tau, therefore increasing the proportion of phosphorylated tau.[13]

Thus, different mechanisms could increase the level of phosphorylated tau in different tauopathies. For example, in AD the level of phosphorylated tau could be the result of an increased GSK3 activity, and this kinase activation could be the consequence of the action of Aβ, an antagonist of the insulin receptor[14] that could activate GSK3 kinase. For

progressive supranuclear palsy (PSP), stress kinases such as p38 could be activated and, as a consequence, tau could be phosphorylated.[3] Finally, in FTDP-17, an inhibition of PP2A, as previously indicated, could occur.

To test whether tau phosphorylation is required for tau assembly, a preliminary experiment was carried out. A transgenic tau mouse, bearing three of the mutations present in FTDP-17[15] and able to form tau filaments, was treated with GSK3 kinase inhibitors, and the formation of those filaments was prevented.[16] The results of this experiment suggest that tau phosphorylation could be related to tau assembly, as indicated in Figure 38.1. Tau phosphorylation could favor tau assembly, and if that phosphorylation were prevented by the addition of a compound such as lithium (Li), it would result in an inhibition of a tau kinase such as GSK3, decreasing the aberrant assembly of tau.

In summary, we propose that tau phosphorylation could facilitate tau assembly, although in some cases that phosphorylation might not be sufficient, and additional factors would be necessary to generate aberrant tau polymers.

REFERENCES

1. Grundke-Iqbal I, Iqbal K, Tung YC, et al. Abnormal phosphorylation of the microtubule-associated protein tau (tau) in Alzheimer cytoskeletal pathology. Proc Natl Acad Sci USA 1986; 83: 4913–17

2. Ihara Y, Nukina N, Miura R, Ogawara M. Phosphorylated tau protein is integrated into paired helical filaments in Alzheimer's disease. J Biochem (Tokyo) 1986; 99: 1807–10

3. Gomez-Ramos A, Diaz-Nido J, Smith MA, et al. Effect of the lipid peroxidation product acrolein on tau phosphorylation in neural cells. J Neurosci Res 2003; 71: 863–70

4. Munoz-Montano JR, Moreno FJ, Avila J, Diaz-Nido J. Lithium inhibits Alzheimer's disease-like tau protein phosphorylation in neurons. FEBS Lett 1997; 411: 183–8

5. Munoz-Montano JR, Moreno FJ, Avila J, Diaz-Nido J. Downregulation of glycogen synthase kinase-3beta (GSK-3beta) protein expression during neuroblastoma IMR-32 cell differentiation. J Neurosci Res 1999; 55: 278–85

6. Lucas JJ, Hernandez F, Gomez-Ramos P, et al. Decreased nuclear beta-catenin, tau hyperphosphorylation and neurodegeneration in GSK-3beta conditional transgenic mice. Embo J 2001; 20: 27–39

7. Hernandez F, Borrell J, Guaza C, et al. Spatial learning deficits in transgenic mice that conditionally over-express GSK-3beta in the brain but do not form tau filaments. J Neurochem 2002; 83: 1529–33

8. Barghorn S, Mandelkow E. Toward a unified scheme for the aggregation of tau into Alzheimer paired helical filaments. Biochemistry 2002; 41: 14885–96

9. Perez M, Hernandez F, Gomez-Ramos A, et al. Formation of aberrant phosphotau fibrillar polymers in neural cultured cells. Eur J Biochem 2002; 269: 1484–9

10. Abraha A, Ghoshal N, Gamblin TC, et al. C-terminal inhibition of tau assembly in vitro and in Alzheimer's disease. J Cell Sci 2000; 113: 3737–45

11. Wilson DM, Binder LI. Free fatty acids stimulate the polymerization of tau and amyloid beta peptides. In vitro evidence for a common effector of pathogenesis in Alzheimer's disease. Am J Pathol 1997; 150: 2181–95

12. Goedert M, Crowther RA, Spillantini MG. Tau mutations cause frontotemporal dementias. Neuron 1998; 21: 955–8

13. Goedert M, Jakes R, Qi Z, et al. Protein phosphatase 2A is the major enzyme in brain that dephosphorylates tau protein phosphorylated by proline-directed protein kinases or cyclic AMP-dependent protein kinase. J Neurochem 1995; 65: 2804–7

14. Xie L, Helmerhorst E, Taddei K, et al. Alzheimer's beta-amyloid peptides compete for insulin binding to the insulin receptor. J Neurosci 2002; 22: RC221

15. Lim F, Hernandez F, Lucas JJ, et al. FTDP-17 mutations in tau transgenic mice provoke lysosomal abnormalities and tau filaments in forebrain. Mol Cell Neurosci 2001; 18: 702–14

16. Perez M, Hernandez F, Lim F, et al. Chronic lithium treatment decreases mutant tau protein aggregation in a transgenic mouse model. J Alzheimers Dis 2003; 5: 301–8

Alzheimer's disease: a true tauopathy fueled by amyloid precursor protein dysfunction

A Delacourte

INTRODUCTION

Plaques or tangles?

We know from the pioneer work of Alois Alzheimer[1] that Alzheimer's disease (AD) is characterized by two types of lesion: one is extracellular, corresponding to spherical deposits, and the other is intraneuronal and composed of a fibrillar material named neurofibrillary tangles. These two types of lesion in high number in neocortical regions are the consensus criteria for the neuropathological diagnosis.[2] Biochemical analyses starting in 1984 demonstrated that extracellular amyloid plaques are made of a peptide named amyloid-β (Aβ), of 40–43 amino acid residues.[3] The intraneuronal filamentous lesions, formed by bundles of paired helical filaments, result from the assembly of tau proteins.[4] From the beginning of Alzheimer's research history, researchers have attempted to determine the cause of Alzheimer pathology: plaques or tangles? Or, in molecular terms, Aβ deposition or tau aggregation?[5–9]

Amyloid precursor protein dysmetabolism is central in Alzheimer's disease etiology

At the present time, the initiating cause of neurodegeneration in Alzheimer's disease is still a matter of debate. There is, however, no doubt that amyloid precursor protein (APP) dysfunction is a key event in AD, because mutations altering APP metabolism, such as mutations in APP and presenilin, invariably provoke AD with an early onset. Both familial AD, which is extremely rare, and sporadic AD, have the same distribution and number of amyloid plaques, demonstrating that APP metabolism is central in AD. For sporadic AD, which represents more than 99% of all cases, a number of hypotheses to explain neurodegeneration have been proposed, including the extracellular or intracellular neurotoxicity of Aβ, or a loss of function of APP. In the absence of any genetic mutation, physiopathological processes leading to amyloid deposition and neurodegeneration in sporadic AD remain poorly understood and poorly investigated. The fact is that scientific investment in AD has been inversely proportional to the most represented form of AD and hence, the amyloid cascade hypothesis reflects the major trend of research. This theory relies on aggregated Aβ as the neurotoxic substance provoking the disease.[10] According to this theory, removing Aβ should cure the disease.[11]

Tau pathology is well correlated with cognitive impairment

In parallel, neurofibrillary degeneration, i.e. tau pathology, has been described in the amyloid cascade hypothesis as a late and secondary event, in perfect disagreement with most neuropathological studies. Indeed, all these studies emphasize that neurofibrillary degeneration is also instrumental in the disease.[9,12–17] Our biochemical spatiotemporal analysis of tau pathology in non-demented elderly patients from a prospective and multidisciplinary approach corroborates neuropathological findings.[18] Indeed, neuropathological as well as biochemical approaches show that tau pathology of AD spreads progressively, invariably hierarchically, from the trans-entorhinal cortex to the whole neocortex, along corticocortical connections. The brain regions that are sequentially affected explain the successive types of cognitive impairment that characterize the disease: amnesia following the entorhinal and hippocampal degeneration; aphasia, apraxia and agnosia with the involvement of the neocortex. Of course, amyloid and tau pathology are present before the clinical symptoms, because neuronal plasticity is able to compensate at the first AD stages. Our studies have shown that tau pathology is already distributed in the hippocampal formation and the temporal cortex at the 'pre-clinical' stage of AD.[8]

The questions for this new century

Most of the researchers nowadays are convinced that APP dysfunction as well as tau pathology are important physiopathological factors. However, the precise relationship between these two very different degenerating processes remains a mystery. Understanding the spatiotemporal connection between APP and tau pathology could not only produce a better explanation of AD, but could also open new therapeutic perspectives. Moreover, it is also well established that clinical cognitive impairment is already a late event in the physiopathological development of AD. Therefore, it is essential to investigate both APP and tau pathologies in non-demented patients who have already developed the neuropathological stigmata of the disease. For that purpose, our strategy has been to study the distribution of APP and tau abnormal catabolic products in different brain regions of numerous patients, at different ages and with different cognitive skills or impairments, from perfect memory to dementia, and followed prospectively with a multidisciplinary approach. The aim was to study all possible cases from non-affected to fully affected patients. If the disease spreads along a precise path, we should be able to align all the different pieces of the puzzle along this path.

RELATIONSHIP BETWEEN DEMENTIA, TAU AND Aβ PATHOLOGY

Tau pathology spreading in cortical areas is invariable and hierarchical

The prospective and multidisciplinary study of more than 200 cases, including 70 non-demented patients, showed that tau pathology always extends along ten stages, corresponding to ten brain areas that are successively affected. Paired helical filaments (PHF)-tau pathology, visualized as a triplet of abnormal tau proteins, was systematically found to be present in variable amounts in the entorhinal and hippocampal regions of non-demented patients aged over 75 years. When tau pathology was found in other brain areas, it was always along a stereotyped, sequential, hierarchical pathway. The progression was categorized into ten stages according to the brain regions affected: trans-entorhinal cortex (S1), entorhinal cortex (S2), hippocampus (S3), anterior temporal cortex (S4), inferior temporal cortex (S5), mid-temporal cortex (S6), polymodal association areas (prefrontal, parietal inferior, temporal superior) (S7), unimodal areas (S8), primary motor (S9a) or sensory (S9b, S9c) areas, and all neocortical areas (S10) (Figure 39.1, left). Up to

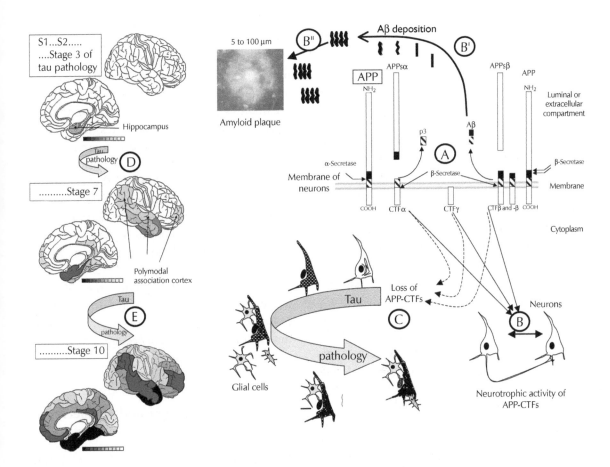

Figure 39.1 The possible synergy of amyloid precursor protein (APP)–tau pathologies in Alzheimer's disease. APP is a transmembrane protein cleaved by different secretases, at the α, β, β' and γ sites (A). The cleavages release several APP carboxy-terminal fragments (APP-CTFs), which probably have a neurotrophic activity (B). Final secretase activities release, in parallel, Aβ peptide (B') that will aggregate into plaques (B''). A decrease of APP-CTFs is observed in Alzheimer's disease, which probably enhances tau pathology and neurodegeneration (C). The stimulated tau degenerating process progresses in brain areas, along corticocortical connections, from stages 1 to 3 (entorhinal then hippocampal formation) to stage 10 (all neocortical areas, via polymodal association areas (stage 7) (D and E)

stage 6, the disease could be asymptomatic. In all cases of our study, stage-7 individuals with two polymodal association areas affected by tau pathology were cognitively impaired.[18]

Distribution of Aβ 42 and 40 species during the course of Alzheimer's disease

Insoluble Aβ 42 and 40 species were fully solubilized and quantified in the main neocortical areas, with a new procedure adapted to human brain tissue. The nature and quantities of Aβ species that aggregate were compared to the extent of tau pathology, as well as to cognitive impairment. In AD, there was a constellation of amyloid phenotypes, extending from cases with exclusively aggregated Aβ 42 to cases with, in addition, large quantities of insoluble Aβ 40 species. Nonetheless, insoluble Aβ 40 detection was often observed late in the amyloid deposition process (starting at stages 4–5). Moreover, we observed that there was no obvious spatial and temporal overlap in the distribution of these two insoluble Aβ species in cortical brain areas. The physical properties were also different. Formic acid-solubilized Aβ 40 aggregates were composed essentially of monomers and dimers, while solubilized Aβ 42 was essentially observed as dimers and multimers. More importantly, Aβ 42 aggregates were observed at the early stages of tau pathology, in non-demented patients, whereas the insoluble Aβ 40 pool was found at the last stages of AD, in demented patients.

All together, it was interesting to note that, during the progression of the disease, Aβ aggregates increased in quantity and heterogeneity, in close parallel with the extension of tau pathology. Unexpectedly, however, there was no spatial overlap between Aβ aggregation that was widespread and heterogeneously distributed in cortical areas, and tau pathology that was progressing sequentially, stereotypically and

hierarchically. Therefore, these observations demonstrate that Aβ 42 aggregation, and not Aβ 40, is the marker that is close to Alzheimer etiology. It should be the main target for the early biological diagnosis of AD and modeling. Furthermore, the spatial mismatch between Aβ and tau pathologies in cortical areas was obvious. First of all, the neocortical areas that first accumulate Aβ, or contain more Aβ, were not always the same. Generally, but not always, the occipital cortex was more prone to develop amyloid deposits. Remarkably, this region was the last to develop a tau pathology. In contrast, the hippocampal region, which is affected early by tau pathology, was not especially affected by amyloid deposition. These observations confirm the findings of Braak and Braak.[14] Together, this Aβ/tau mismatch demonstrates that neurodegeneration is not a direct consequence of extracellular Aβ neurotoxicity (considering that toxicity is mediated through the cell body). Hence, there is a synergistic effect of APP dysfunction on the neuron-to-neuron propagation of tau pathology. This is demonstrated by the fact that tau pathology can be found in the hippocampal area without Aβ deposits. However, the extension of PHF-tau in the polymodal association areas was always found in the presence of Aβ deposits, as if these species, directly or indirectly, were necessary to stimulate the progression of tau pathology.[19]

Distribution of N-truncated Aβ species in Alzheimer's disease

During our quantification of Aβ 42 aggregated species in non-demented individuals, we noticed that the 4-kDa band, corresponding to Aβ monomers, was extremely heterogeneous, as shown by immunological tools against the amino-terminal region of Aβ.[19] This led us to analyze these species with a proteomic approach. We were more than surprised to observe that amino-truncated species represented more than 60% of all Aβ species, not only in full-blown AD, but also, and more unexpectedly, at the earliest stage of Alzheimer pathology. At this stage (non-demented patients with diffuse Aβ deposits), Aβ oligomers consisted exclusively of Aβ 42 species, most of them being amino-truncated. Thus, our results strongly suggest that amino-truncated Aβ 42 species are instrumental in the amyloidosis process. Since vaccination has been proposed to remove amyloid deposits, the possible cause of AD, and because vaccination against the 'physiological' Aβ peptide provoked severe adverse events, a vaccine specifically targeting these pathological amino-truncated species of Aβ-42 are likely to be doubly beneficial, by inducing the production of specific antibodies against pathological Aβ products that are, in addition, involved in the early and basic mechanisms of amyloidosis in humans.[20] Moreover, the early implication of the amino-truncated Aβ 42 peptides in amyloidosis supports the usefulness of these species for an early, specific and accurate biological diagnosis of AD. Preliminary data show their specific presence, detected by mass spectra, in the cerebrospinal fluid (CSF) of patients who developed AD (personal communication from E. Vanmechelen, Innogenetics). Overall, our results show that amyloidosis must be completely revisited with this new concept of truncated Aβ as the cause of amyloidosis in sporadic AD.

Relationship of brain lesion distribution to mild cognitive impairment

Because our prospective study of more than 200 patients led us to collect all data on cognitive status as well as the extent of tau and Aβ pathology, it was interesting to determine whether there was a relationship between brain lesions and mild cognitive impairment (MCI). The table of all our patients, presented in reference 18, showed in fact that all MCI patients had a tau pathology, but not necessarily Aβ pathology. Furthermore, all patients with a mild tau pathology did not have MCI, probably because the tau burden can be compensated for in some patients. These results agree with those of a recent paper of the Mesulam group,[21] showing that tau pathology is more closely related to cognitive impairment than is Aβ. However, longitudinal studies have shown that the additional presence of N-truncated Aβ deposits in the brain or in the CSF in patients with MCI and tau pathology is a predictor of emerging AD (E. Vanmechelen, in preparation).

Plaques and tangles: which are the closest to cognitive impairment?

Together, neuropathological and biochemical results show that tau pathology is closer to cognitive impairment than Aβ deposition. There is an almost general agreement on that point, and this is logical, because tau pathology shows the neuronal networks that are affected. This correlation concerns a rather late stage of the disease. The question of the origin of neurodegeneration, which concerns the very first steps of the disease, is a different issue that was addressed by searching the earliest molecular defects linked to Aβ and tau aggregation.

RELATIONSHIP BETWEEN TAU PATHOLOGY AND AMYLOID PRECURSOR PROTEIN DYSMETABOLISM

The parallelism and the synergy between tau and Aβ aggregation led us to search an APP molecular event linking the two degenerating processes. Therefore, we quantified all APP metabolic products in relationship to the different stages of tau pathology.

We did not observe significant changes in full-length APP in Alzheimer patients. However, we found that APP carboxy terminal fragments (APP-CTFs), which are released after the action of secretases (α-, β- and γ-secretase activities) upstream of the production of Aβ were significantly modified and decreased at an early stage of AD (Figure 39.1). A significant decrease of the five main APP-CTFs electrophoretic bands was observed, which correlated well with the progression of tau pathology, in most cases with infraclinical AD and with AD (either familial or non-familial). Furthermore, solubility properties and the ratio between the five bands were also modified, in both the Triton-soluble and/or -insoluble fractions. This modification directly observed on APP-CTFs upstream of Aβ products and its relationship with tau pathology could reflect the basic etiological APP dysfunction mechanisms of sporadic AD.[22] This abnormal processing of APP-CTFs could be directly responsible for the production of N-truncated Aβ species and amyloidosis.

CONCLUSION

The facts that tau pathology is a neuron-to-neuron spreading phenomenon, and that the neocortical involvement is always found in the presence of Aβ deposits, demonstrate that: AD is a real tauopathy; there is a synergy between amyloidosis and tauopathy; and the early transformation and decrease of APP-CTFs, in parallel with tau pathology, is in favor of a loss of APP function as the central cause of AD. AD could be explained by the loss of APP-CTFs trophic activities, provoking the extent of tau pathology. APP-CTFs are likely modulating transcription factors.[23] They can be considered as 'survival factors'. Their lack could stimulate the tau degenerating process. Conversely, the microtubule network also has a major importance in regulating the transport and metabolism of APP and associated molecules. Thus, it is also possible that APP dysfunction in sporadic AD is an early consequence of an altered microtubule network, implicating microtubule-associated tau proteins. Therefore, AD is most likely to be the result of a convergence of a tau pathology that occurs frequently in aging, and a defect of APP metabolism, which fuels the spreading of the tauopathy in neocortical areas. Our results suggest that both tau and APP pathologies are targets for diagnosis and therapy.

REFERENCES

1. Alzheimer A, Stelzmann RA, Schnitzlein HN, Murtagh FR. An English translation of Alzheimer's 1907 paper, 'Uber eine eigenartige Erkankung der Hirnrinde'. Clin Anat 1995; 8: 429–31

2. Hyman BT, Trojanowski JQ. Consensus recommendations for the postmortem diagnosis of Alzheimer disease from the National Institute on Aging and the Reagan Institute Working Group on diagnostic criteria for the neuropathological assessment of Alzheimer disease. J Neuropathol Exp Neurol 1997; 56: 1095–7

3. Glenner GG. Amyloid beta protein and the basis for Alzheimer's disease. Prog Clin Biol Res 1989; 317: 857–68

4. Brion JP. Neurofibrillary tangles and Alzheimer's disease. Eur Neurol 1998; 40: 130–40

5. Hardy J, Selkoe DJ. The amyloid hypothesis of Alzheimer's disease: progress and problems on the road to therapeutics. Science 2002; 297: 353–6

6. Bierer LM, Hof PR, Purohit DP, et al. Neocortical neurofibrilllary tangles correlate with dementia severity in Alzheimer's disease. Arch Neurol 1995; 52: 81–8

7. Braak H, Braak E. Staging of Alzheimer-related cortical destruction. Int Psychogeriatr 1997; 9 (Suppl 1): 257–61; discussion 269–72

8. Delacourte A, Sergeant N, Champain D, et al. The biochemical spreading of tau and amyloid beta precursor protein pathologies in aging and sporadic Alzheimer's disease. Brain Aging 2001; 1: 33–42

9. Bierer LM, Hof PR, Purohit DP, et al. Neocortical neurofibrillary tangles correlate with dementia severity in Alzheimer's disease. Arch Neurol 1995; 52: 81–8

10. Hardy J, Selkoe DJ. The amyloid hypothesis of Alzheimer's disease: progress and problems on the road to therapeutics. Science 2002; 297: 353–6

11. Schenk D. Amyloid-beta immunotherapy for Alzheimer's disease: the end of the beginning. Nat Rev Neurosci 2002; 3: 824–8

12. Braak H, Braak E. Evolution of neuronal changes in the course of Alzheimer's disease. J Neural Transm Suppl 1998; 53: 127–40

13. Duyckaerts C, Colle MA, Dessi F, et al. The progression of the lesions in Alzheimer disease: insights from a prospective clinicopathological study. J Neural Transm Suppl 1998; 53: 119–26

14. Braak H, Braak E. Staging of Alzheimer's disease-related neurofibrillary changes. Neurobiol Aging 1995; 16: 271–8; discussion 278–84

15. Fewster PH, Griffin-Brooks S, MacGregor J, et al. A topographical pathway by which histopathological lesions disseminate through the brain of patients with Alzheimer's disease. Dementia 1991; 2: 121–32

16. Mesulam MM. Neuroplasticity failure in Alzheimer's disease: bridging the gap between plaques and tangles. Neuron 1999; 24: 521–9

17. Price JL, Morris JC. Tangles and plaques in nondemented aging and 'preclinical' Alzheimer's disease. Ann Neurol 1999; 45: 358–68

18. Delacourte A, David JP, Sergeant N, et al. The biochemical pathway of neurofibrillary degeneration in aging and Alzheimer's disease. Neurology 1999; 52: 1158–65

19. Delacourte A, Sergeant N, Champain D, et al. Non-overlapping but synergetic tau and APP pathologies in sporadic Alzheimer's disease. Neurology 2002; 59: 398–407

20. Sergeant N, Bombois S, Ghestem A, et al. Truncated beta-amyloid peptide species in preclinical Alzheimer's disease as new targets for the vaccination approach. J Neurochem 2003; 85: 1581–91

21. Guillozet AL, Weintraub S, Mash DC, Mesulam MM. Neurofibrillary tangles, amyloid, and memory in aging and mild cognitive impairment. Arch Neurol 2003; 60: 729–36

22. Sergeant N, David J, Champain D, et al. Progressive decrease of APP carboxy-terminal fragments, associated with tau pathology stages in Alzheimer's disease. J Neurochem 2002; 81: 663–72

23. Cao X, Sudhof TC. A transcriptively active complex of APP with Fe65 and histone acetyltransferase tip60. Science 2001; 293: 115–20

Neurofibrillary degeneration: a promising target for the treatment of Alzheimer's disease and other tauopathies

K Iqbal, A del C Alonso, E El-Akkad, C-X Gong, N Haque,

S Khatoon, H Tanimukai, I Tsujio, I Grundke-Iqbal

INTRODUCTION

Alzheimer's disease (AD) is multifactorial, but its pathogenesis is characterized by neurofibrillary degeneration and β-amyloidosis.[1,2] Whereas neurofibrillary degeneration is associated with the clinical expression of AD, i.e. dementia, the β-amyloidosis alone in the absence of neurofibrillary degeneration does not produce the disease. Hereditary cerebral hemorrhage with amyloidosis of the Dutch type (HCHWA-D) and sporadic cerebral amyloid angiopathy (CAA) are characterized by extensive β-amyloidosis without any dementia.[3,4] Some of the normal aged individuals have as much β-amyloid plaques in the brain as typical cases of AD.[5–8] Furthermore, there are several other neurodegenerative conditions, such as Guam parkinsonism–dementia complex, dementia pugilistica, frontotemporal dementia with parkinsonism linked to chromosome-17 (FTDP-17) and progressive supranuclear palsy, which are characterized by neurofibrillary degeneration of the Alzheimer type and dementia, but in the absence of β-amyloidosis. Moreover, the discovery of mutations in the tau gene and their co-segregation with the disease in the inherited FTDP-17 has confirmed that abnormalities in tau protein as a primary event

can lead to neurodegeneration and dementia.[9–11] Neither β-amyloidosis nor neurofibrillary degeneration is unique to AD, but disorders with the latter lesion called tauopathies (e.g. FTDP-17, dementia pugilistica, Pick disease, corticobasal degeneration) are associated with dementia. The neurofibrillary degeneration of the Alzheimer type is seen only sparsely in aged animals and in experimentally induced conditions. Thus, all these findings taken together suggest that neurofibrillary degeneration plays a pivotal role in the pathogenesis of AD and related tauopathies and that inhibition of this lesion is a promising therapeutic target for these diseases. Identification of specific therapeutic pharmacological targets requires understanding of the molecular mechanism by which this lesion might cause neurodegeneration.

PATHOGENESIS OF NEUROFIBRILLARY DEGENERATION

Microtubule-associated protein (MAP) tau, which promotes the assembly and maintains the structure of microtubules in a normal mature neuron, is a family of six isoforms that differ from one another in having three or four microtubule binding repeats (R) of 31–32 amino acids each, and two, one or no amino terminal inserts (N) of 29 amino acids each.[12,13] Tau is abnormally hyperphosphorylated in AD and in this form is the major protein subunit of paired helical filaments (PHF).[14–18] In AD brains the levels of tau, but not the mRNA for this protein,[19] are 4–8 fold increased as compared to age-matched control brains and this increase is in the form of the abnormally hyperphosphorylated tau.[20,21] This abnormally hyperphosphorylated tau is found in the AD brain in two subcellular pools: polymerized into neurofibrillary tangles of PHF mixed with straight filaments (SF); and in a non-fibrillized form in the cytosol.[16,22,23] The tau polymerized into neurofibrillary tangles is apparently inert and behaves like normal tau in promoting microtubule assembly only on enzymatic dephosphorylation *in vitro*, when released from PHF/tangles.[24,25] Whereas the cytosolic abnormally hyperphosphorylated tau (AD p-tau), which can be as much as 40% of the total abnormal tau in the AD brain,[23] does not interact with tubulin/microtubules but instead sequesters normal tau, MAP1 and MAP2 and cause inhibition and disassembly of microtubules *in vitro*.[26–28] Furthermore, the association between AD p-tau and normal tau is not saturable and *in vitro* results in the formation of tangles of filaments of about 2.1 mm.[27] The association between AD p-tau and MAP1 or MAP2 is weaker than that between the AD p-tau and normal tau, and does not result in the formation of filaments.[28] This toxic property of the AD p-tau appears to be solely due to its abnormal hyperphosphorylation, because dephosphorylation by alkaline phosphatase, protein phosphatase (PP)-2A, PP-2B and, to a lesser degree, by PP-1, converts the abnormal tau into a normal-like protein in promoting the microtubule assembly *in vitro*.[24–29]

The six human tau isoforms, τ4RL (4R, 2N), τ4S (4R, 1N), τ4 (4R, no N), τ3RL (3R, 2N), τ3RS (3R, 1N), and τ3, also called fetal tau (3R, no N), are differentially sequestered by AD p-tau, *in vitro*.[30] The association of AD p-tau to normal tau is τ4RL > τ4RS > τ4R and τ3RL > τ3RS > τ3, and, to human brain recombinant tau it is τ4RL > τ3RL. AD P-tau also inhibits the assembly and disrupts microtubules pre-assembled with each tau isoform with an efficiency that corresponds directly to the degree of interaction with these isoforms. *In vitro* hyperphosphorylation of recombinant tau converts it into an AD p-tau-like state in sequestering normal tau and inhibiting microtubule assembly. The preferential sequestration of 4R taus and taus with amino terminal inserts explains both: why fetal brain (fetal tau is with 3R and no N) is protected from Alzheimer neurofibrillary pathology; and why intronic mutations seen in certain inherited cases of FTDP-17, which result in alternate splicing of tau mRNA, and consequently in an increase in the 4R : 3R ratio, lead to neurofibrillary degeneration and the disease.

The abnormal hyperphosphorylation of tau makes it resistant to proteolysis by the calcium-activated neutral protease,[25,29] and probably it is for this reason that the levels of tau are several-fold increased in AD.[20,21] It is likely that, to neutralize the AD p-tau's ability to sequester normal MAPs and cause disassembly of microtubules, the affected neurons promote the self-assembly of the abnormal tau into tangles of PHF. The fact that the tangle-bearing neurons seem to survive for many years[31] is consistent with such a self-defense role of the formation of tangles. The AD p-tau readily self-assembles into tangles of PHF/SF *in vitro* under physiological conditions of protein concentration, pH, ionic strength and reducing conditions.[32] Furthermore, dephosphorylation inhibits the self-assembly of AD p-tau into PHF/SF, and the *in vitro* abnormal hyperphosphorylation of each of the six recombinant human brain tau isoforms promotes their assembly into tangles of PHF/SF. Thus, all these studies taken together demonstrate the pivotal involvement of abnormal hyperphosphorylation in neurofibrillary degeneration.

INVOLVEMENT OF PROTEIN PHOSPHATASES IN THE ABNORMAL HYPERPHOSPHORYLATION OF TAU

The state of phosphorylation of a phosphoprotein is a function of the balance between the activities of the protein kinases and the protein phosphatases that regulate its phosphorylation. Tau, which is phosphorylated only at serine/threonine residues, is a substrate for several protein kinases such as glycogen synthase kinase-3, cyclin-dependent protein kinase-5, protein kinase A, calcium and calmodulin-dependent protein kinase-II and stress-activated protein kinases (for review see references 2 and 33). However, to date, the activities of none of these protein kinases have been reproducibly shown to be upregulated in the AD brain. In contrast, the activities of protein phosphatase (PP)-2A and PP-1 are compromised by about 20–30% in the AD brain,[34,35] and the phosphorylation of tau that suppresses its microtubule binding and assembly activities in adult mammalian brain is regulated by PP-2A but not by PP-2B.[36,37] PP-2A also regulates the activities of several tau kinases in the brain. Inhibition of PP-2A activity by okadaic acid in metabolically active rat brain slices results in abnormal hyperphosphorylation of tau at several of the same sites as in AD, not only directly, by a decrease in dephosphorylation but also indirectly, by promoting the activities of CaM kinase II,[9] MAP kinase kinase (MEK1/2), extracellular regulated kinase (ERK 1/2) and P70S6 kinase.[38,39]

PP-2A and PP-1 make up more than 90% of the serine/threonine protein phosphatase activity in mammalian cells.[40] The intracellular activities of these enzymes are regulated by endogenous inhibitors. PP-1 activity is regulated mainly by a 18.7-kDa heat-stable protein called inhibitor-1 (I-1).[41,42] In addition, a structurally related protein, DARPP-32 (dopamine and cAMP-regulated phosphoprotein of apparent molecular weight 32 000) is expressed predominantly in the brain.[43] I-1 and DARPP-32 are activated on phosphorylation by protein kinase A and inactivated at basal calcium level by PP-2A. Thus, inhibition of PP-2A activity would keep I-1 and DARPP-32 in active form and thereby result in a decrease in PP-1 activity. In the AD brain a reduction in PP-2A activity might decrease the PP-1 activity by allowing the upregulation of the I-1/DARPP-32 activity. PP-2A is inhibited in the mammalian tissue by two heat-stable proteins: the I_1^{PP2A}, a 30-kDa cytosolic protein that inhibits PP-2A with a ki of 30 nmol/l, and the I_2^{PP2A}, a 39-kDa nuclear protein that inhibits PP-2A at a ki of 23 nmol/l.[44,45] Both I_1^{PP2A} and I_2^{PP2A} have been cloned from the human kidney[45,46] and brain.[47] I_1^{PP2A} has been found to be the same protein as the putative histocompatibility leukocyte antigen class II-associated protein (PHAP-1). This protein, which has also been described as mapmodulin, pp32 and LANP[48] is 249 amino acids long and has an apparent molecular weight of 30 kDa on sodium dodecyl sulfate–polyacrylamide gel electrophoresis (SDS-PAGE). I_2^{PP2A}, which is the same as TAF-1β or PHAPII, is a nuclear protein that is a homolog of the human SETα protein.[49] In a preliminary study we have found that the level of I_1^{PP2A} is about 20% increased in AD brains as compared with age-matched control brains. The decrease in PP-

2A activity in the AD brain could in part be due to a decline in prolyl isomerase Pin 1 activity.[50,51]

THERAPEUTIC TARGETS TO INHIBIT ALZHEIMER'S DISEASE THROUGH INHIBITION OF NEUROFIBRILLARY DEGENERATION

The most promising therapeutic approaches to inhibit neurofibrillary degeneration and consequently AD are: to inhibit sequestration of normal MAPs by the AD p-tau; and to inhibit the abnormal hyperphosphorylation of tau. The latter can be carried out either by inhibiting the activity of a PP-2A inhibitor or restoring the PP-2A activity in the affected areas of the brain or by inhibiting the activity of one or more tau kinase activities that are critically involved in converting normal tau into an abnormal state whereby it sequesters normal MAPs. Memantine, a low-to-moderate-affinity NMDA receptor antagonist, which improves mental function and the quality of daily living of patients with moderate-to-severe AD[52,53] restores the okadaic acid-induced inhibition of PP-2A activity and the abnormal hyperphosphorylation of tau at Ser-262 in hippocampal slice cultures from adult rats.[54]

Development of therapeutic targets requires: a compelling scientific rationale for a therapeutic target; and the availability of a practical outcome measure(s). Tau is primarily a neuronal protein and its level in cerebrospinal fluid (CSF) is a reliable measure of the rate of neuronal degeneration. The CSF level of this protein, both as total tau and as tau abnormally hyperphosphorylated at Ser-396/404, is markedly elevated in AD.[55] The differential diagnosis between AD and vascular dementia, the two major causes of age-associated dementia, can be made in living patients by determining the ratio of abnormally hyperphosphorylated tau to total tau in the lumbar CSF.[55] Thus, levels of CSF total tau and abnormally hyperphosphorylated tau offer excellent outcome measures to test the efficacy of therapeutic agents towards total neurodegeneration and neurofibrillary degeneration, respectively. These outcome measures can be used to test drugs that inhibit neurofibrillary degeneration either by inhibiting the sequestration of normal MAPs by the AD p-tau or by inhibiting the abnormal hyperphosphorylation of tau.

In conclusion, given the pivotal and the primary role of neurofibrillary degeneration in AD and related tauopathies, identification of the rational therapeutic targets for this lesion, and the availability of the CSF total tau and abnormally hyperphosphorylated tau as outcome measures, it is now feasible to develop a new generation of drugs that can inhibit and/or prevent AD and related tauopathies.

ACKNOWLEDGEMENTS

We are grateful to Janet Biegelson and Sonia Warren for secretarial assistance. Studies in our laboratories were supported in part by the New York State Office of Mental Retardation and Developmental Disabilities and NIH grant AG19158, Alzheimer's Association (Chicago, IL) grant IIRG-00-2002 and a grant from the Institute for the Study of Aging (ISOA), New York.

REFERENCES

1. Finch C, Tanzi RE. Genetics of aging. Science 1997; 278: 407–11

2. Iqbal K, Grundke-Iqbal I. Metabolic hypothesis, mechanism and therapeutic targets of Alzheimer neurofibrillary degeneration. Neurosci News 2000; 3: 14–20

3. Coria F, Castaño B, Frangione B. Brain amyloid in normal aging and cerebral amyloid angiopathy is antigenically related to Alzheimer's disease beta-protein. Am J Pathol 1987; 129: 422

4. Levy E, Carman MD, Fernandez-Madrid IJ, et al. Mutation of the Alzheimer's disease amyloid gene in hereditary cerebral hemorrhage, Dutch type. Science 1990; 248: 1124–6

5. Alafuzoff I, Iqbal K, Friden H, et al. Histopathological criteria for progressive dementia disorders: clinical–pathological correlation and classification by multivariate data analysis. Acta Neuropathol (Berlin) 1987; 74: 209–25

6. Arrigada PA, Growdon JH, Hedley-White ET, Hyman BT. Neurofibrillary tangles but not senile plaques parallel duration and severity of Alzheimer's disease. Neurology 1992; 42: 631–9

7. Dickson DW, Crystal HA, Mattiace LA, et al. Identification of normal and pathological aging in prospectively studied non-demented elderly humans. Neurobiol Aging 1991; 13: 179–89

8. Katzman R, Terry RD, DeTeresa R, et al. Clinical, pathological and neurochemical changes in dementia: a subgroup with preserved mental status and numerous neocortical plaques. Ann Neurol 1988; 23: 138–44

9. Hutton M, Lendon CL, Rizzu P, et al. Association of missense and 5′-splice-site mutations in tau with the inherited dementia FTDP-17. Nature 1998; 393: 702–5

10. Poorkaj P, Bird TD, Wijsman E, et al. Tau is a candidate gene for chromosome 17 fronto-temporal dementia. Ann Neurol 1998; 43: 815–25

11. Spillantini MG, Murrell JR, Goedert M, et al. Mutation in the tau gene in familial multiple system tauopathy with presenile dementia. Proc Natl Acad Sci USA 1998; 95: 7737–41

12. Goedert M, Spillantini MG, Jakes R, et al. Multiple isoforms of human microtubule-associated protein tau: sequences and localization in neurofibrillary tangles of Alzheimer's disease. Neuron 1989; 3: 519–26

13. Weingarten MD, Lockwood AH, Hwo SY, Kirschner MW. A protein factor essential for microtubule assembly. Proc Natl Acad Sci USA 1975; 72: 1858–62

14. Grundke-Iqbal I, Iqbal K, Quinlan M, et al. Microtubule-associated protein tau: a component of Alzheimer paired helical filaments. J Biol Chem 1986; 261: 6084–9

15. Grundke-Iqbal I, Iqbal K, Tung YC, et al. Abnormal phosphorylation of the microtubule associated protein tau in Alzheimer cytoskeletal pathology. Proc Natl Acad Sci USA 1986; 83: 4913–17

16. Iqbal K, Grundke-Iqbal I, Zaidi T, et al. Defective brain microtubule assembly in Alzheimer's disease. Lancet 1986; 2: 421–6

17. Iqbal K, Grundke-Iqbal I, Smith AJ, et al. Identification and localization of a tau peptide to paired helical filaments of Alzheimer disease. Proc Natl Acad Sci USA 1989; 86: 5646–50

18. Lee VMY, Balin BJ, Otvos L Jr, Trojanowski JQ. A68: a major subunit of paired helical filaments and derivitized forms of normal tau. Science 1991; 251: 675–8

19. Mah VH, Eskin TA, Kazee AM, et al. In situ hybridization of calcium/calmodulin dependent protein kinase II and tau mRNAs; species differences and relative preservation in

Alzheimer's disease. Brain Res Mol Brain Res 1992; 12: 85–94

20. Khatoon S, Grundke-Iqbal I, Iqbal K. Brain levels of microtubule-associated protein tau are elevated in Alzheimer's disease: a radio-immuno-slot-blot assay for nanograms of the protein. J Neurochem 1992; 59: 750–3

21. Khatoon S, Grundke-Iqbal I, Iqbal K. Levels of normal and abnormally phosphorylated tau in different cellular and regional compartments of Alzheimer disease and control brains. FEBS Lett 1994; 351: 80–4

22. Bancher C, Brunner C, Lassmann H, et al. Accumulation of abnormally phosphorylated tau precedes the formation of neurofibrillary tangles in Alzheimer's disease. Brain Res 1989; 477: 90–9

23. Köpke E, Tung YC, Shaikh S, et al. Microtubule associated protein tau: abnormal phosphorylation of non-paired helical filament pool in Alzheimer disease. J Biol Chem 1993; 268: 24374–84

24. Iqbal K, Zaidi T, Bancher C, Grundke-Iqbal I. Alzheimer paired helical filaments: restoration of the biological activity by dephosphorylation. FEBS Lett 1994; 349: 104–8

25. Wang JZ, Gong CX, Zaidi T, et al. Dephosphorylation of Alzheimer paired helical filaments by protein phosphatase-2A and -2B. J Biol Chem 1995; 270: 4854–60

26. Alonso A del C, Zaidi T, Grundke-Iqbal I, Iqbal K. Role of abnormally phosphorylated tau in the breakdown of microtubules in Alzheimer disease. Proc Natl Acad Sci USA 1994; 91: 5562–6

27. Alonso A del C, Grundke-Iqbal I, Iqbal K. Alzheimer's disease hyperphosphorylated tau sequesters normal tau into tangles of filaments and disassembles microtubules. Nature Med 1996; 2: 783–7

28. Alonso A del C, Grundke-Iqbal I, Barra HS Iqbal K. Abnormal phosphorylation of tau and the mechanism of Alzheimer neurofibrillary degeneration: sequestration of MAP1 and MAP2 and the disassembly of microtubules by the abnormal tau. Proc Natl Acad Sci USA 1997; 94: 298–303

29. Wang JZ, Grundke-Iqbal I, Iqbal K. Restoration of biological activity of Alzheimer abnormally phosphorylated by dephosphorylation with protein phosphatase-2A, -2B and -1. Mol Brain Res 1996; 38: 200–8

30. Alonso A del C, Zaidi T, Novak HS, et al. Interaction of tau isoforms with Alzheimer's disease abnormally hyperphosphorylated tau and in vitro phosphorylation into the disease-like protein. J Biol Chem 2001; 276: 37967–73

31. Morsch R, Simon W, Coleman PD. Neurons may live for decades with neurofibrillary tangles. J Neuropathol Exp Neurol 1999; 58: 188–97

32. Alonso A del C, Zaidi T, Novak M, et al. Hyperphosphorylation induces self-assembly of tau into tangles of paired helical filaments/straight filaments. Proc Natl Acad Sci USA 2001; 98: 6923–8

33. Iqbal K, Alonso A del C, Gondal JA, et al. Mechanism of neurofibrillary degeneration and pharmacologic therapeutic approach. J Neural Transm 2000; 59: 213–22

34. Gong CX, Singh TJ, Grundke-Iqbal I, Iqbal K. Phosphoprotein phosphatase activities in Alzheimer disease brain. J Neurochem 1993; 61: 921–7

35. Gong CX, Shaikh S, Wang JZ, et al. Phosphatase activity towards abnormally phosphorylated τ: decrease in Alzheimer disease brain. J Neurochem 1995; 65: 732–8

36. Bennecib M, Gong CX, Grundke-Iqbal I, Iqbal K. Inhibition of PP-2A upregulates CaMKII in rat forebrain and induces hyperphosphorylation of tau at Ser 262/356. FEBS Lett 2001; 490: 15–22

37. Gong CX, Lidsky T, Wegiel J, et al. Phosphorylation of microtubule-associated protein tau is regulated by protein phosphatase

2A in mammalian brain. J Biol Chem 2000; 275: 5535–44

38. An WL, Cowburn RF, Li L, et al. Up-regulation of phosphorylated/activated p70 S6 kinase and its relationship to neurofibrillary pathology in Alzheimer's disease. Am J Pathol 2003; 163: 591–607

39. Pei JJ, Gong CX, An WL, et al. Okadaic-acid-induced inhibition of protein phosphatase 2A produces activation of mitogen-activated protein kinases ERK1/2, MEK1/2, and p70 S6, similar to that in Alzheimer's disease. Am J Pathol 2003; 163: 845–58

40. Oliver CJ, Shenolikar S. Physiologic importance of protein phosphatase inhibitors. Frontiers Biosci 1998; 3: 961–72

41. Cohen P, Alemany S, Hemmings BA, et al. Protein phosphatase-1 and protein phosphatase-2A from rabbit skeletal muscle. Methods Enzymol 1988; 159: 390–408

42. Cohen P. The structure and regulation of protein phosphatases. Ann Rev Biochem 1989; 58: 453–508

43. Walaas SI, Greengard P. Protein phosphorylation and neuronal function. Pharmacol Rev 1991; 43: 299–349

44. Li M, Guo H, Damuni Z. Purification and characterization of two potent heat-stable protein inhibitors of protein phosphatase 2A from bovine kidney. Biochemistry 1995; 34: 1988–96

45. Li M, Makkinje A, Damuni Z. Molecular identification of I_1^{PP2A}, a novel potent heat-stable inhibitor protein of protein phosphatase 2A. Biochemistry 1996; 35: 6998–7002

46. Li M, Makkinje A, Damuni Z. The myeloid leukemia-associated protein SET is a potent inhibitor of protein phosphatase 2A. J Biol Chem 1996; 271: 11059–62

47. Tsujio T, Xu J, Kotula L, et al. The structures and activities of the endogenous inhibitors of PP-2A in brain. Neurobiol Aging 2002; 23: S498

48. Ulitzur N, Rancano C, Pfeffer SR. Biochemical characterization of mapmodulin, a protein that binds microtubule-associated proteins. J Biol Chem 1997; 272: 30577–82

49. von Lindern M, van Baal S, Wiegant J, et al. *can*, a putative oncogene associated with myeloid leukemogenesis, may be activated by fusion of its 3' half to different genes: characterization of the *set* gene. Mol Cell Biol 1992; 12: 3346–55

50. Zhou XZ, Kops O, Werner A, et al. Pin1-dependent prolyl isomerization regulates dephosphorylation of cdc25c and tau proteins. Mol Cell 2000; 6: 873–83

51. Liou YC, Sun A, Ryo A, et al. Role of the prolyl isomerase Pin 1 in protecting against age-dependent neurodegeneration. Nature 2003; 424: 556–61

52. Winblad B, Poritis N. Memantine in severe dementia: results of the 9M-Best Study (benefit and efficacy in severely demented patients during treatment with memantine). Int J Geriatr Psychiatry 1999; 14: 135–46

53. Reisberg B, Ferris S, Mobius HJ, et al. Long-term treatment with the NMDA antagonist Memantine: results of a 24-week, open-label extension study in Alzheimer's disease. Neurobiol Aging 2002; 23: S555

54. Li L, Sengupta A, Grundke-Iqbal I, Iqbal K. Memantine restores the okadaic acid-induced changes in the activities of protein phosphatase-2A and calcium, calmodulin-protein kinase II and hyperphosphorylation of tau in rat hippocampal slices in culture. Neurobiol Aging 2002; 23: S111

55. Hu YY, He SS, Wang X, et al. Levels of nonphosphorylated and phosphorylated tau in CSF of Alzheimer disease patients: an ultra-sensitive bienzyme-substrate-recycle ELISA. Am J Pathol 2002; 160: 1269–78

Chapter 41

Neuropathology and tau

KA Jellinger

INTRODUCTION

Many neurodegenerative diseases, previously classified according to clinical and morphological criteria, are characterized by distinct brain lesions that have in common the formation of filamentous deposits of abnormal proteins. This allows a biochemical re-classification of neurodegenerative diseases. A group of heterogeneous dementias and movement disorders are hallmarked by prominent intracellular accumulations of abnormal filaments formed by the microtubule-associated protein tau that appears to share common mechanisms of disease. They are summarized as neurodegenerative tauopathies (Table 41.1). Despite their diverse phenotypic manifestation, brain dysfunction and degeneration are linked to the progressive accumulation of tau inclusions in neurons and glia, implicating their pathogenic importance. Some of these disorders are due to various mutations of the tau gene,[1,2] while novel tau polymorphisms have been observed in various frontotemporal dementias,[3] thus broadening the molecular genetic aspects of the tauopathies.[4,5] These findings have opened up new ways for understanding the role of tau abnormalities in neurodegeneration.

After a brief summary of the human tau gene, the neuropathology of several prototypical tauopathies, some novel tauopathies and transgenic mice and other animal models are reviewed in this chapter.

STRUCTURE AND MOLECULAR GENESIS OF TAU

Tau proteins are low-molecular-weight, microtubule-associated proteins in the central and peripheral nervous system, where they are expressed predominantly in axons. Human tau proteins are encoded by a single gene consisting of 16 exons on chromosome 17q21, and the central nervous system (CNS) isoforms are generated by alternative mRNA splicing of 11 of these isoforms. In the adult human brain, there are six tau isoforms that differ by the presence of either three (3-R) or four (4-R) carboxy-terminal tandem repeat sequences of 31 or 32 amino acids, which are encoded by exons 9–12. The triplets of 3- and 4-R tau isoforms differ as a result of alternative splicing of exons 2 and 3 to generate isoforms with, or without, 29 or 58 amino acid inserts. In the human brain, the ratio of 3-R and 4-R tau is about 1, and all six

Table 41.1 Neurodegenerative diseases with filamentous tau pathology

---

Alzheimer's disease (+ amyloid deposition)

* Amyotrophic lateral sclerosis/parkinsonism–dementia complex

* Argyrophilic grain disease

* Corticobasal degeneration

Creutzfeldt–Jakob disease

* Dementia pugilistica

* Diffuse neurofibrillary tangles with calcification

Familial British dementia

Down's syndrome

* Frontotemporal dementia with parkinsonism linked to chromosome 17

* Guamanian amyotrophic lateral sclerosis/parkinsonism–dementia complex

Gerstmann–Sträussler–Scheinker disease

Hallervorden–Spatz disease (pantothenate kinase-related neurodegeneration)

Myotonic dystrophy

Niemann–Pick disease, type C

Non-Guamanian motor neuron disease with neurofibrillary tangles

* Pick's disease

* Postencephalitic parkinsonism

Prion protein cerebral amyloid angiopathy

* Progressive subcortical gliosis

* Progressive supranuclear palsy

Subacute sclerosing panencephalitis

* Tangle predominant dementia

---

* Diseases in which tau-positive neurofibrillary pathology is the most predominant neuropathological feature

isoforms appear in the postnatal period. Tau binds to and stabilizes microtubules, promotes their polymerization and contributes to their binding. Tau contains multiple phosphorylation sites that weaken its affinity to build microtubules, leading to detachment, formation of intracellular aggregates and neuronal dysfunction. Tau phosphorylation that negatively regulates the microtubule binding and function is regulated by protein kinases, mainly GSK-3β and cdk5, and phosphatases, e.g. PP1 and PP2A,

the inhibition of which results in increased tau phosphorylation, resulting in decreased tau binding to microtubules, causing their selective destruction and the degeneration of axons.[4]

FILAMENTOUS PATHOLOGY OF ABNORMALLY PHOSPHORYLATED TAU

Filamentous neuronal and glial tau inclusions associated with degeneration of affected brain areas are the morphological hallmarks of tauopathies. Western blot binding has distinguished different patterns of insoluble and soluble tau from different tauopathies. Tau from the Alzheimer's disease (AD) brain forming both paired helical filaments (PHF) and straight filaments in neurofibrillary tangles (NFT) and some cases of frontotemporal dementia and parkinsonism linked to chromosome 17 (FTDP-17) runs in three major bands of 68, 64 and 60 kDA, and a minor band of 72 kDA. In progressive supranuclear palsy (PSP) and corticobasal degeneration (CBD), in argyrophilic grain disease (AGD),[6,7] in hippocampal neurofibrillary degeneration in atypical dementia cases,[8] and in some FTDP-17 mutations, two 68- and 64-kDA insoluble tau bands are detected, and immunohistochemistry shows selective aggregation of 4-R tau. In contrast, in FTDP-17 mutations that affect mRNA splicing, predominantly 4-R tau is expressed throughout the brain. Only 4-R tau is deposited in filamentous forms. In Pick disease and some FTDP-17 mutants that do not affect splicing, the two 64- and 60-kDA insoluble tau bands predominate, while recent studies in Pick disease detected a spectrum of major phosphorylated 3- and 4-R tau isoforms in brain tissue.[9] Different immunoreactivities to the microtubule-binding domain (MBD) of tau-positive structures indicate variable post-translational modifications among tauopathies.[10] Intense labeling of NFTs in AD differed from inclusions in PSP and CBD, which required formic acid treatment, while Pick bodies showed an intermediate pattern, since tau lacks the insertion of exon 10, and a smaller proportion of tau is phosphorylated at Ser262 than in other abnormal structures.[11] This suggests that tau accumulated in AD and Pick disease is processed more markedly than in PSP and CBD, which may be important for the pathogenesis of these disorders.

Hyperphosphorylation is believed to be an early event in the pathway that leads from soluble to insoluble and filamentous tau protein. Pathological co-localization of sulfated glycosaminoglycans (GAGs) and RNA with hyperphosphorylated tau protein is suggested to be relevant for its assembly.[4] α-Synuclein (AS) can induce fibrillation of tau, and co-incubation of tau and AS synergistically induces fibrillation of both proteins.[12] The *in vivo* relevance of these findings is grounded in the co-occurrence of AS and tau inclusions in the human brain, especially in neuronal populations vulnerable to both NFTs and Lewy bodies, e.g. in familial and sporadic AD and in dementia with Lewy bodies (DLB),[13,14] as well as in oligodendroglia of transgenic mice expressing human AS plus P301L mutant tau.[4]

NEUROPATHOLOGY OF HUMAN TAUOPATHIES

Sporadic tauopathies

Alzheimer's disease

AD, the most frequent cause of dementia in advanced age, is characterized morphologically by deposition of hyperphosphorylated tau protein containing PHFs in neurons (NFTs), in dendrites (neuropil threads) and in neuritic plaques associated with extracellular deposition of β-amyloid peptide (Aβ) in senile plaques and cerebral vasculature (cerebral amyloid angiopathy). Although these changes are non-specific, they represent the major histopathological hallmarks of AD. Both lesions start before clinical symptoms become apparent, and clinically manifested AD is considered a late stage of these processes, starting much earlier. According to the amyloid cascade hypothesis, accumulation of Aβ in the brain is the primary influence driving AD pathogenesis, and tau pathology with formation of NFTs is proposed to be derived from an imbalance between Aβ production and clearance.[15] Others have suggested that tau is essential to Aβ-induced neurotoxicitiy and that tau pathology is initiated before, and independent of, amyloidosis or amyloid precursor protein (APP) dysfunction, amplifying tau pathology.[16]

The neuritic lesions associated with conformational changes of tau protein[17] show a distinct, predictable non-random spreading from the (trans-) entorhinal allocortex in the mediobasal temporal lobe, progressing via the hippocampus to neocortical association areas and later to subcortical nuclei.[18] This pattern correlates with early memory disorders due to deafferentation of the hippocampus by dissection of the γ-aminobutyric acid (GABA)ergic 'perforant pathway' followed by disturbance of higher cortical functions due to diffuse tau pathology involving the whole brain.[16] Tau extension is different from the phases of Aβ deposits beginning in the neocortex and later progressing to allocortical areas, expanding anterogradely into regions receiving projections from already affected areas.[19] Little is known about the relationship between APP, Aβ and tau pathologies, which is the missing link in the development of AD, but recent data indicate non-overlapping but synergistic tau and Aβ pathologies in sporadic AD, while rare familial AD is determined by various genetic factors (presenilins 1 and 2, APP mutation, apolipoprotein E (apoE), etc.) resulting in excessive production and accumulation of neurotoxic and fibrillogenic Aβ due to abnormal proteolytic processing of APP. Parahippocampal tau pathology is more frequent in persons with both mild cognitive impairment (MCI) or pre/subclinical forms of AD and/or full-blown AD than in those who are cognitively normal,

and NFT density is significantly correlated with memory deficits and cognitive impairment. This indicates that: tau pathology and/or synaptic dysfunction, either by diffusible oligomeric assemblies of Aβ or by tau protein[20] in the ventromedial temporal lobe, develop prior to the onset of dementia; NFTs constitute a pathological substrate of memory loss not only in AD but also in normal aging and MCI;[21] and tangles and neuronal loss, particularly in the neocortex, but not amyloid load, predict cognitive status in AD.[22] Although the Nun study showed that only 17–20% of cognitively normal seniors were free of considerable AD lesions and all the others showed severe AD pathology,[23] the available data suggest that NFT pathology is one of the major morphological substrates of cognitive impairment and that substantial involvement of the hippocampus is often the key step in the development of dementia. However, the notion that AD is a heterogeneous disorder with various phenotypes awaits further clarification, based on strong molecular information and clinical relevance of brain lesions.

Progressive supranuclear palsy

Progressive supranuclear palsy (Steele–Richardson–Olszewski syndrome), the second most common neurodegenerative extrapyramidal disorder after Parkinson's disease, is a sporadic, rarely familial, late-onset atypical parkinsonian syndrome with supranuclear gaze palsy and frontal lobe dementia; its prevalence is 3–6 per 100 000.[24] It shows overexpression of 4-R tau associated with a polymorphous tandem repeat allele, located in intron 9 of the tau gene, with prevalence of the tau genotypes A0/A0 and the presence of the H1/H1 genotype as a modest genetic predisposition marker.[24] The brain shows atrophy of the midbrain and superior cerebellar peduncle.[25] The histological features are multisystem neuronal loss and gliosis with widespread globose tangles and neuropil threads composed of 12–15-nm straight tubules containing a 64- and 68-kDA 4-R tau doublet with a sequence encoded by exon 10, thus differing from NFTs in both AD and CBD.[26] Swollen achromatic neurons in cortex and basal ganglia contain tau aggregates with straight filaments, which are also present in 'tufted' or thorn-shaped astrocytes throughout the neuraxis. Cortical involvement differs from that in AD, with the highest density of tau pathology in prefrontal and angular gyri, and the major location in the deeper cortical layers as compared to bimodal distribution in AD. ApoE ε4 has been found as a determinant for AD pathology in PSP.[27]

Corticobasal degeneration

Corticobasal degeneration is an uncommon sporadic, late-onset progressive neurodegenerative disorder, clinically characterized by levodopa-non-responsive rigidity with focal cortical signs, e.g. apraxia and aphasia, and frontal lobe dementia. Neuropathology reveals depigmentation of the substantia nigra and asymmetrical frontoparietal atrophy with neuronal loss, spongiosis, and gliosis. Histological hallmarks are prominent neuronal and glial intracytoplasmic tau inclusions (ballooned/achromatic neurons) in the cortex, basal ganglia, brain stem and cerebellum, with extensive accumulation of tau-immunoreactive thread-like processes throughout the brain. In the white matter, astroglial plaques and numerous inclusions involve both astrocytes and oligodendroglia (coiled bodies). The tau filaments include both PHF-like filamentous and straight tubules which, in both CBD and PSP, are composed of predominant 4-R tau doublets (64 and 68 kDa).[28] Although the isoforms in CBD may differ from those in PSP, and an H1/H1 tau genotype would be supportive of CBD, recent biochemical and genetic data suggest a substantial overlap between both disorders. Current neuropathological criteria for CBD[29] alone do not allow it to be distinguished from familial tauopathies; additional genetic and molecular information is necessary.

Argyrophilic grain disease

AGD, a recently recognized disorder with unclear genetic features and a relationship to dementia and other disorders, is morphologically characterized by spindle- or comma-shaped argyrophilic grains particularly in the neurons of the allocortex (hippocampus, amygdala) and ambient gyrus,[25,30] accompanied by coiled bodies in the white matter and ballooned neurons in the limbic lobe. Recent studies have revealed predominance of 4-R tau;[6,7,31] the frequency of the extended haplotype is not different from that in PSP and CBD,[6,32] but is different from AD and Pick's disease.[33] AGD occurs in PSP and CBD more frequently than in dementia controls, including AD.[32] It lacks relationship with apoE,[34,35] shows similar frequencies in H1 and H2 tau haplotypes to those in healthy controls, and is genetically associated with polymorphisms in α_2-macro-globulins and low-density lipoprotein receptor-related protein genes.[36]

In some cases of dementia not fitting the current criteria for AD, NFTs in the CA2 sector of the hippocampus showed 4-R tau pathology. Most of these represented pure or mixed cases of AGD, with similar apoE allele frequency to that in controls and increased frequency of the extended H 1 haplotype, but the biological basis for this type of lesion is unknown.[8]

A novel leukoencephalopathy was reported recently, with severe frontal atrophy, nigral cell loss, tau deposits in white matter glia composed of straight filaments of 10 nm, and numerous argyrophilic threads in gray and white matter.[37]

Frontotemporal dementia

Frontotemporal dementia (FTD) morphogically shows frontotemporal atrophy with neuronal loss, microvacuolar (spongiform) changes and gliosis with or without tau or ubiquitin pathology. The Constantinidis classification of Pick's disease[38] distinguishes type A (classic Pick's disease with Pick's bodies and cells); and type B (frontal and parietal atrophy, ballooned neurons but no Pick's bodies). Most cases are now considered as CBD or FTDP-17, while type C is a heterogeneous phenotype without Pick bodies or tau pathology, now classified as dementia lacking distinctive histopathology (DLDH).

An updated classification of FTD recommends:[39] when neuropathology includes tau-positive lesions, neuron loss, gliosis and predominantly insoluble 3-R tau, the likely diagnoses are Pick's disease or FDTP-17; in the presence of tau-positive lesions, neuron loss, gliosis and predominantly insoluble 4-R tau, the likely diagnosis is CBD, PSP or FTDP-17; tau-positive inclusions, neuron loss, gliosis and insoluble 3- + 4-R tau, suggest NFT dementia or FTD-17; frontotemporal neuronal loss and gliosis without tau/ubiquitin-positive inclusions, and no insoluble tau or tau with reduced solubility, suggest frontotemporal lobe degeneration (FTLD), also known as DLDH; frontotemporal neuronal loss and gliosis with ubiquitin-positive, tau-negative inclusions and without detectable insoluble tau, with or without motoneuron disease (MND), but with MND-type inclusions, suggests FTLD with MND, or FTLD with MND-type inclusions without MND.

Pick's disease

Pick's disease is a rare variant FTD that accounts for 1–2% of all elderly dementia cases. Its classical type shows frontotemporal lobar and limbic atrophy with marked neuronal loss, spongiosis and gliosis, achromatic (Pick) cells and intraneuronal globose inclusions (Pick bodies) in the hippocampus, in particular in dentate granule neurons, in the cerebral cortex and in selected brain stem nuclei. Ultrastructurally, they are composed of wide, straight and long-period twisted filaments, made up of 3-R tau doublets (60 and 64 kDa), and a minor 68-kDa band.[4,25,30] Tau-positive glial inclusions, NFTs and a network of dystrophic neurites may be present. In sporadic Pick's disease cases, in addition to 4-R tau deposits, isolated straight and twisted filaments are also formed from 3- and 4-R tau isoforms, and tau phosphorylation-dependent and exon 10-specific epitopes are found. This indicates that Pick's disease is characterized by accumulation of Pick bodies in the hippocampal region and cortex as well as of 3-R and 4-R microtubule-binding tau pathology that distinguish this disorder from other tauopathies.[9]

FTD, in contrast to Pick's disease, characterized by frontotemporal neuronal loss, gliosis and spongiform changes but no disease-specific lesions, has been referred to as DLDH. Similar brain pathology was seen in a familial FTD pedigree known as hereditary dysphasic disinhibition dementia (HDDD2) with linkage to chromosome 17q21-22 but no tau mutation. Biochemical analysis demonstrated reduction in soluble tau in most brains with DLDH and in some HDDD2 brains, which differs from previous FTD cases containing substantial amounts of pathological insoluble tau.[41,42] These findings suggest a definition of DLDH as a sporadic or familial 'tau-less' tauopathy with reduced levels of soluble tau and no insoluble or fibrillary tau inclusions, and a phenotypic heterogeneity of HDDD2 which parallels that of other hereditary FTDs caused by tau gene mutation.[1,3] No tau mutations have been identified in sporadic FTD cases.[43]

Famlial tauopathies – FTDP-17 syndromes

This group of autosomal dominantly inherited neurodegenerative diseases linked to chromosome 17q21-22 shows diverse, but overlapping clinical and morphological features. It is characterized by abundant filamentous tau pathology in neurons and glia, without Aβ deposits or other disease-specific brain lesions in the majority of cases.[2] Two classes of tau mutation have been found in up to 10–40% of familial FTD cases: those directly affecting the microtubule binding sites of tau and those that alter tau splicing.[1,4] The majority of the currently known tau mutations are located in exons 9–13. Recent studies have detected a P301L mutation in 11% of familial FTD cases. The H1 haplotype was not over-represented, but the P301L mutation appeared in the background of the H2 tau haplotype. Further single nuclear polymorphisms in intron 9 and deletions in other introns upstream from exon 10 were increased in FTD cases with an increase in exon 10-containing tau transcripts.[3] These data indicate that sequence variations in regulatory regions of tau may have consequences leading to tau dysfunction and neurodegeneration.

ANIMAL MODELS OF TAUOPATHIES

A number of experimental and transgenic animal models produced by overexpressing human tau protein show axonopathy due to somatodendritic tau expression associated with tau-immunoreactive spheroids and/or NFTs in the brain and spinal cord, in the absence of Aβ production. The axonal inclusions are composed of 10–20-nm tau-positive straight filaments. These models link neurofibrillary degeneration to neuronal loss and thus provide

in vivo models that may give further insights into the pathogenetic role of tau in neurodegeneration and provide new approaches to therapy.[4,44,45]

CONCLUSION

The accumulation of filamentous tau inclusions is a common feature of a wide variety of neurodegenerative disorders that either are distinguished by distinct topographic or cell-type specific patterns of inclusions, or show various overlaps. The biochemical and ultra-structural characteristics of tau abnormalities, which are frequently related to tau polymorphisms, haplotypes and splicing in exons 9 to 13, also show significant phenotype overlap. The mutations lead to specific cellular alterations, including altered expression, function and biochemistry of tau which may be influenced by other genetic and epigenetic factors. It remains to be established which are the initial steps leading to abnormal hyperphosphorylation and generation of filamentous tau, and their impact on cellular dysfunction. Whereas the cascade of pathogenic events in sporadic tauopathies is unclear, at least in familial forms, genetic and/or environmental factors could initiate a cascade of events that leads to abnormal phosphorylation of tau and dysfunction of microtubules and neurons through incompletely defined pathways (Figure 41.1). Further studies into the mechanisms of dysfunction of tau and other proteins and their impact on neuronal dysfunction will provide better insight into the mechanisms of neurodegeneration, their clinicopathological correlations and possible novel strategies for disease prevention and treatment.

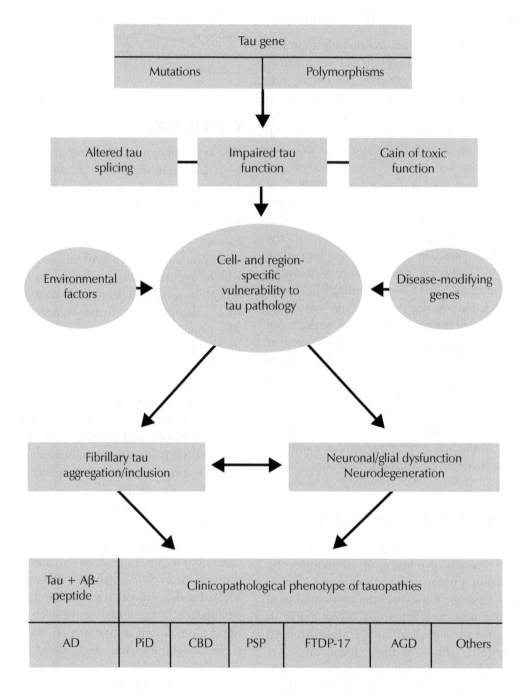

Figure 41.1 Disease pathways in tauopathies leading to specific clinicopathological phenotypes (modified from reference 4). AD, Alzheimer's disease; PiD, Pick's disease; CBD, corticobasal degeneration; PSP, progressive supranuclear palsy; FTDP-17, frontotemporal dementia and parkinsonism linked to chromosome 17; AGD, argyrophilic grain disease

REFERENCES

1. Hutton M. Missense and splice site mutations in tau associated with FTDP-17: multiple pathogenic mechanisms. Neurology 2001; 56 (11 Suppl 4): S21–5

2. Spillantini MG, Van Swieten JC, Goedert M. Tau gene mutations in frontotemporal dementia and parkinsonism linked to chromosome 17 (FTDP-17). Neurogenetics 2000; 2: 193–205

3. Sobrido MJ, Miller BL, Havlioglu N, et al. Novel tau polymorphisms, tau haplotypes, and splicing in familial and sporadic frontotemporal dementia. Arch Neurol 2003; 60: 698–702

4. Lee VM, Goedert M, Trojanowski JQ. Neurodegenerative tauopathies. Annu Rev Neurosci 2001; 24: 1121–59

5. Tolnay M, Probst A. Tau protein pathology in Alzheimer's disease and related disorders. Neuropathol Appl Neurobiol 1999; 25: 171–87

6. Togo T, Sahara N, Yen SH, et al. Argyrophilic grain disease is a sporadic 4-repeat tauopathy. J Neuropathol Exp Neurol 2002; 61: 547–56

7. Tolnay M, Sergeant N, Ghestem A, et al. Argyrophilic grain disease and Alzheimer's disease are distinguished by their different distribution of tau protein isoforms. Acta Neuropathol (Berl) 2002; 104: 425–34

8. Ishizawa T, Ko LW, Cookson N, et al. Selective neurofibrillary degeneration of the hippocampal CA2 sector is associated with four-repeat tauopathies. J Neuropathol Exp Neurol 2002; 61: 1040–7

9. Zhukareva V, Mann D, Pickering-Brown S, et al. Sporadic Pick's disease: a tauopathy characterized by a spectrum of pathological tau isoforms in gray and white matter. Ann Neurol 2002; 51: 730–9

10. de Silva R, Lashley T, Gibb et al. Pathological inclusion bodies in tauopathies contain distinct complements of tau with three or four microtubule-binding repeat domains as demonstrated by new specific monoclonal antibodies. Neuropathol Appl Neurobiol 2003; 29: 288–302

11. Arai T, Ikeda K, Akiyama H, et al. Different immunoreactivities of the microtubule-binding region of tau and its molecular basis in brains from patients with Alzheimer's disease, Pick's disease, progressive supranuclear palsy and corticobasal degeneration. Acta Neuropathol (Berl) 2003; 105: 489–98

12. Giasson BI, Forman MS, Higuchi M, et al. Initiation and synergistic fibrillization of tau and alpha-synuclein. Science 2003; 300: 636–40

13. Iseki E, Togo T, Suzuki K, et al. Dementia with Lewy bodies from the perspective of tauopathy. Acta Neuropathol (Berl) 2003; 105: 265–70

14. Trembath Y, Rosenberg C, Ervin JF, et al. Lewy body pathology is a frequent co-pathology in familial Alzheimer's disease. Acta Neuropathol (Berl) 2003; 105: 484–8

15. Hardy J, Allsop D. Amyloid deposition as the central event in the aetiology of Alzheimer's disease. Trends Pharmacol Sci 1991; 12: 383–8

16. Delacourte A, Sergeant N, Champain D, et al. Nonoverlapping but synergetic tau and APP pathologies in sporadic Alzheimer's disease. Neurology 2002; 59: 398–407

17. Ghoshal N, Garcia-Sierra F, Wuu J, et al. Tau conformational changes correspond to impairments of episodic memory in mild cognitive impairment and Alzheimer's disease. Exp Neurol 2002; 177: 475–93

18. Braak H, Braak E. Neuropathological staging of Alzheimer-related changes. Acta Neuropathol (Berl) 1991; 82: 239–59

19. Thal DR, Rub U, Orantes M, Braak H. Phases of A beta-deposition in the human brain and its relevance for the development of AD. Neurology 2002; 58: 1791–800

20. Selkoe DJ. Alzheimer's disease is a synaptic failure. Science 2002; 298: 789–91

21. Guillozet AL, Weintraub S, Mash DC, Mesulam MM. Neurofibrillary tangles, amyloid, and memory in aging and mild cognitive impairment. Arch Neurol 2003; 60: 729–36

22. Giannakopoulos P, Herrmann FR, Bussiere T, et al. Tangle and neuron numbers, but not amyloid load, predict cognitive status in Alzheimer's disease. Neurology 2003; 60: 1495–500

23. Riley KP, Snowdon DA, Markesbery WR. Alzheimer's neurofibrillary pathology and the spectrum of cognitive function: findings from the Nun Study. Ann Neurol 2002; 51: 567–77

24. Burn JB, Lees AJ. Progressive supranuclear palsy: where are we now? Lancet Neurol 2002; 1: 359–69

25. Dickson DW. Sporadic tauopathies: Pick's disease, corticobasal degeneration, progressive supranuclear palsy and argyrophilic grain disease. In Esiri MM, Lee VM-Y, Trojanowski JQ, eds. The Neuropathology of Dementia, 2nd edn. Cambridge, UK: Cambridge University Press, 2004: 227–56

26. Berry RW, Sweet AP, Clark FA, et al. Tau epitope display in progressive supranuclear palsy and corticobasal degeneration. J Neurocytol 2004; 33: 287–95

27. Tsuboi Y, Josephs KA, Cookson N, Dickson DW. APOE E4 is a determinant for Alzheimer type pathology in progressive supranuclear palsy. Neurology 2003; 60: 240–5

28. Buee L, Bussiere T, Buee-Scherrer V, et al. Tau protein isoforms, phosphorylation and role in neurodegenerative disorders. Brain Res Brain Res Rev 2000; 33: 95–130

29. Dickson DW, Bergeron C, Chin SS, et al. Office of Rare Diseases neuropathologic criteria for corticobasal degeneration. J Neuropathol Exp Neurol 2002; 61: 935–46

30. Saito Y, Nakahara K, Yamanouchi H, Murayama S. Severe involvement of ambient gyrus in dementia with grains. J Neuropathol Exp Neurol 2002; 61: 789–96

31. Ferrer I, Barrachina M, Tolnay M, et al. Phosphorylated protein kinases associated with neuronal and glial tau deposits in argyrophilic grain disease. Brain Pathol 2003; 13: 62–78

32. Togo T, Dickson DW. Ballooned neurons in progressive supranuclear palsy are usually due to concurrent argyrophilic grain disease. Acta Neuropathol (Berl) 2002; 104: 53–6

33. Zhukareva V, Shah K, Uryu K, et al. Biochemical analysis of tau proteins in argyrophilic grain disease, Alzheimer's disease, and Pick's disease: a comparative study. Am J Pathol 2002; 161: 1135–41

34. Jellinger KA. Dementia with grains (argyrophilic grain disease). Brain Pathol 1998; 8: 377–86

35. Togo T, Cookson N, Dickson DW. Argyrophilic grain disease: neuropathology, frequency in a dementia brain bank and lack of relationship with apolipoprotein E. Brain Pathol 2002; 12: 45–52

36. Ghebremedhin E, Schultz C, Thal DR, et al. Genetic association of argyrophilic grain disease with polymorphisms in alpha-2 macroglobulin and low-density lipoprotein receptor-related protein genes. Neuropathol Appl Neurobiol 2002; 28: 308–13

37. Powers JM, Byrne NP, Ito M, et al. A novel leukoencephalopathy associated with tau deposits primarily in white matter glia. Acta Neuropathol 2003; 106: 181–4

38. Constantinidis J. Pick dementia. Anatomo-clinical correlations and pathophysiological considerations. In Rose FC, ed. Modern Approaches to the Dementias. Part I: Etiology and Pathophysiology, Interdisciplinary Topics in Gerontology. Basel, Switzerland: Karger, 1985; 19: 72–97

39. Trojanowski JQ, Dickson D. Update on the neuropathological diagnosis of frontotemporal dementias. J Neuropathol Exp Neurol 2001; 60: 1123–6

40. Dickson DW. Neuropathology of Pick's disease. Neurology 2001; 56 (11 Suppl 4): 16–20

41. Zhukareva V, Sundarraj S, Mann D, et al. Selective reduction of soluble tau proteins in sporadic and familial frontotemporal dementias: an international follow-up study. Acta Neuropathol (Berl) 2003; 105: 469–76

42. Zhukareva V, Vogelsberg-Ragaglia V, Van Deerlin VM, et al. Loss of brain tau defines novel sporadic and familial tauopathies with frontotemporal dementia. Ann Neurol 2001; 49: 165–75

43. Poorkaj P, Grossman M, Steinbart E, et al. Frequency of tau gene mutations in familial and sporadic cases of non-Alzheimer dementia. Arch Neurol 2001; 58: 383–7

44. Götz J. Tau and transgenic animal models. Brain Res Brain Res Rev 2001; 35: 266–86

45. Lee VM, Kenyon TK, Trojanowski JQ. Transgenic animal models of tauopathies. Biochim Biophys Acta 2005; 1739: 251–9

Chapter 42

Conformational analysis of tau and tau aggregates by fluorescence spectroscopy

M von Bergen, L Li, E-M Mandelkow, E Mandelkow

INTRODUCTION

The neurofibrillary tangles of Alzheimer's disease (AD) are composed mainly of paired helical filaments (PHF) made up of aggregated and hyperphosphorylated tau protein. This axonal microtubule-associated protein normally serves to stabilize microtubules; it is highly soluble in most conditions, but in the disease state it begins to aggregate. The reasons for this unusual behavior are not well understood, but several approaches have been developed to mimic the process *in vitro* using recombinant tau protein. One problem is how to induce the aggregation of a soluble protein; in the case of tau this can be achieved by polyanionic cofactors. Another problem is how to monitor the aggregation in a time-resolved mode in order to determine the aggregation kinetics. Electron microscopy is useful, because it reveals the nature of the aggregates, but it has a poor time resolution and is usually not quantitative. In the past we have used the fluorescence change of the dye thioflavin S, which occurs upon PHF aggregation, but the caveat is that this is an external additive. In order to find intrinsic signals for monitoring aggregation we have recently turned to modifications of the protein. One particularly useful marker is the amino acid

residue tryptophan (Trp) which can be inserted into the tau sequence *ad libitum* by site-directed mutagenesis. Tau contains no intrinsic Trp; therefore, the inserted Trp residues provide unique fluorescence signals that report on their immediate vicinity. This property can be exploited to probe the accessibility to solvent, the packing of the protein, the pathway of protein folding and conformational changes.

Tau is encoded by a single gene on chromosome 17, giving rise to six isoforms by alternative splicing[1] (Figure 42.1). The C-terminal half contains three or four pseudo-repeats of about 31 residues each; repeat R2 may be present or absent, depending on the isoform. This domain is important for the physiological role of tau, the attachment to microtubules,[2] but it also contributes to the formation of the pathological PHFs.[3] The N-terminal domain is termed the 'projection domain' because it does not bind to microtubules by itself, but rather projects away from the microtubule surface.[4] Over the past few years we have analyzed some of the requirements that are important for PHF aggregation. One is that cross-linking of tau into dimers via the disulfide link at Cys322 accelerates PHF formation,[5] indicating that a close apposition of this region is important for the interactions. The

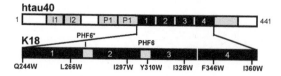

Figure 42.1 Diagram of tau and tryptophan mutants. Top: isoform htau40 (largest isoform in the human central nervous system, containing two alternatively spliced inserts near the N-terminus (I1, I2) and four repeats (R1–R4) in the C-terminal half: 441 residue.[13] It contains five Tyr residues (18, 29, 197, 310, 397), but no Trp. Bottom: enlarged view of repeat domain (construct K18, four repeats only, 125 residues, Q244–N368). The gray boxes in K18 show the hexapeptide motifs PHF6* ([275]VQIINK[280]) and PHF6 ([306]VQIVYK[311]) whose conversion to β-structure is an early step in paired helical filament assembly.[6,7,9] Mutations Q244W, L266W, I297W, I328W, F346W and I360W are indicated for K18

second is that there are certain motifs in the repeat domain that are prone to form β-sheet interactions, and this type of interaction is responsible for the aggregation of tau into PHFs that have a cross-β structure in their core domain.[6–8] In order to gain further information on the conformation of tau in the soluble and aggregated states we explored novel fluorescence signals. The sequence of Tau contains five Tyr residues, but Trp is completely absent. Here we show that the fluorescence of Trp residues introduced into tau by site-directed mutagenesis allows one to study the aggregation process, the solvent accessibility of different sites and the distance between the added Trp and the intrinsic Tyr residues. The results show that the N- and C-terminal ends of tau become folded into the vicinity of the repeat domain during PHF aggregation.

METHODS

Most methods were described in detail in previous publications.[6,9,10] Human tau isoforms and constructs (Figure 42.1) were expressed in *Escherichia coli* as described.[11] The numbering of the amino acids is that of the isoform htau40 containing 441 residues.[12,13] Aggregation of tau into PHFs was induced by incubating tau isoforms or tau constructs (50–100 µmol/l) at 37°C in phosphate-buffered saline (PBS) pH 7.4 containing the anionic cofactor heparin. The formation of aggregates was ascertained by thioflavin S fluorescence and electron microscopy.[14]. The fluorescence experiments were performed on a Spex Fluoromax spectrophotometer (Polytec, Waldbronn, Germany). For tyrosine excitation spectra, scans ranged from 250 to 300 nm at the emission wavelength of 310 nm; for emission spectra, scans ranged from 290 to 450 nm at the excitation wavelength of 275 nm. For Trp excitation spectra scans ranged from 210 to 310 nm at an emission wavelength of 350 nm; for emission spectra, scans ranged from 300 to 400 nm at an excitation wavelength of 290 nm. Fluorescence quenching experiments were performed on soluble or aggregated proteins by adding aliquots of quenching solutions into the cuvette and exciting the fluorescence at 280 nm. Quenching data were fitted to the Stern–Volmer equation,[15] $F_0/F_c = 1 + K_{SV}[Q]$, where F_0 and F_c are the fluorescence intensity in the absence and in the presence of quencher [Q] at concentration c.

RESULTS

Tau is regarded as a 'natively unfolded' protein, and therefore its crystal structure is not known. The available structural information is based on X-ray solution scattering, circular dichroism, Fourier-transform infrared (FTIR) spectroscopy, quasielastic light scattering, hydrodynamic behavior and reaction with conformation-specific antibodies. The data suggest a largely random coil structure for the soluble protein, partial conversion to the β-structure upon PHF aggregation, and folding-back of the N- or C-terminal domains into the repeat domain in certain conformations.[16–19]

The transition towards the β-structure during aggregation involves the repeat domain of tau, notably the hexapeptide motifs V275-K280 in the second repeat and V306-K311 in the third repeat. Tau has an unusual composition in that it contains few aromatic amino acids; the longest isoform contains three phenylalanines (F8, F346 and F379), five tyrosines (Y18, Y29, Y197, Y310 and Y394) and no tryptophan. All of these lie in the regions common to all isoforms of tau. We therefore generated tau mutants by placing tryptophans into different sites within the repeat domain of tau in order to observe the contribution of this domain to PHF aggregation (Figure 42.1 bottom). The mutants were Q244W, L266W, I297W, Y310W, I328W

and F346W, mostly conservative exchanges in order to minimize effects on tau structure. Note that Y310W is at the center of the hexapeptide motif of the third repeat.

Some typical fluorescence spectra of construct K18-Y310W are shown in Figure 42.2. When tau changes from the soluble state to the polymerized state, there is a pronounced blue shift of approximately 15 nm in the emission maximum (354–339 nm, Figure 42.2b), indicating that residue 310 becomes buried in a hydrophobic pocket within the PHFs. Similar results were obtained with the full-length tau isoforms. Although they contain five intrinsic Tyr residues (Y18, Y29, Y197, Y310, Y394) the newly introduced W310 dominates the fluorescence spectrum and shows a similar blue shift upon aggregation. These results are consistent with an open structure of the repeat domain in the soluble state, and with its burial inside the

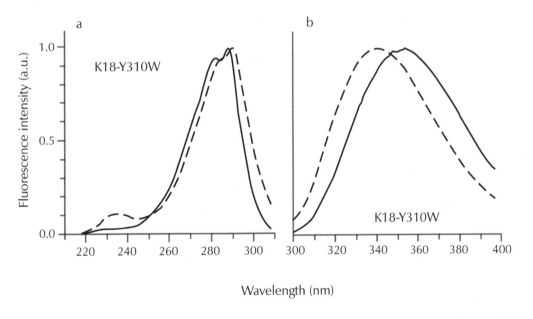

Figure 42.2 Tryptophan fluorescence spectra of repeat domain construct K18-Y310W before and after paired helical filament assembly. Excitation spectra (a) and emission spectra (b) for the mutant K18-Y310W (excitation at 280 nm, emission at 350 nm) are shown. There is a strong blue shift from 354 to 339 nm in the emission maximum changing from the soluble protein (solid line) to the polymerized protein (dashed line)

PHFs during aggregation. All other single-site tryptophan mutations within the microtubule binding domain show blue shifts from the soluble to the aggregated state whose magnitude depends on the site of mutation (Figure 42.3). In separate experiments we ascertained that the mutated proteins had the same aggregation kinetics as the wild-type protein. Thus, the exchange of Tyr310 to Trp does not destroy the capacity of the motif to support aggregation, in contrast to Pro mutations[6]. The fluorescence of W310 can therefore serve as an intrinsic reporter of aggregation (Figure 42.2). For example, the

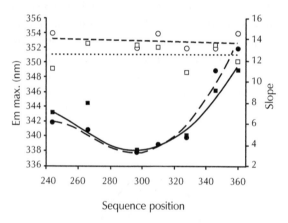

Figure 42.3 Solvent accessibility of Trp in soluble tau and after paired helical filament (PHF) aggregation. Residues of the repeat domain were mutated singly into Trp and probed for their exposure to the solvent before and after PHF aggregation (Q244, L266, I297, Y310, I328, F346, I360 in K18, see Figure 42.1). Quenching of fluorescence of soluble (open squares and dotted line) and aggregated protein (filled squares and solid line) is plotted as slope obtained from Stern–Volmer plots versus protein sequence. After PHF assembly (filled squares, solid curve), a U-shaped curve appears, because the residues near the ends (in R1, R4) are more exposed than those in the middle (in R2, R3). The emission maxima (Em max.) from soluble protein (open circles and dashed line) and from aggregated tau (filled circles and long dashed line) are shown as well. After PHF assembly (filled circles, long dashed curve) the emission maximum shows a blue shift that is most pronounced near the middle of the sequence (R2, R3)

emission maximum of K18 and K19 lies initially around 355 nm and changes towards about 340 nm during PHF formation. Since proteins can often aggregate in different forms, we made sure that the aggregation products were indeed PHFs, by checking all samples by electron microscopy.

Since the formation of PHFs involves local β-structure at the hexapeptide motifs [275]VQIINK[280] and [306]VQIVYK[311] it was important to check whether any of the Trp mutations (Figure 42.1) had an influence on β-structure formation. This was investigated by FTIR spectroscopy where the soluble K18 protein exhibits a maximum at about 1652 wave numbers (indicating mostly random coil structure, data not shown) but it is shifted to lower values upon aggregation (about 1630/cm, a typical behavior for increasing β-structure).[20,21] All of the Trp mutants of K18 gave similar results, and therefore the mutants appear to undergo similar intermediate stages during PHF aggregation. Furthermore, it was important to ensure that the physiological function of tau – stabilization of microtubules – was not impaired by the mutations. This function can be observed by light scattering from assembling microtubule solutions. Tubulin does not self-assemble in these conditions, but assembly is strongly enhanced by htau40 or its Y310W mutant (data not shown). In summary, the Trp mutations in the repeat domain of tau have little effect on the structure and functions of tau that are of importance for PHF aggregation or microtubule assembly. Thus, the mutations are faithful markers of tau conformation and assembly.

We then investigated whether the repeat domain was buried in the core of PHFs upon aggregation. The exposure to solvent before and after aggregation can be monitored by fluorescence quenching by acrylamide. We made seven Trp mutants of K18 distributed over the molecule and measured their accessibility to the solvent. The Stern–Volmer plot[15] displays the ratio of F_0/F_c (without/with quencher at concentration c) as a function of the quencher concentration. All soluble proteins exhibit nearly the same slopes (11–14, Figure 42.3, empty squares) indicating almost maximal accessibility, but the slopes of the polymerized proteins are much lower, varying from 3 to 10 (Figure 42.3, filled squares). Minimal values of the slopes were observed in repeats R2 and R3 (mutations I297W, Y310W, I328W), higher values towards the two ends, R1 and R4 (Q244W, L266W, F346W, I360W). Thus, the quenching experiments indicate that repeats R2 and R3 are more deeply buried in the core of PHFs. These conclusions were confirmed independently by the wavelength shift of the different Trp mutants before and after PHF aggregation. The blue shift was most pronounced for Trp mutants in repeats R2 and R3, showing that the emission maximum is a reliable sensor of the local environment, and that repeats R2 and R3 (notably residue 297) become buried in the PHF structure, whereas the tail (residues 346, 360) remains significantly more accessible to solvent than the first repeat.

In the past it has been difficult to study the aggregation of a soluble protein such as tau, let alone the reverse process of disassembly once the aggregates are formed. This question is closely related to that of PHF stability. We analyzed the stability of PHFs containing the Y310W mutation in the presence of increasing concentrations of guanidine hydrochloride (GuHCl) (Figure 42.4). The emission maximum is 340 nm without GuHCl but rises to 354 nm (the value of soluble tau) as the PHFs become denatured and disintegrate. The concentration of GuHCl at the midpoint of denaturation (C_m) was around 1.1 mol/l for K18 and K19 (data not shown), indicating that the difference of one repeat (R2) has no major influence on the

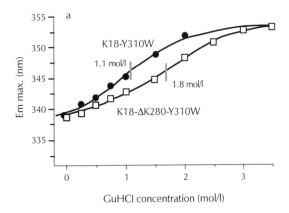

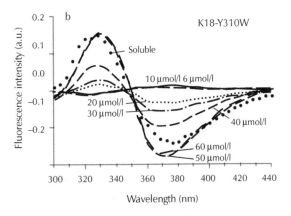

Figure 42.4 Stability of paired helical filament (PHFs). PHFs were first assembled from tau proteins carrying the Y310W mutation, and the emission maximum (Em max.) is plotted vs. increasing concentrations of guanidine hydrochloride (GuHCl) (a). The maximum increases as PHFs become denatured. For K18-Y310W the midpoint of denaturation is at approximately 1.1 mol/l GuHCl, upper curve, filled circles), whereas PHFs made from the mutant K18-ΔK280 are more stable (half point approximately 1.8 mol/l GuHCl, lower curve, open squares). (b) PHFs were made from K18-Y310W and exposed to increasing concentrations of GuHCl. The fluorescence spectra are normalized to their maximum and the difference spectra calculated from the spectrum taken in the absence of GuHCl

stability of these constructs (Figure 42.4a). However, PHFs made from K18-ΔK280 (one of the frontotemporal dementia and parkinsonism linked to chromosome 17 (FTDP-17) mutations) show much higher stability with half maximal denaturation at 1.8 mol/l GuHCl (open squares). This emphasizes the importance of the β-structure around the hexapeptide motifs.[7] Similar stabilities were observed for full-length tau isoforms. The interesting consequence is that these values are relatively low compared with globular folded proteins which require C_m values of about 3–5 mol/l for denaturation. This shows that PHFs are initially not as sturdy as they appear in Alzheimer brain tissue, perhaps because they lack some of the covalent crosslinks that are added with time in the aging brain.[22–25]

One of the strategies to combat neuronal degeneration is to prevent protein aggregation. With the results described above it is possible to test compounds for their ability to dissolve PHFs using the intrinsic fluorescence of Trp. Figure 42.4b shows a dose–response curve of PHFs with increasing GuHCl. The emission maxima become red-shifted during the disintegration of PHFs (Figure 42.4b). The difference spectra with or without GuHCl show maxima at 325 nm (positive) and 380 nm (negative), which increase with GuHCl concentration. This example illustrates how PHFs can be monitored by Trp fluorescence, particularly in cases where other techniques are not suitable.

DISCUSSION

The aggregation of tau represents one of the features of Alzheimer's disease so that it is of importance to study the several aspects of the aggregation mechanism. Progress has been slow, because tau is a highly soluble protein that aggregates very inefficiently, but this barrier has been overcome by several findings: the repeat domain aggregates faster than the intact protein;[26] dimerization of tau accelerates aggregation;[5,26,27] cofactors such as polyanions

or fatty acid micelles promote aggregation;[28–31] and mutations of tau in FTDP-17 dementias promote aggregation.[9,32,33] This makes it possible to form tau aggregates rapidly from recombinant protein and analyze the structure and kinetics. Another problem was the development of assay methods of tau aggregation. Electron microscopy is not well suited for kinetic analysis, although it is important for identifying the 'paired helical' appearance of aggregates. CD or FTIR spectroscopy does not reveal pronounced changes between the soluble and aggregated state, because tau is mostly in a random coil state (Figure 42.5).[34,35] Thioflavin S fluorescence and light scattering have been suitable for kinetic studies,[14,31,33] but they have a limited sensitivity to initial states of aggregation. This prompted a search for other methods, and here we report results obtained with the use of the intrinsic fluorescence of Trp, which has several advantages. Trp is absent from normal tau and is therefore easily detected. Trp senses changes in the local environment by changes in fluorescence. This change allows one to monitor

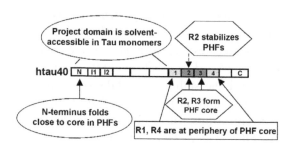

Figure 42.5 Summary of conformational analysis. Soluble tau is natively unfolded and therefore the sequence is solvent accessible throughout. In paired helical filament (PHFs) the repeat domain becomes buried, especially R2 and R3. The N- and C-terminal tails of full-length tau are far from the repeat domain, but fold back during PHF aggregation

solvent accessibility and protein folding during aggregation. Trp can be introduced at many different sites in tau. Fluorescence energy transfer (FRET) from Tyr to Trp enables one to observe changes of distances. Trp as an integral component of tau reports on all molecules, including monomers, oligomers and aggregates. Trp fluorescence can be used to monitor aggregation independently of other compounds such as thioflavin S.

In the case of tau the replacement of Y310 by Trp is particularly interesting, since this lies within the repeat domain and within the PHF6 hexapeptide motif. It reveals the aggregation of PHFs without obstructing the formation of a β-structure. Trp inserted into other sites responds in a similar fashion, but with variations, as seen by solvent accessibility (Figure 42.3). Soluble tau is completely accessible, confirming earlier conclusions from X-ray experiments that tau is a natively unfolded protein.[34] Trp residues inserted in different positions in the repeat domain show a lower solvent accessibility upon PHF aggregation, consistent with the view that the repeat domain becomes packed in PHFs. The tightest packing occurs in R2 and R3 near the hexapeptide motifs, while R1 and R4 are less tightly packed. This agrees with the view that the repeats form the core of PHFs.[12]

An important issue in AD research is that of PHF stability and disaggregation, since the PHF load in cells results from both opposing processes. The stability can be monitored by exposing preformed PHFs to denaturants. One unexpected result was that PHF aggregation is fairly reversible, even in mild conditions (around 1 mol/l GuHCl). Thus, the buildup of PHFs in cells might be prevented if one could avoid stabilization by covalent crosslinking reactions. Some FTDP-17 mutations such as ΔK280 increase the stability of the PHFs since they promote β-structure. Finally, we note that constructs containing tryptophan are suitable for screening compounds that might inhibit PHFs. In automated screens this would avoid the use of exogenous fluorescent probes (such as thioflavin S) which, in certain cases, might interfere with the recording of the aggregation process.

ACKNOWLEDGEMENTS

We thank S. Hübschmann for expert technical assistance. We are grateful to Drs J. Biernat and S. Barghorn for many suggestions and providing the tau isoforms and constructs used in this study. This project was supported in part by the Deutsche Forschungsgemeinschaft.

REFERENCES

1. Goedert M, Wischik CM, Crowther RA, et al. Cloning and sequencing of the cDNA encoding a core protein of the paired helical filament of Alzheimer disease: identification as the micro-tubule-associated protein tau. Proc Natl Acad Sci USA 1988; 85: 4051–5

2. Weingarten MD, Lockwood AH, Hwo SY, Kirschner MW. A protein factor essential for microtubule assembly. Proc Natl Acad Sci USA 1975; 72: 1858–62

3. Kosik KS, Joachim CL, Selkoe DJ. Microtubule-associated protein tau (tau) is a major antigenic

component of paired helical filaments in Alzheimer disease. Proc Natl Acad Sci USA 1986; 83: 4044–8

4. Gustke N, Trinczek B, Biernat J, et al. Domains of tau protein and interactions with microtubules. Biochemistry 1994; 33: 9511–22

5. Schweers O, Mandelkow EM, Biernat J, Mandelkow E. Oxidation of cysteine-322 in the repeat domain of microtubule-associated protein tau controls the in vitro assembly of paired helical filaments. Proc Natl Acad Sci USA 1995; 92: 8463–7

6. von Bergen M, Friedhoff P, Biernat J, et al. Assembly of tau protein into Alzheimer paired helical filaments depends on a local sequence motif [(306)VQIVYK(311)] forming beta structure. Proc Natl Acad Sci USA 2000; 97: 5129–34

7. von Bergen M, Barghorn S, Li L, et al. Mutations of tau protein in frontotemporal dementia promote aggregation of paired helical filaments by enhancing local beta-structure. J Biol Chem 2001; 276: 48165–74

8. Berriman J, Serpell LC, Oberg KA, et al. Tau filaments from human brain and from in vitro assembly of recombinant protein show cross-beta structure. Proc Natl Acad Sci USA 2003; 100: 9034–8

9. Barghorn S, Zheng-Fischhofer Q, Ackmann M, et al. Structure, microtubule interactions, and paired helical filament aggregation by tau mutants of frontotemporal dementias. Biochemistry 2000; 39: 11714–21

10. Li L, von Bergen M, Mandelkow EM, Mandelkow E. Structure, stability, and aggregation of paired helical filaments from tau protein and FTDP-17 mutants probed by tryptophan scanning mutagenesis. J Biol Chem 2002; 277: 41390–400

11. Baumann K, Mandelkow EM, Biernat J, et al. Abnormal Alzheimer-like phosphorylation of tau-protein by cyclin-dependent kinases cdk2 and cdk5. FEBS Lett 1993; 336: 417–24

12. Crowther T, Goedert M, Wischik CM. The repeat region of microtubule-associated protein tau forms part of the core of the paired helical filament of Alzheimer's disease. Ann Med 1989; 21: 127–32

13. Goedert M, Spillantini MG, Jakes R, et al. Multiple isoforms of human microtubule-associated protein tau: sequences and localization in neurofibrillary tangles of Alzheimer's disease. Neuron 1989; 3: 519–26

14. Friedhoff P, Schneider A, Mandelkow EM, Mandelkow E. Rapid assembly of Alzheimer-like paired helical filaments from microtubule-associated protein tau monitored by fluorescence in solution. Biochemistry 1998; 37: 10223–30

15. Eftink MR, Jameson DM. Acrylamide and oxygen fluorescence quenching studies with liver alcohol dehydrogenase using steady-state and phase fluorometry. Biochemistry 1982; 21: 4443–9

16. Carmel G, Mager EM, Binder LI, Kuret J. The structural basis of monoclonal antibody Alz50's selectivity for Alzheimer's disease pathology. J Biol Chem 1996; 271: 32789–95

17. Gamblin TC, Berry RW, Binder LI. Tau polymerization: role of the amino terminus. Biochemistry 2003; 42: 2252–7

18. Ksiezak-Reding H, Chien CH, Lee VM, Yen SH. Mapping of the Alz 50 epitope in microtubule-associated proteins tau. J Neurosci Res 1990; 25: 412–19

19. Jicha GA, Bowser R, Kazam IG, Davies P. Alz-50 and MC-1, a new monoclonal antibody raised to paired helical filaments, recognize conformational epitopes on recombinant tau. J Neurosci Res 1997; 48: 128–32

20. Byler DM, Susi H. Examination of the secondary structure of proteins by deconvolved FTIR spectra. Biopolymers 1986; 25: 469–87

21. Susi H, Byler DM. Fourier transform infrared study of proteins with parallel beta-chains. Arch Biochem Biophys 1987; 258: 465–9

22. Ledesma MD, Bonay P, Colaco C, Avila J. Analysis of microtubule-associated protein tau glycation in paired helical filaments. J Biol Chem 1994; 269: 21614–19

23. Murthy SN, Wilson JH, Lukas TJ, et al. Cross-linking sites of the human tau protein, probed by reactions with human transglutaminase. J Neurochem 1998; 71: 2607–14

24. Tucholski J, Kuret J, Johnson GV. Tau is modified by tissue transglutaminase in situ: possible functional and metabolic effects of polyamination. J Neurochem 1999; 73: 1871–80

25. Morishima M, Ihara Y. Posttranslational modifications of tau in paired helical filaments. Dementia 1994; 5: 282–8

26. Wille H, Drewes G, Biernat J, et al. Alzheimer-like paired helical filaments and antiparallel dimers formed from microtubule-associated protein tau in vitro. J Cell Biol 1992; 118: 573–84

27. DeTure MA, Zhang EY, Bubb MR, Purich DL. In vitro polymerization of embryonic MAP-2c and fragments of the MAP-2 microtubule binding region into structures resembling paired helical filaments. J Biol Chem 1996; 271: 32702–6

28. Goedert M. Tau protein and the neurofibrillary pathology of Alzheimer's disease. Ann NY Acad Sci 1996; 777: 121–31

29. Giaccone G, Pedrotti B, Migheli A, et al. beta PP and Tau interaction. A possible link between amyloid and neurofibrillary tangles in Alzheimer's disease. Am J Pathol 1996; 148: 79–87

30. Kampers T, Friedhoff P, Biernat J, et al. RNA stimulates aggregation of microtubule-associate protein tau into Alzheimer-like paired helical filaments. FEBS Lett 1996; 399: 344–9

31. Goode BL, Denis PE, Panda D, et al. Functional interactions between the proline-rich and repeat regions of tau enhance microtubule binding and assembly. Mol Biol Cell 1997; 8: 353–65

32. Bugiani O, Murrell JR, Giaccone G, et al. Frontotemporal dementia and corticobasal degeneration in a family with a P301S mutation in tau. J Neuropathol Exp Neurol 1999; 58: 667–77

33. Abraha A, Ghoshal N, Gamblin TC, et al. C-terminal inhibition of tau assembly in vitro and in Alzheimer's disease. J Cell Sci 2000; 113: 3737–45

34. Schweers O, Schonbrunn-Hanebeck E, Marx A, Mandelkow E. Structural studies of tau protein and Alzheimer paired helical filaments show no evidence for beta-structure. J Biol Chem 1994; 269: 24290–7

35. Cleveland DW, Hwo SY, Kirschner MW. Purification of tau, a microtubule-associated protein that induces assembly of microtubules from purified tubulin. J Mol Biol 1977; 116: 207–25

Transglutaminase-catalyzed cross-linking of tau in Alzheimer's disease and progressive supranuclear palsy

NA Muma, RA Halverson

INTRODUCTION

Tau is one of the major proteins that contributes to the neuropathology of Alzheimer's disease (AD), progressive supranuclear palsy (PSP), frontotemporal dementia and parkinsonism linked to chromosome 17 (FTDP-17), and other neurodegenerative diseases with neurofibrillary tangles (NFT). Recent studies have demonstrated that some of the FTDP-17 mutations in tau either increase expression of tau protein isoforms with four microtubule binding sites (4R tau), or reduce the binding of tau to microtubules.[1–3] Most importantly, these mutations in tau lead to the formation of NFT and neuronal degeneration. However, the mechanisms underlying the polymerization of tau protein into straight and paired helical filaments (PHF) and the formation of stable NFT in tauopathies are unclear. We hypothesize that cross-linking of tau protein by transglutaminase stabilizes tau microfilaments and thereby promotes their aggregation into NFT in tauopathies.

Several laboratories have described mechanisms that can induce the formation of tau filaments *in vitro*. These include cross-linking of tau with transglutaminase or the interaction of tau with sulfated glycosaminoglycans, arachidonic acid, or RNA.[4–7] All of these mechanisms may contribute independently or in concert with the formation of PHF, while transglutaminase-catalyzed cross-linking may also stabilize the tau filaments in NFT.

Many studies have suggested that transglutaminase-induced cross-linking may play a role in the formation and stabilization of tau filaments in NFT in AD.[4,8,9] This type of covalent bond can cross-link proteins into stable, rigid, insoluble complexes suggesting that transglutaminases could be responsible for converting tau into insoluble filamentous polymers. Our data demonstrate that NFT and PHF tau contains intramolecular and intermolecular cross-links through ε(γ-glutamyl) lysine bonds in AD and PSP.[10,11] In AD, cross-linking of PHF tau occurs before the presence of microscopically detectable NFT.[12]

TAU PROTEINS

Tau is a family of proteins encoded by a single gene whereby alternative splicing and variations in post-translational modifications give rise to multiple isoforms. In the C-terminal end of tau either three (3R tau) or four (4R tau) microtubule-binding domains are alternatively expressed. Insertions of either 58 or 29 amino acids are found in the N-terminal of tau. Tau is a microtubule-associated protein and plays a role in the regulation of polymerization and stability of microtubules.[13]

Several neurodegenerative diseases are characterized by tau-containing NFTs including PSP, AD, Pick's disease, corticobasal degeneration and FTDP-17.[14] Recent reports describe mutations in the tau gene that can cause FTDP-17[1] and PSP.[15] Some of these tau mutations cause increased expression of 4R tau mRNA and protein isoforms.[2] Interestingly, in those cases of FTDP-17, the NFTs are mainly composed of 4R tau isoforms.[1] Data from our laboratory demonstrated that 4R tau is also overexpressed in PSP but not AD.[16] Other FTDP-17 and PSP mutations such as R5L, P301L and P301S, result in tau protein with reduced binding to microtubules.[15] Together, these studies have demonstrated that perturbations in tau protein can lead to formation of NFTs and neuronal degeneration. These mechanisms are not likely to be involved in the formation of NFT in AD, as our data have demonstrated that 4R tau expression is not increased in AD, and mutations in tau have not been associated with AD.[16] Increased expression of 4R tau does occur in PSP,[16] which may impact on NFT formation in PSP as in FTDP-17. However, increased expression of 4R tau either in cells in culture or in transgenic mice does not result in the formation of tau filaments or NFT. Numerous lines of investigation directly and indirectly suggest that transglutaminase-induced ε(γ-glutamyl)lysine cross-linking of tau is important in these pathological processes.

TAU IN NEUROFIBRILLARY TANGLES

Tau in NFT is abnormally phosphorylated, which could prevent tau from efficiently polymerizing and stabilizing microtubules.[17] Abnormally phosphorylated tau protein would then be floating free in the neuron and available to self-polymerize and aggregate. The mechanism(s) leading to self-assembly of tau *in vivo* are unknown. Other post-translational modifications of tau in NFT are quite likely to be involved. For example, tau filaments in AD are glycated; however, glycation does not appear to inhibit the ability of tau to promote microtubule assembly.[18] Tau filaments can be formed *in vitro*. Tau proteins will form structures resembling straight and PHF tau in the presence of free fatty acids (such as arachidonic acid), RNA, or sulfated glycosaminoglycans *in vitro*.[5-7] Transglutaminase will also cause tau to form filaments.[4] Although these types of mechanistic studies are crucial, it is not known whether any of these reagents that can induce tau filaments *in vitro* are relevant to filament formation in human disease. However, transglutaminase-induced cross-links are present in tau filaments in AD, and PSP and glycosaminoglycans are found in NFT in AD. It is therefore possible that transglutaminase and/or glycosaminoglycans are important in the formation of tau microfilaments. Further, transglutaminase-induced cross-linking of tau could also stabilize tau microfilaments, leading to the formation of NFT.

TRANSGLUTAMINASES

Transglutaminases are a family of calcium-activated enzymes that catalyze the covalent cross-linking of peptide-bound glutamine residues of proteins to the γ-amino-group of lysine residues. The resulting isopeptide bonds can occur intra- or intermolecularly leading to conformational changes, dimers or multimeric complexes. Polyamines can also be added to proteins through the actions of transglutaminases. There are nine transglutaminase isoforms coded for by genes on six different chromosomes. Transglutaminases are found in a variety of mammalian tissues including the central and peripheral nervous systems. In the human brain, transglutaminase activity has been demonstrated in the frontal and temporal cortex, the hippocampus and the cerebellum.[19,20] The transglutaminases expressed in the human brain are factor XIIIa, transglutaminase 2 (also known as tissue transglutaminase) and transglutaminase 1 and 3.[9]

Transglutaminase enzymes are found both intra- and extracellularly in tissues such as skeletal tissue, where they are involved in cartilage matrix stabilization, fibrin during blood clot formation, and the cornified envelopes of terminally differentiated skin keratinocytes.[21] Transglutaminases are inducible enzymes, with increased activity during development, terminal differentiation and apoptosis.[22] Alterations in the abundance of ε(γ-glutamyl) lysine cross-links are found in pathological tissues such as atherosclerotic plaques, tumors and lens tissue in cataract formation.[23,24]

The activity of transglutaminase enzymes is highly regulated. Transglutaminases are calcium-dependent enzymes containing a cysteine in their active site, that is unmasked only in the presence of calcium; thus calcium is their universal activator.[20] Dysregulation of calcium homeostasis in AD and PSP could result in abnormal activation of transglutaminase enzymes, leading to pathological cross-linking of proteins. A loss of calcium homeostasis is a common characteristic of neurodegenerative diseases,[25] and the regulation of intracellular calcium is altered and levels are increased in aging.[26]

NEUROFIBRILLARY TANGLES AND TRANSGLUTAMINASES

The hypothesis that NFT contain transglutaminase-induced ε(γ-glutamyl) lysine cross-links was first proposed by Selkoe and collaborators.[19,27] Early studies investigated the cross-linking of neurofilament and microtubule proteins, which at the time were candidate substrates for PHF formation. These studies demonstrated the presence of transglutaminases in postmortem human brain of normal individuals and in those with AD. Transglutaminases are present in human hippocampal neurons and co-localize with PHF in hippocampal neurons.[28] Immunolabeling with anti-transglutaminase antibodies was more intense in AD hippocampus compared to that in age-matched controls.[28] Tau is an excellent substrate for ε(γ-glutamyl) lysine cross-linking by transglutaminases.[11,29] Amine donor and acceptor sites on human tau 23 and 40 (using the Goedert numbering system) were identified in an in vitro study.[30] Not all of the glutamine and lysine residues in tau could act as acceptor or donor sites. However, many of the amine acceptor and donor sites on human tau are located in, and adjacent to, the microtubule-binding repeat regions.

In AD and PSP, PHF tau protein is cross-linked, as demonstrated using immunoprecipitation and Western blots.[10,11] Using double-label immunofluorescence, we demonstrated co-localization of tau and the transglutaminase-catalyzed cross-link in NFT in both AD and PSP.[10,12] These lysine–glutamine cross-links could impact on tau filament and NFT formation in several ways (Figure 43.1). Cross-linked tau may not bind as well to microtubules, resulting in an increase in free tau available for polymer formation. Cross-links may make tau protein resistant to degradation, leading to an increase in tau protein levels available for PHF

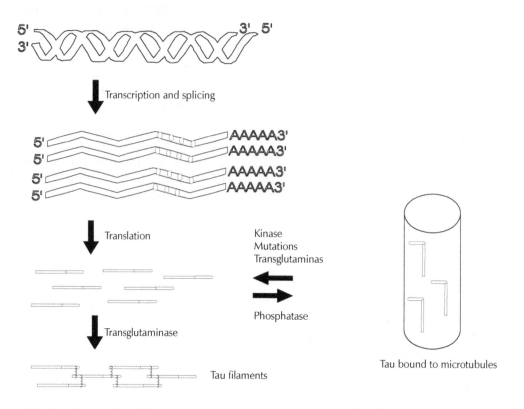

Figure 43.1 Hypothetical effects of transglutaminase-catalyzed cross-links on tau filaments

formation. Alternatively, cross-linking may be the mechanism by which tau assembles into polymers.[4] Finally, cross-links may stabilize PHF tau in NFT formed by some other mechanism.

TRANSGLUTAMINASE ISOFORMS IN TAUOPATHIES

The transglutaminase isoforms expressed in normal human brain or in the PSP and AD brain have not been fully clarified. It is important to determine which transglutaminase isoform is involved in the cross-linking of tau in tauopathies, to model the cross-linking of tau in

cells and target the inhibition of the appropriate transglutaminase isoform. Transglutaminase isoforms are differentially regulated and show different substrate specificity.[31] Transglutaminase 1, 2 and 3 have been identified in the human brain.[9,32,33] In the rat brain, two isoforms of tissue transglutaminase 2 have been described: a short and a long form.[31,34] The expression of the short transglutaminase 2 mRNA isoform in the human brain has been only recently reported in the AD cortex, but it was not present in the cortex of two control cases.[8] A short human transglutaminase 2 isoform has been identified in human erythroleukemia cells. This short human transglutaminase 2 is similar to the short rat isoform in that the shorter isoform contains a different carboxy-terminus from that in the long isoform. While the long form is constitutively expressed, the short form is induced by cytokines, such as interleukin-1β.[34] Since cytokines, including interleukin-1β, are up-regulated in AD,[35] this is a possible mechanisms regulating the expression of this short transglutaminase form in AD. The short form does not contain a GTP binding site present in the long transglutaminase 2 isoform, suggesting that GTP cannot be inhibitory in the short transglutaminase 2 isoform as it is in the long isoform. The short splice variant is up-regulated following axonal injury.[36] Our studies have demonstrated that the levels of the short splice variant of transglutaminase 2 mRNA are dramatically increased in PSP in the globus pallidus.[37] We have also demonstrated an increase in transglutaminase 1 in the globus pallidus in PSP.[37] There is also a report of an increase in mRNA coding for transglutaminase 1 and 2 in AD.[9] It is not known whether there is an accompanying increase in protein expression of transglutaminase 1 and 2 in AD,[38] or an increase in protein levels of the short isoform of transglutaminase 2 in either AD or PSP.

SIGNIFICANCE

The mechanisms involved in NFT formation, specifically those leading to tau polymerization into filaments are unknown, but they appear to involve transglutaminase protein cross-linking. We have demonstrated that these ε(γ-glutamyl) lysine cross-links are present in tau filaments from AD and PSP brain tissue. In AD, cross-linking of tau is an early event in the formation of PHF and occurs before microscopically detectable NFT are present.[12] High-molecular-weight tau polymers and tau filaments are formed from transglutaminase-induced cross-linking in vitro; however, the mechanisms involved in the regulation of cross-linking by transglutaminase in vivo are unclear. The key to understanding the neurofibrillary pathology is not only to understand the mechanisms by which tau can form filaments in vitro but also to understand the mechanisms by which tau forms filaments in disease. Therefore, it is important to examine the cross-linking of tau in transgenic mice that form NFT, in addition to the studies performed in tissue from human neurodegenerative disease cases. The isoforms of transglutaminase that are expressed in the human brain, and most importantly in the AD and PSP brain, are being delineated. Identification of the transglutaminase isoforms involved in cross-linking tau in tauopathies will allow us to target the appropriate transglutaminase for therapeutic intervention. Second, although we know that PHF tau protein contains transglutaminase-catalyzed cross-links, the functional consequences resulting from this cross-linking of tau protein are unclear. One of the advantages to studies in animal models is the ability to look at the development of pathology over time, since studies in humans are limited to a single static time point. One can liken studies in animal models to a movie film in which we can observe early abnormalities leading to pathological changes of versus a single snap shot in humans in which we observe a single time point often only at the end of the disease course. A current hypothesis on neuronal cell death in neurodegenerative diseases with neurofibrillary pathology implicates tau as a central player.[1] The NFT and neuropil threads displace cellular organelles and may interfere with normal neuronal function. Conversely, loss of functional tau protein may also lead to neuronal dysfunction and cell death. Preventing the cross-linking of tau by transglutaminase may prevent the sequestration or stabilization of tau into filaments and thereby prevent synaptic loss and cell death. Understanding the formation and stabilization of NFT will lead to novel substrates and new avenues for research and drug discovery in disorders with NFT such as AD, PSP and FTDP-17.

ACKNOWLEDGEMENTS

This work was supported by grants from The Society for Progressive Supranuclear Palsy, and the National Institutes of Health (NS043053).

REFERENCES

1. Poorkaj P, Bird TD, Wijsman E, et al. Tau is a candidate gene for chromosome 17 frontotemporal dementia. Ann Neurol 1998; 43: 815–25

2. Hutton M, Lendon CL, Rizzu P, et al. Association of missense and 5'-splice-site mutations in tau with the inherited dementia FTDP-17. Nature 1998; 393: 702–5

3. Spillantini MG, Bird TD, Ghetti B. Frontotemporal dementia and parkinsonism linked to chromosome 17: a new group of tauopathies. Brain Pathol 1998; 8: 387–402

4. Appelt DM, Balin BJ. The association of tissue transglutaminase with human recombinant tau results in the formation of insoluble filamentous structures. Brain Res 1997; 745: 21–31

5. Goedert M, Jakes R, Spillantini MG, et al. Assembly of microtubule-associated protein tau into Alzheimer-like filaments induced by sulphated glycosaminoglycans [see comments]. Nature 1996; 383: 550–3

6. Kampers T, Friedhoff P, Biernat J, et al. RNA stimulates aggregation of microtubule-associated tau into Alzheimer-like paired helical filaments. FEBS Lett 1996; 399: 344–9

7. Wilson DM, Binder LI. Free fatty acids stimulate the polymerization of tau and amyloid β peptides: in vitro evidence for a common effector of pathogenesis in Alzheimer's disease. Am J Pathol 1997; 150: 2181–95

8. Citron BA, SantaCruz K, Davies PJA, Festoff BW. Intro-exon swapping of transglutaminase mRNA and neuronal tau aggregation in Alzheimer's disease. J Biol Chem 2001; 276: 3295–301

9. Kim S-Y, Grant P, Lee J-H, et al. Differential expression of multiple transglutaminases in human brain. J Biol Chem 1999; 274: 30715–21

10. Zemaitaitis MO, Lee JM, Troncoso JC, Muma NA. Transglutaminase-induced cross-linking of tau proteins in progressive supranuclear palsy. J Neuropathol Exp Neurol 2000; 59: 983–9

11. Norlund MA, Lee JM, Zainelli GM, Muma NA. Elevated transglutaminase-induced bonds in PHF tau in Alzheimer's disease. Brain Res 1999; 851: 154–63

12. Singer SM, Zainelli GM, Norlund MA, et al. Transglutaminase bonds in neurofibrillary tangles and paired helical filament tau early in Alzheimer's disease. Neurochem Int 2002; 40: 17–30

13. Drubin D, Kobayashi S, Kirschner M. Association of tau protein with microtubules in living cells. Ann NY Acad Sci 1985; 257–68

14. Feany MB, Dickson DW. Neurodegenerative disorders with extensive tau pathology: a comparative study and review. Ann Neurol 1996; 40: 139–48

15. Poorkaj P, Muma NA, Zhukareva V, et al. An R5L tau mutation in a subject with a progressive supranuclear palsy phenotype. Ann Neurol 2002; 52: 511–16

16. Chambers CB, Lee JM, Troncoso JC, et al. Overexpression of four-repeat tau mRNA

isoforms in progressive supranuclear palsy but not in Alzheimer's disease. Ann Neurol 1999; 46: 325–32

17. Gustke N, Steiner B, Mandelkow E-M, et al. The Alzheimer-like phosphorylation of tau protein reduces microtubule binding and involves Ser-Pro and Thr-Pro motifs. FEBS Lett 1992; 307: 199–205

18. Wang JZ, Grundke-Iqbal I, Iqbal K. Glycosylation of microtubule-associated protein tau: an abnormal post-translational modification in Alzheimer's disease. Nat Med 1992; 2: 871–5

19. Selkoe DJ, Abraham C, Ihara Y. Brain transglutaminase: in vitro crosslinking of human neurofilament proteins into insoluble polymers. Proc Natl Acad Sci USA 1982; 79: 6070–4

20. Hand D, Perry MJ, Haynes LW. Cellular transglutaminases in neural development [published erratum appears in Int J Dev Neurosci 1994; 12: 527]. Int J Dev Neurosci 1993; 11: 709–20

21. Aeschlimann D, Kaupp O, Paulsson M. Transglutaminase-catalyzed matrix cross-linking in differentiating cartilage: identification of osteonectin as a major glutaminyl substrate. J Cell Biol 1995; 129: 881–92

22. Fesus L. Biochemical events in naturally occurring forms of cell death. FEBS Lett 1993; 328: 1–5

23. Roch AM, Noel P, Alaoui SE, et al. Differential expression of isopeptide bonds N^ε(-glutamyl)lysine in benign and malignant human breast lesions: an immunohistochemical study. Int J Cancer 1991; 48: 215–20

24. Bowness MJ, Venditti M, Tarr AH, Taylor JR. Increase in epsilon (gamma-glutamyl) lysine crosslinks in atherosclerotic aortas. Atherosclerosis 1994; 111: 247–53

25. Querfurth HW, Selkoe DJ. Calcium ionophore increases amyloid beta peptide production by cultured cells. Biochemistry 1994; 33: 4550–61

26. Ouanounou A, Zhang L, Charlton MP, Carlen PL. Differential modulation of synaptic transmission by calcium chelators in young and aged hippocampal CA1 neurons: evidence for altered calcium homeostasis in aging. J Neurosci 1999; 19: 906–15

27. Selkoe DJ, Ihara Y, Salazar FJ. Alzheimer's disease: insolubility of partially purified paired helical filaments in sodium dodecyl sulfate and urea. Science 1982; 215: 1243–5

28. Appelt DM, Kopen GC, Boyne LJ, Balin BJ. Localization of transglutaminase in hippocampal neurons – implications for Alzheimer's disease. J Histochem Cytochem 1996; 44: 1421–7

29. Miller ML, Johnson GVW. Transglutaminase cross-linking of the τ protein. J Neurochem 1995; 65: 1760–70

30. Murthy SNP, Wilson JH, Lukas TJ, et al. Cross-linking sites of the human tau protein, probed by reactions with human transglutaminase. J Neurochem 1998; 71: 2607–14

31. Monsonego A, Friedmann I, Shani Y, et al. GTP-dependent conformational changes associated with the functional switch between $G\alpha$ and cross-linking activities in brain-derived tissue transglutaminase. J Mol Biol 1998; 282: 713–20

32. Yamada T, Yoshiyama Y, Kawaguchi N, et al. Possible roles of transglutaminase in Alzheimer's disease. Dementia Geriatr Cogn Disord 1998; 9: 103–10

33. Akiyama H, Kondo H, Ikeda K, et al. Immunohistochemical detection of coagulation factor XIIIa in post-mortem human brain tissue. Neurosci Lett 1995; 202: 29–32

34. Monsonego A, Shani Y, Friedmann I, et al. Expression of GTP-dependent and GTP-independent tissue-type transglutaminase in cytokine-treated rat brain astrocytes. J Biol Chem 1997; 272: 3724–32

35. Cacabelos R, Alvarez XA, Franco-Maside A, et al. Serum tumor necrosis factor (TNF) in Alzheimer's disease and multi-infarct dementia. Methods Find Exp Clin Pharmacol 1994; 16: 29–35

36. Festoff BW, SantaCruz K, Arnold PM, et al. Injury-induced 'switch' from GTP-regulated to novel GTP-independent isoform of tissue transglutaminase in the rat spinal cord. J Neurochem 2002; 81: 708–18

37. Zemaitaitis MO, Kim SY, Halverson RA, et al. Transglutaminase activity, protein, and mRNA expression are increased in progressive supranuclear palsy. J Neuropathol Exp Neurol 2003; 62: 173–84

38. Kim SY, Jeitner TM, Steinert PM. Transglutaminases in disease. Neurochem Int 2002; 40: 85–103

Chapter 44

The impact of extracellular amyloid-β (Aβ) peptides on cortical neurotransmitters and of intracellular Aβ accumulation on protein expression

AC Cuello, KFS Bell, V Echeverria, E Lopez, A Ribeiro-da-Silva, M Szyf

INTRODUCTION

The extracellular accumulation and aggregation of amyloid-β (Aβ) peptides unquestionably play a major role in Alzheimer's disease (AD) neuropathology. However, in addition to the role of extracellular Aβ, the impact of intracellular Aβ deposits in central nervous system (CNS) neurons should also be taken into account. In recent years, studies have provided evidence demonstrating the *in vitro* intracellular synthesis of Aβ[1,2] as well as the intracellular presence of this amyloidogenic peptide in both AD-like transgenic models and human AD postmortem material.[3-7] Major advances in the development of suitable cellular and transgenic animal models now allow investigations involving the differential effects of intracellular versus extracellular Aβ burden. This chapter discusses the observable effect of intracellular Aβ accumulation on protein expression and subcellular organelle organization, as well as the effect of extracellular Aβ aggregation on transmitter-specific synapses and the formation of dystrophic neurites.

THE IMPACT OF INTRACELLULAR Aβ ACCUMULATION ON PROTEIN EXPRESSION AND SUBCELLULAR ORGANELLE ORGANIZATION

While Aβ peptides appear to be largely generated via the endocytotic recycling of the amyloid precursor protein (APP),[8-10] other reports have shown that a good proportion of Aβ peptides may be generated intracellularly.[11-13] Using wild-type human APP$_{751}$ stably transfected P19 cell lines, our laboratory observed a several-fold increase in APP synthesis and a subsequent intracellular visualization of Aβ-immunoreactive (IR) material at the light microscopy level, following retinoic acid-induced neural differentiation.[14] At the electron microscopy level, the Aβ-IR material is localized to endocytotic vesicles and compartments involved in protein synthesis and packaging, such as the rough endoplasmic reticulum and the Golgi apparatus,[15] thereby suggesting that a portion of the Aβ-IR material is the product of intracellular synthesis. These Aβ-bearing cells display perturbations of the mitochondrial morphology at the ultrastructural level, a phenomenon that is accompanied by reduced mitochondrial membrane potential.[16] These cells also display an increased level of phosphorylated mitogen-activated protein (MAP) kinases.[14]

Our laboratory has also generated a number of transgenic rat lines which express human APP$_{751}$ with the Swedish and Indiana mutations alone (coded $_{UKUR28}$) or simultaneously with the PS1 Finn mutation (coded $_{UKUR25}$). The modest transgene expression seen in these rats results in a phenotype of marked accumulation of Aβ-IR material within numerous large pyramidal neurons of the cerebral cortex, and nearly all pyramidal neurons of the CA2 and CA3 regions of the hippocampus.[6] As was observed in the P19 cell line displaying intracellular Aβ-IR material, the phenotype is accompanied by an up-regulation of the phosphorylation of the MAP kinase, ErkII, but interestingly not other kinases capable of phosphorylating tau, such as CDK5 or GSK3.[17] An increased immunoreactivity to the monoclonal antibody PHF$_1$ was observed by both Western blots and immunohistochemistry in neurites of the CA2 and CA3 regions, thus indicating an increased tau phosphorylation at the MAP kinase sites.

We have analyzed in detail the morphology of the Golgi, lysosomal and lipofuscin compartments in pyramidal neurons of the hippocampus and cerebral cortex in doubly transgenic $_{UKUR25}$ rats (APP$_{Swe+Ind}$ and PS1$_{Finn}$), as compared to their non-transgenic littermates. This study revealed that neurons expressing intracellular Aβ material had a significant expansion of these three compartments in terms of number, surface area or both.[18] The observed increase in Golgi apparatus number and surface area is somewhat puzzling, since shrinkage and disorganization of this compartment have been reported in advanced cases of AD.[19,20] It is conceivable, however, that this type of Golgi anomaly occurs at late stages of AD progression,

where neurons are in a pre-necrotic or pre-apoptotic situation but not in the early stage of intracellular Aβ pathology, as in this transgenic rat line. The marked expansion of the lysosomal system is in line with the changes observed by Nixon and collaborators, in neuronal cell populations at early stages of AD.[21,22] The observed lysosomal up-regulation could perhaps be in response to an intracellular Aβ-induced neurotoxicity. Lipofuscin material accumulates as a result of the build-up of potentially toxic molecules that cannot easily be degraded or eliminated. Typically, lipofuscin-body abundance is a good indicator of 'neuronal aging'. Therefore, the elevated size and number of lipofuscin bodies seen in our study probably stems from the increased activation of the lysosomal pathway. These alterations indicate that the intracellular Aβ burden has a negative impact on both cell structure and subcellular morphology.

Further evidence of intracellular Aβ-induced cellular disruption arises from the proteomic analysis of the hippocampus in the $_{UKUR25}$ doubly transgenic rats. This analysis revealed a marked change in the expression of a large number of proteins, most of which were related to neuronal plasticity[23,24]. Furthermore, at later stages of pathology, these rats develop mild, yet significant learning impairments, as seen through performance in the Morris water maze task.[25] Taken together, these findings suggest that the abnormal accumulation of intracellular Aβ fragments is capable of disrupting cell structure and biochemistry as well as CNS function, prior to the presence of extracellular Aβ burden. While the results are not at a level which could explain the profound cognitive deficits visible in AD, they do suggest that the visible impairments may result from the combined impact of intracellular Aβ burden and polymeric extracellular Aβ aggregation on neuronal synaptic function.

THE IMPACT OF EXTRACELLULAR Aβ PEPTIDES ON CORTICAL NEUROTRANSMITTER-SPECIFIC NERVE TERMINALS

A past study in our laboratory, involving early-stage, amyloid pathology in 8-month-old transgenic mice (for mouse characterization see references 26 and 27), demonstrated in the 'random neuropile', a selective loss of cholinergic terminals in the cerebral and hippocampal cortices of doubly transgenic ($APP_{K670N, M671L} + PSI_{M146L}$) mice, an up-regulation of cholinergic presynaptic boutons in the single mutant $APP_{K670N, M671L}$ (tg2576) mice and no detectable change in PSI_{M146L} transgenic mice.[28] What is particularly interesting with respect to these findings is that the up-regulation in the number of cholinergic terminals occurred at time points immediately preceding the appearance of Aβ-IR extracellular plaques. This up-regulation in cholinergic presynaptic numbers is then followed by a small yet significant loss of vesicular acetylcholine transporter (VAChT)-IR boutons, in both the hippocampus and the cerebral cortex, concomitant with the appearance of plaque pathology.[28] This latter situation provides the first direct link between extracellular Aβ aggregation and a forebrain cholinergic compromise; thus indicating that a cortical Aβ burden is sufficient to unleash a cholinergic compromise, similar to the type so prevalently seen in advanced AD neuropathology[29,30] (for review see reference 31). In fact, Mufson and Dekosky and their collaborators have found that certain patients with mild cognitive impairment display up-regulated levels of cholinergic markers such as choline acetyltransferase.[32–34] The up-regulation of cholinergic terminals, which is visible prior to plaque formation, may result from a number of potential factors. These could include an initial neurotrophic effect of soluble APPα

fragments[35,36] due to increased transgene expression of APP or, alternatively, the increased terminal numbers could be the result of a compensatory mechanism to balance the Aβ-induced inhibition of acetylcholine release.[37] This apparent up-regulation of presynaptic sites would probably be surpassed by the increasing toxicity of accumulating polymeric and aggregated Aβ peptides in the extracellular space. This negative impact of extracellular Aβ-induced toxicity on cholinergic nerve terminals was clearly illustrated in our past study that investigated the 'plaque adjacent' neuropile as opposed to the 'random' neuropile and compared the densities of VAChT-IR (cholinergic) presynaptic boutons with synaptophysin-IR presynaptic boutons (which label all presynaptic bouton populations). In investigating the impact of plaque proximity on bouton density, at early stages of the amyloid pathology in the doubly ($APP_{K670N, M671L} + PSI_{M146L}$) transgenic mouse line, we observed that plaque proximity further reduced the cholinergic presynaptic bouton density by 40.[38] While no observable difference was visible for the synaptophysin-IR boutons in the random neuropile, an increased bouton density of 9.5% was observed in the 'plaque adjacent' neuropile. Plaque size was shown to have a negative correlation with the density of cholinergic nerve terminals in the 'plaque adjacent' neruropile. Finally, the number of cholinergic dystrophic neurites surrounding the true amyloid plaque core (thioflavin-S⁺) was disproportionately large with respect to the incidence of cholinergic boutons in the overall presynaptic bouton population. Both confocal and electron microscopic observations confirmed the preferential infiltration of dystrophic cholinergic boutons into fibrillar amyloid aggregates.[38] We therefore hypothesize that extracellular Aβ aggregation preferentially affects the cholinergic terminations prior to progression onto other neurotransmitter systems. Subsequently, we investigated the nature of the neurotransmitter systems involved in the visibly up-regulated synaptophysin-IR boutons, in the 'plaque adjacent' neuropile of TgCRND8 transgenic mice.[39] This study used a similar approach to investigate the glutamatergic (vesicular glutamate transporter 1, VGluT-1) and γ-aminobutyric acid (GABA)ergic (glutamic acid decarboxylase 65, GAD$_{65}$-IR) presynaptic bouton populations in both the 'plaque adjacent' neuropile and the 'peri-plaque' neuropile area. This study[40] revealed a subsequent participation of both the glutamatergic and GABAergic presynaptic bouton populations, following the involvement of the cholinergic system, in the neurotransmitter-specific amyloid pathology (Figure 44.1). The participation of the glutamatergic terminals is particularly striking when the incidence of dystrophic neurites bordering Aβ-IR plaques is examined quantitatively with the aid of a computer-assisted image analysis system. A positive relationship was found between plaque size and the area occupied by glutamatergic dystrophic neurites in the peri-plaque neuropile area. Interestingly, the GABAergic dystrophic neurites did not display any such correlation,

suggesting perhaps that this neurotransmitter system may be more resistant to the Aβ-induced neurotoxicity than both the cholinergic and the glutamatergic terminals.[40]

CONCLUDING REMARKS

The investigations summarized here implicate the participation of both intracellular and extracellular Aβ fragments, in AD pathology. The abnormal intracellular Aβ accumulation both in cells and in transgenic animal models leads to disruption in neuronal morphology as well as in expression of functionally relevant proteins. Furthermore, long-term intracellular Aβ accumulation in the transgenic rat leads to moderate cognitive impairments. Whether intracellular accumulation of Aβ acts alone or in concert with extracellular Aβ fragments to play a role in the AD pathophysiology remains unclear; however, for our laboratory it remains a working hypothesis.

While the mechanistic pathway leading to cholinergic basal forebrain attrition is unknown, our findings presented here demonstrate that a cortical amyloid burden is sufficient to initiate a cholinergic presynaptic involvement in transgenic mice. The transgenic overexpression of

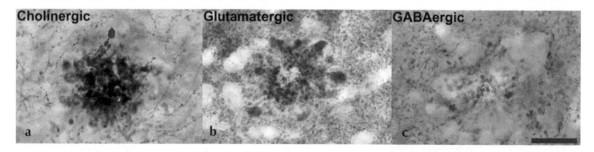

Figure 44.1 Immunohistochemical detection of neurotransmitter-specific dystrophic neurites, surrounding amyloid plaques in the frontal cortex of the TgCRND8 mouse model of Alzheimer's disease-like pathology. Note the abundance of cholinergic (a) and glutamatergic (b) dystrophic neurites as compared to the relatively minor involvement of the γ-aminobutyric acid (GABA)ergic (c) elements. Dystrophic neurites surround the Aβ-immunoreactivity plaque. Scale bar = 20 μm

APP-derived peptides leads to an initial up-regulation at the pre-plaque stage, followed by a gradual synaptic loss coinciding with the progression of extracellular Aβ pathology. Our studies in transgenic models are the first to indicate a synaptic involvement of both the GABAergic and glutamatergic systems. Our findings suggest that amyloid pathology progresses in a time-dependent and neurotransmitter-specific manner, whereby the cholinergic system is the first to be affected, followed by the glutamatergic system and finally, the somewhat more resilient GABAergic system.

While the mechanisms involved in AD pathogenesis remain to be elucidated, the findings of our laboratory suggest that investigations into the combined and independent actions of intra- and extracellular Aβ accumulation are of critical importance in understanding the disease progression (Figure 44.2).

ACKNOWLEDGEMENTS

This research was supported by funds from the Canadian Institutes of Health Research to A. Claudio Cuello (grant no. MOP-37996). The authors would like to thank Professors Karen Duff, Karen Hsiao and Don Westaway for their generous donation of transgenic mouse lines and Dr Shigemoto and Dr Edwards for their kind donation of the anti-VGluT-1 and anti-VAChT antibodies, respectively. K.F.S. Bell is a recipient of a CIHR Doctoral Research Awards.

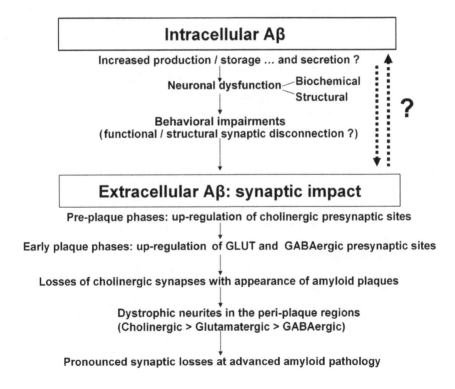

Figure 44.2 A schematic flow chart of the hypothesis discussed within the text. Aβ, amyloid-β; GLUT, glutamate; GABA, γ-aminobutyric acid

REFERENCES

1. Wilson CA, Doms RW, Lee VM. Intracellular APP processing and A beta production in Alzheimer disease. J Neuropathol Exp Neurol 1999; 58: 787–94

2. Echeverria V, Cuello AC. Intracellular A-beta amyloid, a sign for worse things to come? Mol Neurobiol 2002; 26: 299–316

3. Bancher C, Grundke-Iqbal I, Iqbal K, et al. Immunoreactivity of neuronal lipofuscin with monoclonal antibodies to the amyloid beta-protein. Neurobiol Aging 1989; 10: 125–32

4. Borchelt DR, Thinakaran G, Eckman CB, et al. Familial Alzheimer's disease-linked presenilin 1 variants elevate Abeta1-42/1-40 ratio in vitro and in vivo. Neuron 1996; 17: 1005–13

5. Chui DH, Tanahashi H, Ozawa K, et al. Transgenic mice with Alzheimer presenilin 1 mutations show accelerated neurodegeneration without amyloid plaque formation. Nat Med 1999; 5: 560–4

6. Echeverria V, Ducatenzeiler A, Alhonen J, et al. Rat transgenic models with a phenotype of intracellular Abeta accumulation in hippocampus and cortex. J Alzheimers Dis 2004; 6: 209–19

7. Gouras GK, Tsai J, Naslund J, et al. Intraneuronal Abeta42 accumulation in human brain. Am J Pathol 2000; 156: 15–20

8. Cataldo AM, Barnett JL, Pieroni C, Nixon RA. Increased neuronal endocytosis and protease delivery to early endosomes in sporadic Alzheimer's disease: neuropathologic evidence for a mechanism of increased beta-amyloidogenesis. J Neurosci 1997; 17: 6142–51

9. Koo EH, Squazzo SL. Evidence that production and release of amyloid beta-protein involves the endocytic pathway. J Biol Chem 1994; 269: 17386–9

10. Perez RG, Squazzo SL, Koo EH. Enhanced release of amyloid beta-protein from codon 670/671 'Swedish' mutant beta-amyloid precur-sor protein occurs in both secretory and endocytic pathways. J Biol Chem 1996; 271: 9100–7

11. Cook DG, Forman MS, Sung JC, et al. Alzheimer's A beta(1-42) is generated in the endoplasmic reticulum/intermediate compartment of NT2N cells. Nat Med 1997; 3: 1021–3

12. Greenfield JP, Tsai J, Gouras GK, et al. Endoplasmic reticulum and trans-Golgi network generate distinct populations of Alzheimer beta-amyloid peptides. Proc Natl Acad Sci USA 1999; 96: 742–7

13. Hartmann T, Bieger SC, Bruhl B, et al. Distinct sites of intracellular production for Alzheimer's disease A beta40/42 amyloid peptides. Nat Med 1997; 3: 1016–20

14. Grant SM, Morinville A, Maysinger D, et al. Phosphorylation of mitogen-activated protein kinase is altered in neuroectodermal cells overexpressing the human amyloid precursor protein 751 isoform. Mol Brain Res 1999; 72: 115–20

15. Grant SM, Ducatenzeiler A, Szyf M, Cuello AC. Abeta immunoreactive material is present in several intracellular compartments in transfected, neuronally differentiated, P19 cells expressing the human amyloid beta-protein precursor. J Alzheimers Disease 2000; 2: 207–22

16. Grant SM, Shankar SL, Chalmers-Redman RM, et al. Mitochondrial abnormalities in neuroectodermal cells stably expressing human amyloid precursor protein (hAPP751). Neuroreport 1999; 10: 41–6

17. Echeverria V, Ducatenzeiler A, Dowd E, et al. Altered mitogen-activated protein kinase signaling, tau hyperphosphorylation and mild spatial learning dysfunction in transgenic rats expressing the beta-amyloid peptide intra-cellularly in hippocampal and cortical neurons. Neuroscience 2004; 129: 583–92

18. Lopez EM, Bell KF, Ribeiro-da-Silva A, Cuello AC. Early changes in neurons of the hippocampus and neocortex in transgenic rats

expressing intracellular human a-beta. J Alzheimers Dis 2004; 6: 421–31

19. Salehi A, Ravid R, Gonatas NK, Swaab DF. Decreased activity of hippocampal neurons in Alzheimer's disease is not related to the presence of neurofibrillary tangles. J Neuropathol Exp Neurol 1995; 54: 704–9

20. Stieber A, Mourelatos Z, Gonatas NK. In Alzheimer's disease the Golgi apparatus of a population of neurons without neurofibrillary tangles is fragmented and atrophic. Am J Pathol 1996; 148: 415–26

21. Adamec E, Mohan PS, Cataldo AM, et al. Up-regulation of the lysosomal system in experimental models of neuronal injury: implications for Alzheimer's disease. Neuroscience 2000; 100: 663–75

22. Nixon RA, Cataldo AM, Mathews PM. The endosomal–lysosomal system of neurons in Alzheimer's disease pathogenesis: a review. Neurochem Res 2000; 25: 1161–72

23. Vercauteren FGG, Bergeron JJM, Bell A, et al. Changes in the rat hippocampal proteome caused by Alzheimer's disease linked mutations in amyloid precursor protein and presenilin 1. Soc Neurosci Abstr 2002; Program No. 295.4

24. Vercauteren FG, Clerens S, Roy L, et al. Early dysregulation of hippocampal proteins in transgenic rats with Alzheimer's disease-linked mutations in amyloid precursor protein and presenilin 1. Brain Res Mol Brain Res 2004; 132: 241–59

25. Dowd E, Dunnett SB, Cuello AC. Poor spatial learning in transgenic rats that accumulate Aβ intracellularly in the hippocampus and cortex but do not develop extracellular plaques. Soc Neurosci Abstr 2002; Prog No. 881.5

26. Hsiao KK, Borchelt DR, Olson K, et al. Age related CNS disorder and early death in transgenic FVB/N mice overexpressing Alzheimer amyloid precursor proteins. Neuron 1995; 15: 1203–18

27. Duff K, Eckman C, Zehr C, et al. Increased amyloid-beta42(43) in brains of mice expressing mutant presenilin 1. Nature 1996; 383: 710–13

28. Wong TP, Debeir T, Duff K, Cuello AC. Reorganization of cholinergic terminals in the cerebral cortex and hippocampus in transgenic mice carrying mutated presenilin-1 and amyloid precursor protein transgenes. J Neurosci 1999; 19: 2706–16

29. Bowen DM, Smith CD. Neurotransmitter related enzymes and indices of hypoxia in senile dementia and other abiotrophies. Brain 1976; 99: 459–96

30. Davies P, Maloney AJF. Selective loss of central cholinergic neurons in Alzheimer's disease. Lancet 1976; 2: 1403

31. Price DL, Koliatsos VE, Clatterbuck RC. Cholinergic systems: human diseases, animal models and prospects for therapy. In Cuello AC, ed. Progress in Brain Research. London: Elsevier, 1993; 98: 51–60

32. DeKosky ST, Ikonomovic MD, Styren SD, et al. Upregulation of choline acetyltransferase activity in hippocampus and frontal cortex of elderly subjects with mild cognitive impairment. Ann Neurol 2002; 51: 145–55

33. Ikonomovic MD, Mufson EJ, Cochran EJ, et al. Acetylcholinesterase changes in people with mild cognitive impairment: implications for hippocampal plasticity. Soc Neurosci Abstr 2002; Program No. 882.6

34. Ikonomovic MD, Mufson EJ, Wuu J, et al. Cholinergic plasticity in hippocampus of individuals with mild cognitive impairment: correlation with Alzheimer's neuropathology. J Alzheimers Dis 2003; 5: 39–48

35. Mattson MP, Cheng B, Culwell AR, et al. Evidence for excitoprotective and intraneuronal calcium-regulating roles for secreted forms of the beta-amyloid precursor protein. Neuron 1993; 10: 243–54

36. Mattson MP. Secreted forms of beta-amyloid precursor protein modulate dendrite outgrowth and calcium responses to glutamate in cultured

embryonic hippocampal neurons. J Neurobiol 1994; 25: 439–50

37. Kar S, Seto D, Gaudreau P, Quirion R. Beta-amyloid-related peptides inhibit potassium-evoked acetylcholine release from rat hippocampal slices. J Neurosci 1996; 16: 1034–40

38. Hu L, Wong TP, Cote SL, Bell KF, Cuello AC. The impact of Abeta-plaques on cortical cholinergic presynaptic boutons in Alzheimer's disease-like transgenic mice. Neuroscience 2003; 121: 421–32

39. Chishti MA, Yang DS, Janus C, et al. Early-onset amyloid deposition and cognitive deficits in transgenic mice expressing a double mutant form of amyloid precursor protein 695. J Biol Chem 2001; 276: 21562–70

40. Bell KFS, de Kort GJ, Steggerda S, et al. Structural involvement of the glutamatergic presynaptic boutons in a transgenic mouse model expressing early onset amyloid pathology. Neurosci Lett 2003; 353: 143–7

Chapter 45

Activation of *Wnt* signaling protects from amyloid-β-peptide neurotoxicity

NC Inestrosa, MS Urra, J Scheu, GG Farias, A Fisher, M Bronfman, RA Fuentealba

INTRODUCTION

Wnt signaling is essential in cell adhesion and regulation of cell fate determination during development.[1,2] Recently, it has been implicated in oncogenic processes and in neurodegenerative disorders such as autism, schizophrenia and Alzheimer's disease (AD). The activation of the canonical *Wnt* pathway results in the inhibition of glycogen synthase kinase-3β (GSK-3β), a key modulator of this signaling pathway.[3] According to the classical view of *Wnt* signal transduction,[4] in the presence of an extracellular *Wnt* ligand, membrane-anchored receptors of the Frizzled protein family transduce its signal to the intracellular space and activate Dishevelled, which in turn inactivates GSK-3β activity. As a result of GSK-3β inactivation, intracellular levels of β-catenin increase, allowing it to pass to the nucleus, where it binds to components of the high-mobility family of transcription factors (T-cell factor/lymphoid enhancer-binding factor (Tcf/LEF)) and activates the expression of *Wnt* target genes. Alternatively, in the absence of a *Wnt* ligand, the activity of GSK-3β is switched on and thus it phosphorylates β-catenin for ubiquitin–proteosome-mediated degradation.[5,6] As a net result, β-catenin levels are diminished within the cytosol and therefore the expression of *Wnt*-target genes such as cyclin D1 and engrailed is switched off (Figure 45.1). Our recent findings indicate that *Wnt*/β-catenin signaling may play a role in AD pathology.

ACTIVATION OF *Wnt*/β-CATENIN SIGNALING PATHWAY PREVENTS Aβ-DEPENDENT NEUROTOXICITY

Previous studies in our laboratory have suggested a relationship between amyoid-β (Aβ)-induced neurotoxicity and destabilization of β-catenin.[7,8] Other studies have indicated that inhibition of the GSK-3β by lithium protects rat neurons from Aβ insults.[9,10] Taken together, this evidence led us to suggest that a sustained loss of *Wnt* signaling function may be involved in the Aβ-dependent neurodegeneration observed in AD.[7] We have demonstrated that a direct activation of the *Wnt* pathway by its endogenous *Wnt-3a* ligand overcame the neurotoxic effects induced by Aβ in rat hippocampal neurons[10] and this effect was prevented by Frzb-1, a secreted Wnt-antagonist protein[11] (Table 45.1). Also, we have shown that rat hippocampal neurons exposed to Aβ fibrils induce the destabilization of endogenous levels of β-catenin and this effect

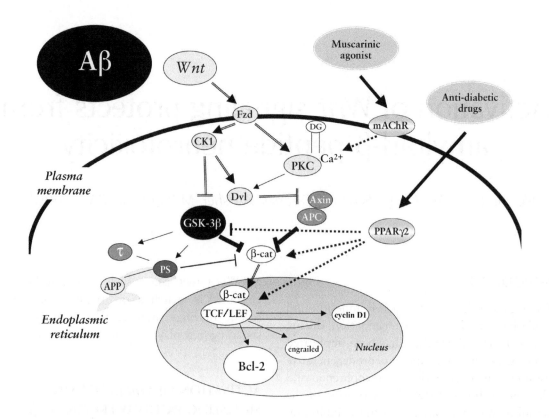

Figure 45.1 Schematic representation of *Wnt*/β-catenin signaling and its interaction with other cell signaling pathways. (a) Dashed lines indicate *Wnt* signaling activation by the muscarinic acetylcholine receptor (mAChR) and the peroxisome proliferator activated receptor γ (PPARγ)-mediated pathways. FzdR, Frizzled receptor; Dvl, Dishevelled; APC, adenomatous poliposis coli; β-cat, β-catenin; GSK-3β, glycogen synthase kinase-3β; Aβ, amyloid-β peptide; APP, amyloid precursor protein; τ, tau protein; PS, presenilin; TCF/LEF, T-cell factor/lymphoid enhancer-binding factor; CK1, casein kinase 1; PKC, protein kinase C; DG diacylglycerol

Table 45.1 Frzb-1 prevents *Wnt-3a* neuroprotection of amyloid-β (Aβ) fibrils in rat hippocampal neurons. Cell survival (MTT reduction assay) of rat hippocampal neurons exposed to Aβ fibrils (10 μmol/l) for 24 h in the presence of *Wnt-3a* with or without Frzb-1-conditioned media

	Cell survival (%)
pcDNA	100
Wnt-3a	116.6 ± 1.4
pcDNA + Aβ	72.1 ± 2.0
Wnt-3a + Aβ	104.6 ± 6.5
Wnt-3a/Frzb-1 + Aβ	79.4 ± 2.0

Values represent mean ± SEM in relation to control (cells not exposed to Aβ)

is prevented by pre-treating neurons with lithium[10] or by a *Wnt-3a*-conditioned medium (A. Alvarez, unpublished results). Additionally, our recent results demonstrated that Frzb-1 conditioned medium reversed the β-catenin stabilization induced by *Wnt-3a* medium in rat hippocampal neurons treated with 5 μmol/l Aβ fibrils (Figure 45.2). These results suggest that *Wnt*/β-catenin signaling plays an important role in neuroprotection against Aβ toxicity and this event is probably a crucial process involved in development of Aβ neurodegeneration observed early in the onset of AD.

In order to determine how *Wnt-3a*-conditioned medium prevents the toxic effects of Aβ, we investigated whether the expression of

anti-apoptotic genes is regulated by this signaling pathway. As a *Wnt* target candidate, we focused on *bcl-2*. This protein and its mRNA levels are induced by lithium, both *in vivo* and *in vitro*, and mediates neuroprotection against Aβ and glutamate toxicity in neuronal cells.[12–14] Also, the β-catenin analog plakoglobin[15] induces *bcl-2* expression.[16] Currently, we have demonstrated that lithium (Figure 45.3) and *Wnt-3a*-conditioned media cause a time-dependent increase in *bcl-2* mRNA levels in primary rat hippocampal neurons. Our results suggest that *bcl-2* might be a *Wnt*-regulated gene and that the *Wnt*/β-catenin/*bcl-2* cascade could be a target for amyloid-mediated toxicity. Accordingly, it has been demonstrated that Aβ decreases neuronal bcl-2 protein levels *in vitro*[17] and that bcl-2 immunoreactivity is reduced in tangle-bearing neurons of AD patients.[18] Collectively, these findings and our previous results[8,10,19] strongly suggest that amyloid inhibits *Wnt* signaling in neurons, and that this sustained loss of function could be responsible for the neuronal death observed in the AD brain.

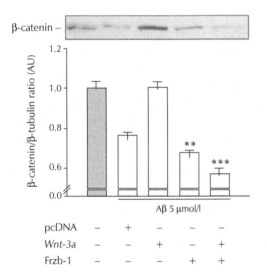

Figure 45.2 Frzb-1 reverses *Wnt*-3a-induced stabilization of β-catenin levels in the rat hippocampal neurons exposed to amyloid-β (Aβ) fibrils. Hippocampal neurons were treated for 8 h with control, *Wnt*-3a and Frzb-1 conditioned media in the presence of 5 μmol/l Aβ fibrils. The cytoplasmic cell extracts were separated by 10% sodium dodecyl sulfate (SDS)-polyacrylamide gel electrophoresis and probed with a monoclonal antibody against β-catenin. The graph shows the densitometric analysis of the β-catenin/β-tubulin ratio, represented as arbitrary units (AU)

ACTIVATION OF SIGNAL TRANSDUCTION PATHWAYS THAT CROSS-TALK WITH *Wnt* SIGNALING LEADS TO PROTECTION AGAINST AMYLOID-β NEUROTOXICITY

The emerging role of *Wnt*/β-catenin signaling as a therapeutic target for treatment of AD led us to study potential *Wnt* signaling interacting pathways that improve cell survival against Aβ toxicity. Attending to the relevance of expanding novel approaches for clinical treatment and therapies, we are currently evaluating the contribution of the M1 muscarinic acetylcholine receptor (mAChR) and of the peroxisome proliferator activated receptor γ (PPARγ)-

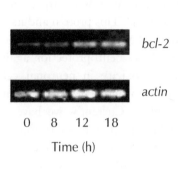

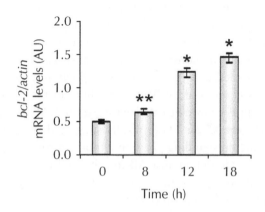

Figure 45.3 *Wnt* signaling activation increases the *bcl-2* mRNA levels in primary hippocampal neurons. Lithium induces a time-dependent increase of *bcl-2* transcripts. *Bcl-2* and *actin* mRNA levels were determined by semiquantitative reverse transcriptase–polymerase chain reaction on primary neurons exposed to 10 mmol/l LiCl for 0, 8, 12 and 18 h. The graph shows the densitometric analysis of a representative experiment. Data correspond to *bcl-2*/actin ratio, represented as arbitrary units (AU)

dependent cell signaling on *Wnt*/β-catenin pathway activation (Figure 45.1).

PPARs are members of the nuclear hormone receptor superfamily of ligand-activated transcriptional factors that bind to the per-oxisome proliferator-responsive element as a heterodimer with the *9-cis* retinoic acid receptor.[20] PPARγ function has been mainly described in regulation of adipocyte differentiation,[21] but recent studies have shown that some anti-inflammatory drugs that are PPARγ agonists have neuroprotective actions in different animal models of neurodegeneration, where it involves the prevention of glia and microglia activation.[22,23] Although PPARγ has been restricted to tissues other than the brain, the observation that PPARγ protein levels change in the temporal cortex of AD patients suggested that it might play a role in AD pathophysiology.[24] At present, it has become clear that anti-inflamatory drugs directly promote neuroprotection in primary neurons exposed to different pro-apoptotic stimuli *in vitro*.[25,26] In our laboratory, we have determined that PPARγ is

expressed in rat hippocampal neurons *in vitro* and that its activation with the anti-diabetic thiazolidinedione drug troglitazone (TGZ) attenuates Aβ-dependent neurotoxicity (Table 45.2). This effect correlates with the modulation of β-catenin levels, inhibition of GSK-3β activity and increased mRNA levels of the *Wnt* target genes *engrailed-1*, *cyclin D1* and *PPARδ* (C.N. Inestrosa, unpublished results). These findings suggest that TGZ-mediated neuroprotection is at least partially dependent on *Wnt*/β-catenin signaling activation and clearly demonstrate that PPARγ activation turns on this signaling pathway. Accordingly, thiazolidinedione drugs have been shown to have a potent insulin-sensitizing action[27] that might be mediated through PPARγ-mediated inhibition of GSK-3β,[28] and some studies have suggested that treatment for insulin resistance may reduce the risk or retard the development of AD.[29]

Another cell signaling pathway in susceptible neuronal populations of Alzheimer's patients that might participate early in the neuro-protection against Aβ toxicity, such as those of

Table 45.2 Activation of M1 muscarinic acetylcholine receptor by its agonist AF267B enhanced survival of hippocampal neurons exposed to amyloid-β (Aβ) fibrils. Hippocampal neurons were treated with 5 μmol/l Aβ fibrils, in the presence or absence of AF267B (10 μmol/l), troglitazone (TGZ) (10 μmol/l) or GW9662 (10 μmol/l) for 24 h. Additionally hippocampal neurons were treated with 5 μmol/l Aβ fibrils, 10 μmol/l AF267B and 10 μmol/l PNZ for 24 h. Cell viability was determined by using the MTT reduction assay

	Cell survival (%)	Cytoplasmic β-catenin
Control	100	100
Aβ	52.3 ± 7.6	33.9 ± 0.7
Aβ-AF267B	94.4 ± 5.8	72.9 ± 6.9
Aβ-AF267B-PNZ	63.0 ± 4.7	65.2 ± 7.9
Aβ-TGZ	95.7 ± 6.5	ND
Aβ-GW9662	14.1 ± 6.5	ND

Values represent the mean ± SEM in relation to control cells

the cholinergic system, is the M1 mAChR-mediated transduction pathway. mAChR activation modulates learning and plays a major role in cognitive processes, including short-term memory.[30] In relation to AD, it is well known that M1 agonists increase the non-amyloidogenic processing of the amyloid precursor protein (APP), reducing Aβ production.[31] Additionally, this activation also protects cells from apoptotic effects caused by several types of damage.[32] Although the precise mechanisms by which M1 mAChR activation promotes neuroprotection remain unclear, mAChR-induced activation of protein kinase C (PKC) through G protein signaling pathways has been demonstrated. Interestingly, it has been shown that PKC protects from apoptosis induced by Aβ.[19,33] It has also been shown that PKC inhibits GSK-3β activity,[34] a crucial *Wnt* signaling component that regulates cytoplasmic β-catenin levels. We present evidence indicating that the activation of M1 mAChR by its agonist AF267B protects hippocampal neurons from Aβ toxicity (Table 45.2), inhibits GSK-3β activity measured with a specific substrate, GS2 (Figure 45.4) and prevents the decrease in cytoplasmic β-

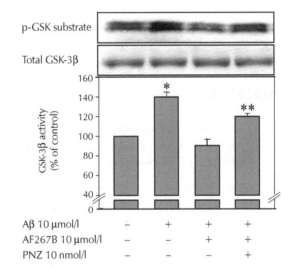

Figure 45.4 The glycogen synthase kinase-3β (GSK-3β) activity elicited by amyloid β (Aβ)-neurotoxicity is inhibited by M1 muscarinic acetylcholine receptor (mAChR) activation. Hippocampal cultures were co-treated with 5 μmol/l Aβ with or without 10 μmol/l AF267B in the presence or absence of 10 nmol/l pirenzepine (PNZ). Endogenous glycogen synthase kinase (GSK)-3β was immunoprecipitated in order to assay the kinase activity. GSK-3β activity was measured by scintillation counting and expressed as a percentage in relation to the control activity of untreated neurons. Bars represent the mean ± SEM. * $p < 0.001$; ** $p < 0.005$ Student's *t* test

catenin levels induced by Aβ treatment (Table 45.2). The protective effect of AF267B against Aβ-toxicity was reversed by co-incubation with pirenzepine (PNZ), an M1 mAChR antagonist (Table 45.2). These results indicate that stimulation of M1 mAChR turns on the Wnt pathway, preventing the Aβ-induced effect on cytoplasmic β-catenin levels. Finally, we analyzed the connection between both signaling pathways and found that activation of M1 mAChR led to inactivation of GSK-3β by Ser-9 phosphorylation through PKC, in transgenic mice that overexpress GSK-3β (G. Farias, unpublished data). These data suggest a link between Wnt/β-catenin and the M1 mAChR signaling pathway that leads to neuroprotection against Aβ toxicity.

Overall, our findings clearly demonstrate that the Wnt/β-catenin signaling pathway is a direct target of Aβ-induced toxicity and that direct or indirect activation of Wnt/β-catenin is neuroprotective against Aβ injury. In this regard, we postulate that modulation of this pathway through the activation of cross-talking signaling cascades should be considered as a promising therapeutic strategy for AD treatment.

ACKNOWLEDGEMENTS

This work was supported by Grants from FONDAP-Biomedicine (No. 13980001) and the Millennium Institute of Fundamental and Applied Biology (MIFAB).

REFERENCES

1. Patapoutian A, Reichardt LF. Roles of Wnt proteins in neural development and maintenance. Curr Opin Neurobiol 2000; 10: 392–9

2. Peifer M, Polakis P. Wnt signaling in oncogenesis and embryogenesis – a look outside the nucleus. Science 2000; 287: 1606–9

3. Chen RH, Ding WV, McCormick F. Wnt signaling to β-catenin involves two interactive components. Glycogen synthase kinase-3β inhibition and activation of protein kinase C. J Biol Chem 2000; 275: 17894–9

4. Wodarz A, Nusse R. Mechanisms of Wnt signaling in development. Annu Rev Cell Dev Biol 1998; 14: 59–88

5. Yost C, Torres M, Miller JR, et al. The axis-inducing activity, stability, and subcellular distribution of β-catenin is regulated in Xenopus embryos by glycogen synthase kinase 3. Genes Dev 1996; 10: 1443–54

6. Aberle H, Bauer A, Stappert J, et al. β-catenin is a target for the ubiquitin–proteasome pathway. EMBO J 1997; 16: 3797–804

7. De Ferrari GV, Inestrosa NC. Wnt signaling function in Alzheimer's disease. Brain Res Brain Res Rev 2000; 33: 1–12

8. Inestrosa N, De Ferrari GV, Garrido JL, et al. Wnt signaling involvement in β-amyloid-dependent neurodegeneration. Neurochem Int 2002; 41: 341–4

9. Alvarez G, Munoz-Montano JR, Satrustegui J, et al. Lithium protects cultured neurons against β-amyloid-induced neurodegeneration. FEBS Lett 1999; 453: 260–4

10. De Ferrari GV, Chacon MA, Barria MI, et al. Activation of Wnt signaling rescues neurodegeneration and behavioral impairments induced by β-amyloid fibrils. Mol Psychiatry 2003; 8: 195–208

11. Jones SE, Jomary C. Secreted Frizzled-related proteins: searching for relationships and patterns. Bioessays 2002; 24: 811–20

12. Chen RW, Chuang DM. Long term lithium treatment suppresses p53 and Bax expression but increases Bcl-2 expression. A prominent role in neuroprotection against excitotoxicity. J Biol Chem 1999; 274: 6039–42

13. Chen G, Zeng WZ, Yuan PX, et al. The mood-stabilizing agents lithium and valproate robustly increase the levels of the neuroprotective protein bcl-2 in the CNS. J Neurochem 1999; 72: 879–82

14. Wei H, Leeds PR, Qian Y, et al. β-amyloid peptide-induced death of PC 12 cells and cerebellar granule cell neurons is inhibited by long-term lithium treatment. Eur J Pharmacol 2000; 392: 117–23

15. Zhurinsky J, Shtutman M, Ben-Ze'ev A. Differential mechanisms of LEF/TCF family-dependent transcriptional activation by β-catenin and plakoglobin. Mol Cell Biol 2000; 20: 4238–52

16. Hakimelahi S, Parker HR, Gilchrist AJ, et al. Plakoglobin regulates the expression of the anti-apoptotic protein BCL-2. J Biol Chem 2000; 275: 10905–11

17. Paradis E, Douillard H, Koutroumanis M, et al. Amyloid β peptide of Alzheimer's disease downregulates Bcl-2 and upregulates bax expression in human neurons. J Neurosci 1996; 16: 7533–9

18. Satou T, Cummings BJ, Cotman CW. Immunoreactivity for Bcl-2 protein within neurons in the Alzheimer's disease brain increases with disease severity. Brain Res 1995; 697: 35–43

19. Garrido JL, Godoy JA, Alvarez A, et al. Protein kinase C inhibits amyloid β peptide neurotoxicity by acting on members of the Wnt pathway. FASEB J 2002; 16: 1982–4

20. Kersten S, Desvergne B, Wahli W. Roles of PPARs in health and disease. Nature 2000; 405: 421–4

21. Tontonoz P, Hu E, Spiegelman BM. Stimulation of adipogenesis in fibroblasts by PPARγ2, a lipid-activated transcription factor. Cell 1994; 79: 1147–56

22. Breidert T, Callebert J, Heneka MT, et al. Protective action of the peroxisome proliferator-activated receptor-γ agonist pioglitazone in a mouse model of Parkinson's disease. J Neurochem 2002; 82: 615–24

23. Feinstein DL, Galea E, Gavrilyuk V, et al. Peroxisome proliferator-activated receptor-γ agonists prevent experimental autoimmune encephalomyelitis. Ann Neurol 2002; 51: 694–702

24. Kitamura Y, Shimohama S, Koike H, et al. Increased expression of cyclo-oxygenases and peroxisome proliferator-activated receptor-γ in Alzheimer's disease brains. Biochem Biophys Res Commun 1999; 254: 582–6

25. Uryu S, Harada J, Hisamoto M, Oda T. Troglitazone inhibits both post-glutamate neurotoxicity and low-potassium-induced apoptosis in cerebellar granule neurons. Brain Res 2002; 924: 229–36

26. Aoun P, Simpkins JW, Agarwal N. Role of PPAR-γ ligands in neuroprotection against glutamate-induced cytotoxicity in retinal ganglion cells. Invest Ophthalmol Vis Sci 2003; 44: 2999–3004

27. Lehmann JM, Moore LB, Smith-Oliver TA, et al. An antidiabetic thiazolidinedione is a high affinity ligand for peroxisome proliferator-activated receptor γ (PPARγ). J Biol Chem 1995; 270: 12953–6

28. Jiang G, Dallas-Yang Q, Li Z, et al. Potentiation of insulin signaling in tissues of Zucker obese rats after acute and long-term treatment with PPARγ agonists, Diabetes 2002; 51: 2412–19

29. Watson GS, Craft S. The role of insulin resistance in the pathogenesis of Alzheimer's disease: implications for treatment. CNS Drugs 2003; 17: 27–45

30. Anagnostaras SG, Murphy GG, Hamilton SE, et al. Selective cognitive dysfunction in acetylcholine M1 muscarinic receptor mutant mice. Nat Neurosci 2003; 6: 51–8

31. Nitsch RM, Slack BE, Wurtman RJ, Growdon JH. Release of Alzheimer amyloid precursor derivatives stimulated by activation of muscarinic acetylcholine receptors. Science 1992; 258: 304–7

32. De Sarno P, Shestopal SA, King TD, et al. Muscarinic receptor activation protects cells from apoptotic effects of DNA damage, oxidative stress, and mitochondrial inhibition. J Biol Chem 2003; 278: 11086–93

33. Xie J, Guo Q, Zhu H, et al. Protein kinase C iota protects neural cells against apoptosis induced by amyloid β-peptide. Brain Res Mol Brain Res 2000; 82: 107–13

34. Cook D, Fry MJ, Hughes K, et al. Wingless inactivates glycogen synthase kinase-3β via an intracellular signalling pathway which involves a protein kinase C. EMBO J 1996; 15: 4526–36

Chapter 46

Human prion diseases

T Pan, R Li, B-S Wong, S-C Kang, P Gambetti, M-S Sy

INTRODUCTION

Creutzfeldt–Jakob disease (CJD), Gerstmann–Sträussler–Scheinker disease (GSS) and fatal familial insomnia (FFI) belong to a group associated with fatal, neurodegenerative, sub-acute, transmissible spongiform encephalopathy (TSE) in humans.[1,2] Overall, TSE diseases are rare in humans, with an incidence of approximately one case/million people per year, and have remained stable over the past few decades.[1,3] Epidemiological studies have so far failed to provide any link between gender, occupational exposures, geographical locations, environmental factors and the frequency of disease. The exception is in cases where there is a familial link between the affected individuals.[1–3]

Cases of CJD and GSS have been known since the 1930s.[4,5] However, owing to their rarity, these diseases had not received much attention for decades, until the 1950s when a new disease, kuru, was discovered.[6] 'Kuru' means 'to tremble' in the Fore language of the east highland of Papua New Guinea, thus, kuru vividly describes the clinical symptoms of the disease.[6] The disease occurs mostly in women and children. It was postulated that kuru was caused by some genetic factors in association with unknown social and environmental factors. A major advance in the understanding of kuru was the serendipitous discovery that the spongiform histopathology seen in the brain of kuru patients was similar to that found in scrapie, a TSE in sheep and goats.[6,7]

Scrapie has existed in Britain since the 1750s.[8] While earlier attempts by Gajdusek and colleagues to transmit kuru from human to primates were unsuccessful, based on this new lead, Gajdusek and Gibbs were able to transmit first kuru, then CJD and then GSS from human to non-human primates.[2,9] It was speculated that natural transmission of kuru might have occurred through cannibalism, which was practiced during the funeral ceremony by the Fore people. Cessation of cannibalism since the 1950s has gradually eliminated the disease in that region of the world. The incubation period of kuru could be as long as 4–5 decades.[1,2]

HUMAN TRANSMISSIBLE SPONGIFORM ENCEPHALOPATHY DISEASES

Recently, human TSE diseases have been classified according to the pathogenic mechanisms of the disease.[1] Therefore, human TSE diseases are classified as inherited, infectious and of a sporadic nature.[1] Infectious human TSE disease was most vividly demonstrated in kuru. Physicians in a variety of medical procedures have also inadvertently transmitted diseases, which are commonly referred to as the iatrogenic CJD.[1] The recently emerged variant CJD (vCJD) mostly in Great Britain is believed to be acquired from cattle affected by bovine spongiform encephalopathy (BSE).[10,11] Approximately 10–15% of human TSE is inherited. Most of the cases of human TSE diseases occur sporadically, and the pathogenic mechanisms remain unknown[3] (Table 46.1).

It has been known since 1936 that scrapie is a transmissible disease. However, the nature of the etiological agent remained elusive and controversial for half a century.[12] Accumulated findings in the 1950s and 1960s revealed that the infectious agent in scrapie was highly unusual for being resistant to agents that destroy nucleic acids, but was sensitive to agents that destroy

protein. The infectious agent was also very small, tended to co-purify with proteins and was highly resistant to heat inactivation.[2,13] In 1967, Griffith proposed that the agent for TSE is a self-replicating protein rather than a conventional bacterium or virus.[14] However, Prusiner made the fundamental discovery that led to the current understanding of these diseases.[2,13] In 1982, Prusiner and colleagues isolated and tentatively identified the infectious pathogen, which they named **pro**teinaceous **in**fectious particle or prion.[2,13] Since then the name prion disease has been used synonymously with TSE. Unexpectedly, it was later found by the same group that the prion is an aberrant form of a protein that is normally expressed, and highly conserved in all mammals.[15,16] It was postulated that all three forms of prion diseases – hereditary, sporadic and infectious – share the same pathogenic mechanism that is based on the conversion of the normal prion protein $(PrP)^C$ into one or more intermediate conformers, which may be

Table 46.1 Transmissible spongiform encephalopahty diseases in humans

Form	%	Disease	Phenotype
Sporadic	85	Creutzfeldt–Jakob disease (CJD) fatal insomnia	disease onset occurs in individuals older than 60 years; patients exhibit cognitive deficits including psychiatric and behavior abnormalities. Short disease duration (5 months) and most patients die within 1 year
Genetic	10–15	Creutzfeldt–Jakob disease fatal familial insomnia Gerstmann–Sträussler–Scheinker disease undefined or mixed	an earlier age of onset and a more protracted course of the disease than the sporadic form
Infectious	>1	kuru iatrogenic CJD variant CJD (vCJD)	the onset, frequency and duration of iatrogenic diseases are much more variable. Patients develop ataxia and movement disorders followed by dementia

designated as PrP^{C*}, and eventually into the pathogenic PrP, commonly called scrapie PrP (PrP^{Sc}).[2,13]

The strongest support for the 'protein only' hypothesis came from genetic engineering experiments. It was discovered that PrP^C 'knock out' mice that did not express the normal PrP^C were resistant to infectious PrP^{Sc}.[17,18] Additional evidence that the normal PrP^C gene is critical for prion diseases came from clinical studies in humans. The identification of the prion gene allowed investigators to search for mutations in the human PrP gene. Since then, more than 20 pathogenic mutations have been found in the coding sequence of the PrP gene in patients with the inherited diseases.[1,2] Most of these mutations are point mutations, with the exception of insertion mutations, which occur at the octapeptide repeat region.[19]

While it is widely accepted that PrP^C is critical for the pathogenesis of prion diseases, the 'protein only hypothesis' is not universally accepted. Some investigators still question whether prion by itself is solely responsible for the pathogenesis of TSE.[20,21] It is also not clear whether PrP^{Sc} is solely responsible for all aspects of the pathogenesis, and that all prion diseases share the same pathogenic mechanism. One transgenic mouse line bearing the human pathogenic mutation developed neurode-generation.[22] However, another transgenic line bearing the same mutation did not.[23] The levels of gene expression in different transgenic mouse lines may explain the discrepancy in these results.

The PrP^C to PrP^{Sc} conversion is based on a change in conformation from the predominant α-helical structure of PrP^C to the predominantly β-sheet structure of PrP^{Sc}.[24] According to the most recent model, the prion protein is inherently unstable, fluctuating between the dominant native state, PrP^C, and other intermediate conformers, one or more of which can self-associate to produce a supramolecular structure, PrP^{Sc}. This structure would then act as a 'seed' recruiting the unstable PrP forms, leading to the formation of new PrP^{Sc}.[2] The conformational changes imposed by PrP^{Sc} also result in drastic alterations in their biochemical properties. One of the most important effects of the change is that, while the N-terminal region of PrP^{Sc} remains sensitive to treatment with proteases, the C-terminal region becomes protease-resistant. In contrast, the entire PrP^C is protease-sensitive.[15,25] The accumulation of proteinase K (PK)-resistant PrP^{Sc} in the brain has provided a very useful diagnostic test for prion diseases (Figure 46.1).[3,26,27] However, sensitivity to PK *in vitro* is relative rather than absolute, and the levels of PK-resistant PrP^{Sc} vary greatly between different prion diseases. In all human prion

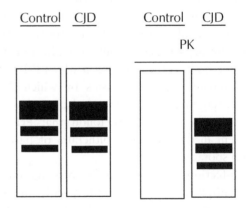

Figure 46.1 Resistance of prion protein (PrP)^{Sc} to proteinase K (PK) digestion. Brain homogenates were prepared from one control, non-Creutzfeldt–Jakob disease (CJD) donor and one CJD donor. Each sample was then divided into two tubes, one treated with PK and the other treated with phosphate-buffered saline. After treatments, proteins in the samples were separated by sodium dodecyl sulfate–polyacrylamide gel electro-phoresis and then immunoblotted with an anti-PrP monoclonal antibody. PK digestion completely eliminated the immunoreactivity in the control sample but not in the CJD sample

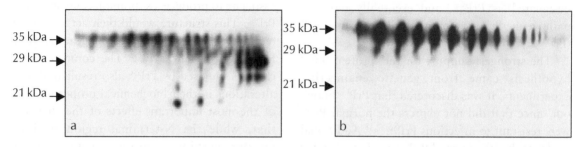

Figure 46.2 Two-dimensional immunoblotting of normal human brain homogenates with an anti-C-terminus-specific monoclonal antibody (Mab) (a) or an anti-N-terminus-specific Mab. Human brain contains multiple full-length prion protein (PrP)^C species and many different N-terminally truncated PrP^C species. Normal human brain homogenate was prepared and then separated by two-dimensional gelelectrophoresis. Separated proteins were then immunoblotted with either Mab 8H4 (a), which reacts with all described PrP^C species, or Mab 8B4 (b), which reacts only with full-length PrP^C species

diseases with the only exception of vCJD, no infectious PrP^{Sc} has ever been convincingly detected in non-central nervous system (CNS) tissues.[11] Therefore, the brain conceivably is the only anatomical site where PrP^C to PrP^{Sc} conversion could occur. Alternatively, other anatomical sites may be able to replicate PrP^{Sc}, but the brain is the only site in which PrP^{Sc} can accumulate. The mechanisms by which PrP^{Sc} selectively target the CNS are also not known. However, a recent study found that PrP^{Sc} is present in the olfactory epithelium of patients with sporadic CJD.[28]

Infectious prions can be propagated in susceptible hosts in a strain-specific manner similar to conventional pathogens.[29,30] Most recent studies have suggested that each of the prion strains represents a PrP^{Sc} molecule with a unique conformation.[31] Human PrP^{Sc} strains have also been proposed, based on the size of the human PrP^{Sc} fragment that is resistant to PK treatment. Essentially, two major strains of PrP^{Sc} have been identified in human prion diseases based on the electrophoretic mobility of the main PrP^{Sc} fragment generated by PK digestion in vitro.[3,26] Type 1 migrates at 21 kDa and type 2

at 19 kDa following gel electrophoresis. More recently, it has been suggested that at least six human prion strains could be identified, based on their electrophoretic mobility.[27]

It is generally believed that, in the human brain, PrP^C species are present in three glycoforms: di-glycosylated, mono-glycosylated and un-glycosylated forms.[15,32] More recently, using a panel of anti-PrP^C monoclonal antibodies that react with different regions of the PrP^C, we found that the expression of PrP^C in the normal brain is far more complex than the three-band pattern previously seen with monoclonal antibodies 3F4.[33–35] By two-dimensional immunoblotting, we observed seven major species of PrP^C, which could be subdivided into multiple subspecies (Figure 46.2). These PrP species were generated as a result of differences in N-linked glycosylation as well as the sites of truncations.[34,35] Based on this evidence we concluded that most of the smaller PrP species are N-terminally truncated PrP species rather than un-glycosylated or mono-glycosylated PrP species.[35] Furthermore, by separating the full-length and truncated PrP^C, the two populations were shown to be glycosylated differentially. We speculated that full-length and truncated PrP^C might have different functions under physiological conditions, and may play different roles in PrP^{Sc} formation.[35,36]

One of the most intriguing findings regarding the inherited form of prion diseases came from studies indicating that a commonly found polymorphism in amino acid residue 129 of the human PrP gene can greatly modulate disease phenotypes.[3] An individual can either be homozygous with methionine (M/M) or valine (V/V) or heterozygous with M and V. Two patients were identified to have an identical mutation in residue 178 with a change from Asp to Asn.[37,38] However, the clinical presentation and histopathology of the two cases differ greatly, depending on whether the amino acid residue on position 129 is either an M or a V.[37,38] Therefore, one single amino acid difference can drastically alter the disease phenotype.

The polymorphism in 129 also plays a critical role in the pathogenesis of vCJD. The origin of vCJD has not been firmly established, but considerable evidence points to BSE.[10,11] In addition, the histopathological changes seen in the vCJD cases are reminiscent of those seen in kuru, suggesting that similar pathological mechanisms are involved in these diseases.[10,11] Interestingly, all vCJD patients were homozygous with M/M at residue 129.[11,39] Either individuals with M/M are uniquely susceptible to vCJD, or this population may represent individuals with the shortest incubation period. A recent study suggests that there is a strong balancing selection against homozygosity at residue 129 in human evolution. The selection pressure was imposed by prehistoric kuru-like epidemics that were caused by the practice of cannibalism.[40] The differences between conventional sporadic CJD and vCJD are summarized in Table 46.2. Most recent studies have suggested that the numbers of vCJD cases have been declining since peaking in 2000, and the incidence of vCJD continues to decline.[41]

FUTURE CHALLENGES

The challenge for human prion diseases is in the diagnosis, cure and eventual prevention. The development of a more reliable and non-invasive diagnostic test is the easiest task. On the other hand, finding a cure for human prion diseases will be much more challenging. Fortunately, human prion diseases have remained very rare over the past few decades. Unless there are drastic changes in the transmissibility of diseases from animals to humans, the rate of

Table 46.2 Differences between sporadic and variant Creutzfeldt–Jakob disease (vCJD)

	Sporadic CJD	vCJD
Polymorphism at residue 129	majority M/M or V/V	all M/M homozygous
Mean age of disease onset	60 years old	29 years old
Mean duration of disease	5 months	14 months
Central nervous system (CNS) histopathology	plaques are present in a small number of patients	presence of unique plaques with a 'daisy'-like appearance
Infectious agent outside the CNS	only in the CNS and olfactory epithelium	in tonsil and appendix

human prion diseases will remain low. However, studying the pathogenic mechanisms of prion diseases will most definitely provide new insights into the pathogenic mechanisms of other more common neurodegenerative diseases, such as Alzheimer's disease and Parkinson's disease.

ACKNOWLEDGEMENTS

This work was supported in part by grants from the National Institutes of Health NS-045981-01 (M.S.S.), AG-14359-07 (P.G.) and an award/contract from the US Department of the Army DAMD17-03-1-0286 (M.S.S.).

REFERENCES

1. Parchi P, Gambetti P. Human prion diseases. Curr Opin Neurol 1995; 8: 286–93

2. Prusiner SB. Prions. Proc Natl Acad Sci USA 1998; 95: 13363–83

3. Parchi P, Giese A, Capellari S, et al. Classification of sporadic Creutzfeldt–Jakob disease based on molecular and phenotypic analysis of 300 subjects. Ann Neurol 1999; 46: 224–33

4. Jakob A. Spastische Pseudosklerose-Encephalomyelopathie mit dissenminierten degenerationsherden. Z Gesamte Neurol Psychiatrie 1921; 64: 147–228

5. Gerstmann J, Straussler E, Scheinker I. Uber eine eigenartige hereditar-familiare erkrankung des zentral-nervensystems zugleich ein beitrag zur frage des vorzeitigen lokalen alterns. Z Neurol 1936; 154: 736–62

6. Gajdusek DC, Zigas V. Degenerative disease of the central nervous system in New Guinea: the endemic occurrence of 'kuru' in the native population. N Engl J Med 1957; 257: 974–78

7. Hadlow W. Scrapie and kuru. Lancet 1959; 2: 289–90

8. Woolhouse ME, Coen P, Matthews L, et al. A centuries-long epidemic of scrapie in British sheep? Trends Microbiol 2001; 9: 67–70

9. Gajdusek DC. Unconventional viruses and the origin and disappearance of kuru. Science 1977; 197: 943–60

10. Bruce ME, Will RG, Ironside JW, et al. Transmissions to mice indicate that 'new variant' CJD is caused by the BSE agent [see Comments]. Nature 1997; 389: 498–501

11. Brown P, Will RG, Bradley R, et al. Bovine spongiform encephalopathy and variant Creutzfeldt–Jakob disease: background, evolution, and current concerns. Emerg Infect Dis 2001; 7: 6–16

12. Culle J, Chelle P-L. La maladie dite tremblante du mouton est-elle inoculable? CR Acad Sci 1936; 203: 1552–4

13. Prusiner SB. Novel proteinaceous infectious particles cause scrapie. Science 1982; 216: 136–44

14. Griffith JS. Self-replication and scrapie. Nature 1967; 215: 1043–44

15. Oesch B, Westaway D, Walchli M, et al. A cellular gene encodes scrapie PrP 27-30 protein. Cell 1985; 40: 735–46

16. Basler K, Oesch B, Scott M, et al. Scrapie and cellular PrP isoforms are encoded by the same chromosomal gene. Cell 1986; 46: 417–28

17. Bueler H, Aguzzi A, Sailer A, et al. Mice devoid of PrP are resistant to scrapie. Cell 1993; 73: 1339–47

18. Prusiner SB, Groth D, Serban A, et al. Ablation of the prion protein (PrP) gene in mice prevents scrapie and facilitates production of anti-PrP antibodies. Proc Natl Acad Sci USA 1993; 90: 10608–12

19. Goldfarb LG, Brown P, McCombie WR, et al. Transmissible familial Creutzfeldt–Jakob disease associated with five, seven, and eight extra octapeptide coding repeats in the PRNP gene. Proc Natl Acad Sci USA 1991; 88: 10926–30

20. Manuelidis L, Sklaviadis T, Manuelidis EE. Evidence suggesting that PrP is not the infectious agent in Creutzfeldt–Jakob disease. Embo J 1987; 6: 341–7

21. Farquhar CF, Somerville RA, Bruce ME. Straining the prion hypothesis [Letter; Comment]. Nature 1998; 391: 345–6

22. Hsiao K, Baker HF, Crow TJ, et al. Linkage of a prion protein missense variant to Gerstmann–Straussler syndrome. Nature 1989; 338: 342–5

23. Manson JC, Jamieson E, Baybutt H, et al. A single amino acid alteration (101L) introduced into murine PrP dramatically alters incubation time of transmissible spongiform encephalopathy. EMBO J 1999; 18: 6855–64

24. Pan KM, Baldwin M, Nguyen J, et al. Conversion of alpha-helices into beta-sheets features in the formation of the scrapie prion proteins. Proc Natl Acad Sci USA 1993; 90: 10962–6

25. Bolton DC, McKinley MP, Prusiner SB. Identification of a protein that purifies with the scrapie prion. Science 1982; 218: 1309–11

26. Parchi P, Castellani R, Capellari S, et al. Molecular basis of phenotypic variability in sporadic Creutzfeldt–Jakob disease. Ann Neurol 1996; 39: 767–78

27. Hill AF, Joiner S, Wadsworth JD, et al. Molecular classification of sporadic Creutzfeldt–Jakob disease. Brain 2003; 126: 1333–46

28. Zanusso G, Ferrari S, Cardone F, et al. Detection of pathologic prion protein in the olfactory epithelium in sporadic Creutzfeldt–Jakob disease. [Comment]. N Engl J Med 2003; 348: 711–19

29. Hecker R, Taraboulos A, Scott M, et al. Replication of distinct scrapie prion isolates is region specific in brains of transgenic mice and hamsters. Genes Dev 1992; 6: 1213–28

30. Bruce M, Fraser H, Mcbride P, et al. The basis of strain variations in scrapie. In Prusiner SB, ed. Prion Diseases in Human and Animals. London: Willis Horwood, 1992: 497–508

31. Safar J, Wille H, Itri V, et al. Eight prion strains have PrP(Sc) molecules with different conformations [see Comments]. Nat Med 1998; 4: 1157–65

32. Kascsak RJ, Rubenstein R, Merz PA, et al. Mouse polyclonal and monoclonal antibody to scrapie-associated fibril proteins. J Virol 1987; 61: 3688–93

33. Zanusso G, Liu D, Ferrari S, et al. Prion protein expression in different species: analysis with a panel of new mAbs. Proc Natl Acad Sci USA 1998; 95: 8812–16

34. Pan T, Colucci M, Wong BS, et al. Novel differences between two human prion strains revealed by two-dimensional gel electrophoresis. J Biol Chem 2001; 276: 37284–8

35. Pan T, Li R, Wong BS, et al. Heterogeneity of normal prion protein in two-dimensional immunoblot: presence of various glycosylated and truncated forms. J Neurochem 2002; 81: 1092–101

36. Pan T, Wong BS, Liu T, et al. Cell-surface prion protein interacts with glycosaminoglycans. Biochem J 2002; 368: 81–90

37. Goldfarb LG, Petersen RB, Tabaton M, et al. Fatal familial insomnia and familial Creutzfeldt–Jakob disease: disease phenotype determined by a DNA polymorphism. Science 1992; 258: 806–8

38. Monari L, Chen SG, Brown P, et al. Fatal familial insomnia and familial Creutzfeldt–Jakob disease: different prion proteins determined by a DNA polymorphism. Proc Natl Acad Sci USA 1994; 91: 2839–42

39. Collinge J, Beck J, Campbell T, et al. Prion protein gene analysis in new variant cases of Creutzfeldt–Jakob disease [Letter]. Lancet 1996; 348: 56

40. Mead S, Stumpf MP, Whitfield J, et al. Balancing selection at the prion protein gene consistent with prehistoric kurulike epidemics. Science 2003; 300: 640–3

41. Andrews NJ, Farrington CP, Ward HJ, et al. Deaths from variant Creutzfeldt–Jakob disease in the UK. Lancet 2003; 361: 751–2

Index

T - #0322 - 101024 - C0 - 246/189/22 [24] - CB - 9781841843209 - Gloss Lamination